DATE DUE

8-23-12 li 92276460			

DEMCO

Integrated Behavioral Health in Primary Care

Integrated Behavioral Health in Primary Care

STEP-BY-STEP GUIDANCE FOR ASSESSMENT AND INTERVENTION

Christopher L. Hunter

Jeffrey L. Goodie

Mark S. Oordt

Anne C. Dobmeyer

American Psychological Association • Washington, DC

Published by
American Psychological Association
750 First Street, NE
Washington, DC 20002
www.apa.org

To order
APA Order Department
P.O. Box 92984
Washington, DC 20090-2984
Tel: (800) 374-2721; Direct: (202) 336-5510
Fax: (202) 336-5502; TDD/TTY: (202) 336-6123
Online: www.apa.org/books/
E-mail: order@apa.org

In the U.K., Europe, Africa, and the Middle East, copies may be ordered from
American Psychological Association
3 Henrietta Street
Covent Garden, London
WC2E 8LU England

Typeset in Berkeley by Circle Graphics, Columbia, MD

Printer: McNaughton & Gunn Inc., Saline, MI
Cover Designer: Mercury Publishing Services, Rockville, MD
Technical/Production Editor: Tiffany Klaff

The opinions and statements published are the responsibility of the authors, and such opinions and statements do not necessarily represent the policies of the American Psychological Association.

Library of Congress Cataloging-in-Publication Data

Integrated behavioral health in primary care : step-by-step guidance for assessment and intervention / Christopher L. Hunter . . . [et al.]. — 1st ed.
    p. ; cm.
  Includes bibliographical references and index.
  ISBN-13: 978-1-4338-0428-1
  ISBN-10: 1-4338-0428-X
  1. Mental health services. 2. Integrated delivery of health care. 3. Primary care (Medicine) I. Hunter, Christopher L. II. American Psychological Association.
  [DNLM: 1. Behavioral Medicine. 2. Primary Health Care—methods. 3. Disease Management. WB 103 I61 2009]

RA790.5.I5156 2009
616.89—dc22

                  2008033093

British Library Cataloguing-in-Publication Data
A CIP record is available from the British Library.

Printed in the United States of America
First Edition

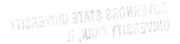

To my soulmate, Christine,
"If ever two were one then surely we." (Anne Bradstreet)
—*Christopher L. Hunter*

To Mary, Alexander, Zachary, and Benjamin,
who provide an endless supply of pleasure and inspiration every day.
—*Jeffrey L. Goodie*

To my wife Ruth and my children Andrew,
Martha Rose, Carol, Ellen, and Catherine.
—*Mark S. Oordt*

To Todd, Genevieve, and Julian.
And in memory of my father, Ferdinand.
—*Anne C. Dobmeyer*

Contents

List of Figures and Tables

Acknowledgments

We acknowledge the help and support we received from the American Psychological Association's Books staff, particularly Susan Reynolds and Margaret Sullivan. We also thank the reviewers of this book, Alexander Blount and Dawn L. Edwards, and our colleagues, Christine Hunter, Sara Kass, Brian Reamy, Scott Schinaman, Pamela Williams, and Brian Unwin, for their valuable advice as we developed this volume.

Integrated Behavioral Health in Primary Care

Introduction

Behavioral health disorders such as depression and anxiety have a significant impact on individuals in the United States, accounting for nearly 15% of the overall disease burden (Murray & Lopez, 1996). As many as 70% of primary care visits are related to behavioral health needs (Fries, Koop, & Beadle, 1993), and over 80% of all psychotropic medications in the United States are prescribed by nonpsychiatric medical providers (Beardsley, Gardocki, Larson, & Hidalgo, 1988). In addition, many common medical problems treated in primary care (e.g., obesity, diabetes, cardiovascular disease, chronic pain conditions) involve behaviors and health habits that initiate, exacerbate, or perpetuate the patient's symptoms and contribute to poor functioning. Physicians, physician assistants, and nurse practitioners provide the vast majority of behavioral health care in primary care settings. These professionals, although well-trained in physical medicine, often lack the training or the time to manage behavioral health problems in an optimal manner.

Over the past decade, professionals in both the mental health and physical health communities have developed a strong interest in the integration of behavioral health services into the primary care medical system (American Psychological Association [APA], 2006; Gray, Brody, & Johnson, 2005). Although numerous books and journal articles have been published in this area, it is notable that with a few exceptions (e.g., Gatchel & Oordt, 2003; O'Donohue, Byrd, Cummings, & Henderson, 2005; Robinson & Reiter, 2007), much of the writing is conceptual and lacks detailed practical information on the specifics of assessment and delivery of services. This volume addresses this unmet need. Our goal is to deliver straightforward information about what services a behavioral health provider (e.g., clinical psychologists, social workers), or any provider who wants to address behavioral health needs, can provide to patients with specific problems in the context of integrated care.

WHAT IS INTEGRATED CARE?

To better meet the behavioral health and overall health care needs of those in primary care, a number of collaborative behavioral health care models have been developed and implemented over the last 20 years with varying degrees of success (Blount, 2003; Blount et al., 2007). The terms *collaborative, coordinated, co-located, care management,* and *integrated* care are often used interchangeably and can lead to confusion regarding the type of service that is being delivered or evaluated. Thus, it is important to provide operational definitions of these terms.

Collaborative care is not a fixed model or specific approach. It is a concept that emphasized opportunities to improve the accessibility and delivery of behavioral health services in primary care through interdisciplinary collaboration (Blount, 2003; Blount et al., 2007; Gagné, 2005; Keesler & Stafford, 2008). It can be done in a range of practice models geared to provide effective patient services across a full spectrum of medical and behavioral health needs.

Models of collaborative care fall on a continuum (Blount, 2003; Blount et al., 2007; Keesler & Stafford, 2008). On one end there is collaboration between primary care providers (PCPs) and behavioral health

The opinions and statements published in this book are the responsibility of the authors, and such opinions and statements do not necessarily represent the policies of the Department of Defense, the United States Department of Health and Human Services, or their agencies.

providers who work in separate systems and facilities, delivering separate care. They exchange information regarding patients on an as-needed basis. This type of collaborative care has been referred to as a *coordinated care model.*

In the middle of the continuum is on-site collaboration, or what has been referred to as a *co-located care model.* In this model behavioral health providers and PCPs deliver separate care in the same block of offices or in the same building, and they may share office staff and waiting rooms; behavioral health providers and PCPs communicate regularly, sometimes face-to-face. PCPs typically refer patients to behavioral health providers and separate treatment records and treatment plans are maintained. Also in the middle of the continuum is the *care management model,* which typically involves a specified process of assessing, planning, facilitation, and advocacy for options to meet the patient's needs. Care managers are often nurses who have special behavioral health training and may be working in or outside of the primary care clinic. Patient education about his or her diagnosis, preference for treatment (e.g., medication or specialty mental health referral), and medication adherence are typical areas of focus. This model usually targets one or two discrete problem presentations, usually depression.

At the other end of the collaborative care continuum is the *integrated care model.* In this model of collaborative care, behavioral health providers and PCPs work together in a shared system, and the behavioral health provider functions as a member of the primary care team to address the full spectrum of problems the patient brings to their PCP. With this model there is one treatment plan targeting the patient's needs, a shared medical record, and the patient is likely to perceive this as part of his or her medical care. It has been argued that optimized integrated care models would involve attention to mission, clinical, physical location, operations, information, and financial and resource integration (Peek, 2008; Strosahl & Robinson, 2008).

The success of these models has been dependent on a variety of factors including the setting, the patient population, and the buy-in from the medical system adopting this care delivery paradigm. Several books (e.g., Blount, 1998; Cummings, Cummings, &

Johnson, 1997; Frank, McDaniel, Bray, & Heldring, 2003; Gatchel & Oordt, 2003; O'Donohue, Byrd, Cummings, & Henderson, 2005; Robinson & Reiter, 2007) do an excellent job of detailing the difference between specialty mental health and collaborative care models, reviewing strategies to establish collaborative care behavioral health services, discussing medical cost offset, and delineating various integrated care models. Readers might consider reviewing these resources for a more in-depth understanding of the rationale behind integrated care.

Research has supported the efficacy of a range of models of collaborative care (Blount, 2003; Blount et al., 2007; Craven & Bland, 2006; Gilbody, Bower, Fletcher, Richards, & Sutton, 2006). Ideally, each collaborative care model should be best matched to the personnel, resources, and desired outcomes. Compared with other collaborative care models, integrated care, which we focus on in this volume, provides the best opportunity to reach the greatest number and variety of patients with evidence-based behavioral health assessments and interventions (Strosahl & Robinson, 2008).

Integrated behavioral health care is a way to bring the skills and expertise for addressing behavioral health needs to a setting in which the patients who can benefit from those services are already receiving care. It normalizes the need for behavioral health support and reduces the stigma associated with it.

Most behavioral health providers have been trained in the traditional specialty mental health care model. In this model, patients either seek help themselves or are referred to a behavioral health provider for problems identified as psychological (e.g., anxiety, depression, interpersonal problems). In specialty mental health care, the practitioner may see the patient in his or her office for brief psychotherapy (e.g., 8–10 sessions) or for long-term therapy of indefinite duration. In either case, sessions last for 45 to 50 minutes on a regularly scheduled basis (e.g., weekly). This type of behavioral health assessment and intervention will not work in an integrated care model. To be an effective primary care team member, the behavioral health provider has to be readily available. The demand for appointments will quickly exceed the behavioral health provider's ability to meet that demand using a specialty mental health model of care. Patients will have extended waiting times for services and, in all likelihood, the behavioral health provider will quickly become an irrelevant team member as a result of not being able to assist the PCP in a timely manner. As such, behavioral health providers have to redefine how they think and what they do to provide behavioral health services that will work in the primary care environment.

BECOMING AN INTEGRATED CARE PROVIDER

We have been teaching behavioral health providers to adapt their training and professional practices to the primary care environment for the past 8 years. Common questions we have received include, "Where do I start?" "What do I do?" Answers to these questions typically elicit the response, "I can't do that in 30 minutes!"

We then explain why, in the primary care setting, the typical conventional model of psychological assessment and intervention will not work. The typical 50-minute interview cannot simply be condensed to fit in a 15- to 30-minute appointment. Time demands and practice expectations are structured differently in the primary care setting; behavioral health services must be adapted to this fast pace. The practicalities of adapting one's assessments and interventions to patient problems in the primary care setting are the main focus of this book.

The strategies we cover are likely to be useful in any integrated care model, but they are particularly germane to the primary care behavioral health (PCBH) model of integrated care. This integrated model (Robinson & Reiter, 2007; Strosahl & Robinson, 2008) has been used by several large health care systems, including Kaiser Permanente, Veterans Administration, Health Resources Service Administration and Bureau of Primary Care through Federally Qualified Health Centers, and the U.S. Air Force and Navy (Strosahl & Robinson, 2008). In this model, the behavioral health provider works as a member of the primary care team and is referred to as a behavioral health consultant (BHC). After consulting with the PCP, the BHC sees patients for an initial 15 to 30 minutes to conduct a focused assessment and to develop a treatment plan. The BHC then pro-

vides feedback to the PCP about the patient's symptoms and functional impairments and details a behavioral health change plan. Based on the PCP's preference and patient needs, the BHC may implement, monitor, or change the intervention, typically using one to four focused 15- to 30-minute appointments. However, when focusing on chronic conditions (e.g., diabetes, obesity, chronic pain), BHCs may periodically meet with patients over months or years to help the PCP manage the patient's health care plan. The BHC also makes recommendations as to how the PCP can support this plan and what the PCP might do to assist the patient in the future. It is fundamental to this model that the BHC is always working as a consultant to the PCP, helping the PCP manage patients' needs. For a more comprehensive review of the PCBH model, see Robinson and Reiter (2007) and Strosahl and Robinson (2008). We use the abbreviation *BHC* throughout this volume when referring to a behavioral health provider working in primary care. However, the strategies we describe are applicable to all providers (i.e., behavioral health providers and PCPs) working in this setting and are not limited to those using a PCBH service model.

THE 5A'S

Our format for assessment and intervention is based on the 5A's model (Whitlock, Orleans, Pender, & Allan, 2002): assess, advise, agree, assist, and arrange. The 5A's format has been strongly recommended for assessment and intervention across a range of problems in primary care (Goldstein, Whitlock, & DePue, 2004). The specific tasks within each of the 5A's vary depending on the nature of the problem as well as its severity and complexity (Whitlock et al., 2002). Nevertheless, the 5A's model can be applied to any patient in any clinic with any problem. We have found this flexible patient-centered model invaluable in providing behavioral health services in the primary care setting. Figure 1 provides an overview of how the 5A's connect and how they lead to a personal action plan.

The *assess* phase involves gathering information on physical symptoms, emotions, thoughts, behaviors, and important environmental variables such as family, friends, or work interactions. From

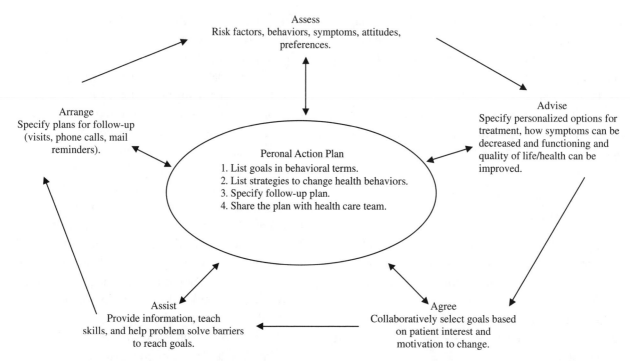

FIGURE 1.   The 5A's model of behavior change in primary care. From "Self-Management Aspects of the Improving Chronic Illness Care Breakthrough Series: Implementation With Diabetes and Heart Failure Teams," by R. E. Glasgow et al., 2002, *Annals of Behavioral Medicine, 24,* pp. 80–87. Copyright 2002 by Erlbaum. Adapted with permission.

a biopsychosocial perspective, the goal is to determine what variables are associated with patients' symptoms and functioning and then, on the basis of patients' values and what they have control over, to determine what they could change or alter that would decrease symptoms and improve functioning.

The *advise* phase involves describing to patients their options for intervention, on the basis of the data gathered in the assessment phase. The goal is to describe the intervention and the expected outcomes.

During the *agree* phase, patients decide on their course of action on the basis of the options discussed. They might also decide that they do not like any of the options and suggest some of their own, or they might take more time to think about their options and discuss them with a significant other.

In the *assist* phase, the BHC's job is to help patients learn new information, develop new skills, solve problems, and overcome environmental or personal barriers to implementing the behavior changes. This is where the formal intervention takes place.

In the *arrange* phase, we specify when or if patients will follow up with the BHC, PCP, or with a

specialty mental health provider. If the patient will be following up with the BHC, we also discuss what will be evaluated or what information or skill will be the focus of the next appointment.

Using the 5A's helps produce a meaningful and personalized health care action plan. The plan is specific, focused on health behavior change, and is an integrated piece of the patient's overall health care plan. Ideally, the plan is then monitored and managed by the entire health care team.

PURPOSE AND ORGANIZATION OF THIS VOLUME

With the increased need for efficient evidence-based care, this volume provides BHCs working in primary care (e.g., psychologists, social workers, psychiatrists, counselors), PCPs, and other medical care providers (e.g., physician assistants, nurses, health care educators) with practical strategies they can use immediately. Our suggestions are drawn from evidence-based data as well as our experience in translating evidence-based care to our clinical settings. Overall, our book is designed to give practical step-by-step guidance to which providers can frequently refer as they target biopsychosocial factors in primary care.

Students may also find this text useful. Undergraduate and graduate courses focused on preparing individuals to work in primary care can use this book as part of a seminar on assessment and intervention in primary care, or as part of a larger class focusing on brief treatments for common behavioral health problems.

The book is divided into two parts. Part I consists of four chapters that lay the foundation for an integrated behavioral health care practice. In chapter 1, we describe how to build and maintain an integrated service, which includes becoming involved, being a team member, building key relationships, being accessible, and learning the primary care culture. In chapter 2, using the 5A's, we outline the steps for an initial consultation appointment. This chapter provides a template for addressing patient problems in the primary care setting and provides the foundation for conducting the initial consultation. In chapter 3, we describe the basic tools of interventions for behavioral health problems that can be implemented in one to four 15- to 30-minute consultation appointments. These include the following nine interventions: relaxation training, goal setting, cognitive disputation, motivational interviewing, problem solving, self-monitoring, antecedent–behavior– consequences analysis, stimulus control, and assertive communication. We have found these nine interventions to be effective for a variety of symptoms and functional impairments. For each intervention, we apply the 5A's format and show how to present the intervention to the patient in plain, easily understandable language. In chapter 4, we discuss the importance of cultural competence in assessment and intervention in behavioral health consultation. Two models of culturally informed functional assessment are described and then adapted to the primary care setting. In addition, we describe the 5A's format in the context of patient-centered, culturally competent care.

In Part II, we apply the foundations presented in chapters 1 through 4 to the most common patient problems the BHC will encounter in the primary care setting. Each of the 11 chapters in Part II is structured as follows:

- description of the problem area;
- review of evidence-based interventions in the problem area;
- adaptation of interventions for the primary care setting;
- use of the 5A's format for assessment and intervention; and
- assessment and intervention tools, such as handouts, worksheets, checklists, and monitoring forms (these tools can also be downloaded from the APA Books Web site (http://www.apa. org/books/resources/Hunter) and tailored to one's particular needs and setting).

For clarity, throughout the volume, the term *specialty mental health* refers to traditional or standard assessment and treatment in an outpatient mental health clinic. The term *behavioral health* refers to activities that are performed within the primary care clinic. Our goal is to provide straightforward, easy-to-use information to assist in addressing particular problems in the primary care setting. We believe readers will find, as we have, that this way of working with patients will result in functional improvement and symptom change over a surprisingly short period.

We have had the opportunity to spend thousands of hours in primary care settings, including family medicine, internal medicine, and obstetrics and gynecology, as part of successful integrated behavioral health services. We have also taught hundreds of behavioral health providers to deliver effective behavioral health care in integrated settings. We hope that by using these evidence-based assessments and interventions, coupled with our shared experiences, you can become more effective in your primary care work and can continue to improve the health of the population.

PART I

FOUNDATIONS OF INTEGRATED BEHAVIORAL HEALTH CONSULTATION SERVICES

CHAPTER 1

BUILDING AN INTEGRATED PRIMARY CARE SERVICE

A traditionally trained behavioral health professional working in a primary care setting is similar to someone who goes to live in a foreign country for the first time. On arriving, one would quickly note that many things are different. The people speak a language that cannot be understood. Customs, mores, and norms are different. Work habits and hours are unfamiliar. People relate to time differently; some things are done more leisurely and some more urgently. Even dealing with money requires some adjustment. If one is not aware of these differences, and is not prepared to accept and to adjust to them, it will not be possible to thrive in the new country or be accepted by its inhabitants. If, however, one embraces this different way of life and does one's best to fit in, it is likely that the uniqueness of the culture and the background one brings will be viewed as a positive factor that enriches the community rather than challenges it.

Mental health providers and physicians are trained differently, think differently, relate to patients and colleagues differently; they also practice under different standards and rules (Bray, 1996). Specialty mental health practitioners work under different time constraints than their physician colleagues, especially those in the primary care setting. Reimbursement systems are typically dissimilar as well. Similar to the ethnocentric foreigner, a mental health provider who attempts to integrate into primary care without adapting to the "culture" of primary care will likely not be accepted by medical peers, making true integration of behavioral health care into the medical practice impossible. Such adaptation is much easier when you have access to a travel guide to explain the culture in sufficient detail.

A TRAVEL GUIDE

Any worthwhile travel guide tells the reader not only about sights to see and places of interest but also about how things work at the destination, such as transportation, tipping, laws, and customs. This chapter is intended to provide similar guidance for the mental health provider entering the primary care world. We review step-by-step strategies on what to consider when building a behavioral health primary care service. Important "cultural shift" information is discussed, including how to "speak primary care language," read medical records and notes, comply with privacy requirements, and handle treatment interruptions. In short, we present strategies you can use to become immersed into the primary care culture and to adapt quickly.

We provide plans and handouts to help the primary care staff understand what you, the behavioral health provider, have to offer. All of the patient handouts and checklists for behavioral health providers in this volume are also available for limited, noncommercial use at an associated Web page (http://www.apa.org/books/resources/Hunter). We also suggest ways to determine staff deficits in the understanding of the role of the behavioral health consultant (BHC), and we describe how to provide useful in-service training to address such deficits. Finally, we review what one should and should not do to develop collegial relationships and how to create opportunities for primary care staff to discuss, formally and informally, personal and professional difficulties with the primary care behavioral health provider consistent with the way primary care providers (PCPs) support their colleagues.

This travel guide will smooth the way toward successful integration into what can be a foreign culture for many mental health professionals. Using this material will help you build a foundation that will pay off tremendously in your primary care service and support a thriving practice in which you can apply the clinical material in this volume with your patients.

THE ROADMAP

Although there is increasing interest in mental health providers working in primary care settings, many health care organizations and individual physicians are still unfamiliar with the concept of integrated primary care. In our experience, the majority of primary care physicians, nurse managers, and clinic administrators become enthusiastic about integrated services as they learn about and experience the benefits. Patients with psychosocial and behavioral health needs are prevalent in primary care (Kroenke & Mangelsdorff, 1989), and therefore many clinic personnel welcome behavioral health expertise within a specific clinical practice. Integrated behavioral health means better care for patients, fewer referrals to specialty mental health providers outside the primary care practice, and better collaboration among professionals.

Several key recommendations can serve as a roadmap for mental health providers to navigate the culture of primary care and build a foundation for integrated behavioral health care. Gatchel and Oordt (2003) categorized these recommendations under the following areas: (a) get your foot in the door, (b) be a team member, (c) build key relationships, (d) be highly available, and (e) learn the primary care culture. Some of the main points from Gatchel and Oordt's (2003) work are summarized here to guide your successful integration into a primary care clinical setting. Most important, however, is that this volume is designed to provide tools and resources to assist you in implementing this material. Handouts for starting and building your practice are included in this chapter (see Figures 1.1–1.4).

Get Your Foot in the Door

The first step in developing a primary care service is to market your services to clinic management. Success begins with effectively selling what you have to offer and how it can benefit the practice and its patients. Despite what may seem to you as the inherent logic of integrating behavioral health services into a medical practice, numerous factors can hamper acceptance, including biases about mental health care, reimbursement issues, financial issues related to overhead and support staff costs, workspace concerns, territorial issues, use of support staff, and simple resistance to changing the customary ways in which mental health services have been used in the past (e.g., through referral to an outside source). You may need to overcome each barrier by demonstrating your worth to the medical staff. A number of arrangements for associations between physicians and nonphysician mental health providers and legal options vary by state. Guidance is available from the American Psychological Association Practice Directorate (see *Models for Multidisciplinary Arrangements: A State-by-State Review of Options*; [APA, 1996]).

Staff model systems in which the salaries of health care providers are paid by the health care organization provide greater flexibility for provision of behavioral health services in primary care than do systems based on a fee-for-service structure. This is because of the complexities and limitations in reimbursement for certain services from third parties. For example, many insurance companies will only reimburse behavioral health providers for mental health care using codes for psychiatric services. This may limit services to the treatment of primary or comorbid mental health disorders and not allow for psychophysiological treatment (e.g., biofeedback therapy), preventive interventions, or behavioral services directed at primary medical disorders. This situation has improved in recent years with the addition of new current procedural terminology (CPT) codes that allow BHCs to bill for services directed at physical health problems (Smith, 2002). These codes, however, are reimbursed at significantly lower rates than would be paid if BHCs were permitted to bill using medical CPT codes. These financial issues must be carefully

A Behavioral Health Consultant can provide a broad range of services including assessment, education and brief intervention for your patients. To help ensure that I provide services that meet the needs of you and your patients, please complete the following survey.

In sections **B** and **C** below, use the following scale to rate your responses:

	Never	Rarely	Sometimes	Often
	1	2	3	4

A. Please circle the number of any item below in which you are unclear on how a behavioral health (BH) provider can help or for which your confidence is low that a BH provider can help.

B. How often in your practice do you see patients who present with the following problems?

C. When working with a patient with this problem, how often might you request assistance from behavioral health consultant?

	B				C			
1. Mental Health Disorders (depression, anxiety/panic, etc.)	1	2	3	4	1	2	3	4
2. Sub-clinical emotional symptoms (sadness, worry, guilt, etc)	1	2	3	4	1	2	3	4
3. Difficulties coping with stress	1	2	3	4	1	2	3	4
4. Marital problems	1	2	3	4	1	2	3	4
5. Child behavior problems	1	2	3	4	1	2	3	4
6. Other family problems	1	2	3	4	1	2	3	4
7. Chronic pain	1	2	3	4	1	2	3	4
8. Tension or migraine headache	1	2	3	4	1	2	3	4
9. Chronic insomnia	1	2	3	4	1	2	3	4
10. Grief and bereavement	1	2	3	4	1	2	3	4
11. Non-compliance with medication	1	2	3	4	1	2	3	4
12. Tobacco use (wanting to quit)	1	2	3	4	1	2	3	4
13. Tobacco use (not wanting to quit)	1	2	3	4	1	2	3	4
14. Overweight/obesity	1	2	3	4	1	2	3	4
15. Sedentary lifestyle impacting health	1	2	3	4	1	2	3	4
16. Stress-related medical conditions	1	2	3	4	1	2	3	4
17. Self-esteem issues	1	2	3	4	1	2	3	4
18. Unhealthy alcohol use	1	2	3	4	1	2	3	4
19. Drug abuse	1	2	3	4	1	2	3	4
20. Over-utilization of healthcare	1	2	3	4	1	2	3	4
21. Coping with chronic/terminal illness	1	2	3	4	1	2	3	4
22. "White-coat" hypertension	1	2	3	4	1	2	3	4
23. Anxiety interfering with medical care	1	2	3	4	1	2	3	4

Please indicate by number the top five items or clinical areas above in which you would like to see services from the behavioral health consultant.

1._____   2._____   3._____   4._____   5._____

Thank you for completing the survey. Please add any comments to the back of this form.

FIGURE 1.1. Provider survey.

considered with respect to the type of setting in which you are trying to work; you should discuss these issues explicitly when approaching clinic management about the services you can offer. You will also need to negotiate overhead cost arrangements in advance of beginning your primary care practice. Overhead costs can be managed in variety of ways, including cost sharing based on the space and administrative services used or by employing separate administrative staff for billing and scheduling behavioral health patients. In public sector health care settings or other staff model practices,

---

Providing the Right Care, for the Right People, at the Right Time

---

Family Medicine Behavioral Health Consultant

Services: Consultation (30 minutes) for assessment and behavioral health treatment planning, recommendations, and interventions.

Referrals: ANYTHING you think might be helped through habit, behavioral, cognitive, or emotional changes.

Goals of Service: To help you and your patients develop practical knowledge and skills to promote and improve physical and emotional health.

The following is a list of common problems for which I may be helpful.

General Mental Health Problems
- ❏ Stress
- ❏ Anxiety/Fears
- ❏ Depression
- ❏ Anger
- ❏ Relationship Problems
- ❏ Grief or Bereavement
- ❏ Diet (weight loss, dietary adherence problems)
- ❏ Exercise
- ❏ Chronic Illness Management:
- ❏ Diabetes, GI Problems, COPD, Medication Adherence

Clinical Health Problems
- ❏ Insomnia
- ❏ Chronic Pain
- ❏ Headache
- ❏ Fibromyalgia
- ❏ Temporomandibular Disorders
- ❏ Low Back Pain
- ❏ Tobacco Use
- ❏ ETOH Use

FIGURE 1.2.   Behavioral health consultant marketing brochure.

Patient Name and ID: _____   **Referring PCP:**_____

Circle Consult Problem: Anxiety, Panic, IBS, Hyperventilation, Depression, Stress, Insomnia, Chronic Pain, GERD, COPD, Diabetes, ETOH Problems, Adherence, Tobacco Cessation, Obesity, Anger, Relational Problems, Bereavement, Memory Problems, Other: _____

*Requesting Provider, please circle requested skills training/patient education:

Anxiety/ Panic/ IBS/ Hyperventilation: 1. Deep Breathing Training; 2. Cue Controlled Relaxation; 3. Modify Thoughts That↑Sx; 4. Educate on Physiology of Autonomic Arousal; 5. Medication Side Effect Education

Depression: 1. Educated on Depression Cycle; 2.↑Exercise; 3.↑Social Support; 4.↑Pleasant Activities; 5. ↑Medical Tx Adherence; 6. Medication S/E Education

Stress Management: 1. Deep Breathing Training; 2. Cue Controlled Relaxation; 3. Modify Thoughts That ↑Sx; 4. ↑Exercise; 5.↑Social Support; 6.↑Pleasant Activities; 7. Assertive Communication

Insomnia: 1. Sleep Behaviors, Stimulus Control, Sleep Hygiene; 2. Relaxation Skills Training

Weight Management: 1. Improving Exercise Habits; 2. Eating Behavior Change; 3. Weight Management Education; 4. Modify Thoughts That Perpetuate Problem

Chronic Pain (musculoskeletal/HA): 1. Pacing Activities; 2. Relaxation Training; 3.↑Exercise; 4.↑Social Support; 5.↑Pleasant Activities; 6. Modify Thoughts; 7. Education on Pain

Medical Illness Management: 1. Depression Cycle Education; 2. Relaxation Skills Training; 3. ↑Social Support; 4.↑Pleasant Activities; 5. Modify Thoughts That Perpetuate Problem

OTHER:_____

FIGURE 1.3.   Consultation request.

> **Stress**
>
> Is STRESS a factor in your patients' well-being?
>
> I can help your patients in the following ways:
>
> - Recognizing the signs and symptoms of stress
> - Identifying triggers for stress reactions
> - Relaxation training
> - Teaching healthy thinking strategies
> - Improving balance between work and leisure
> - Enhancing problem solving skills
>
> Patients can be scheduled for behavioral health consultation appointments at the reception desk or can be seen promptly on the day he or she has an appointment with you. I can be contacted by pager at 555-5555.

FIGURE 1.4.   **Problem of the week sample flyer.**

overhead issues may be less of a concern because costs are shared across the facility. Readers are referred to Gatchel and Oordt (2003) and Robinson and Reiter (2007) for a more extensive discussion of financial issues related to integrated behavioral health care.

Getting your foot in the door requires being as flexible and accommodating as possible. This is most important at the beginning of your collaborative relationship with the medical staff. The services a well-qualified behavioral health provider can offer are greatly needed in primary care, and patients tend to welcome these services (Talcott, Russ, & Dobmeyer, 2001). It is likely, therefore, that you will quickly demonstrate your value to providers, nurses, and other staff, which, in turn, will open new doors for developing your primary care behavioral health service. However, pushing too hard and demanding too much before colleagues are persuaded of your value may obstruct your integration efforts. It is important to remember that you are entering a world and a culture that "belongs" to other professions, and that you are the one who will have to be flexible to gain entrance.

In the optimal situation, you will need your own office space and equipment, medical record management, reception and appointment service, as well as coding and billing support. Initially, however, it may be necessary to accept minimal support to enter the practice. This may include keeping your own appoint-

ment template, providing your own computer, or working in a different office every day. As you become accepted and valued by the staff, you will likely succeed in negotiating more support. With time, behavioral health services commonly become viewed as an indispensable component of how health care is delivered, and colleagues may actually advocate on your behalf with clinic management for improvements to make your work easier and more productive.

BHCs should take steps to identify the priorities and needs of the clinic, and work to establish initial services that address these needs. For example, if the clinic is establishing a new clinical pathway for obesity, the behavioral health provider can offer to contribute by running a weight management group. If providers are struggling to meet the needs of a few patients with chronic medical conditions who are overusing medical services, the behavioral health provider might offer to see these patients as soon as possible. Interviews with the personnel at all levels within the organization can shed light on what their priorities are. Asking personnel what their greatest challenges are in providing good care or which types of patients are most challenging can elicit valuable health care targets for the behavioral health provider to pursue. A brief provider survey may also help identify these areas (see Figure 1.1). When presenting this survey, it may be useful to introduce it as follows:

> I was wondering if you had 5 minutes this week to circle the numbers on this sheet so I can get a better idea of the types of patients you see and how you like to use behavioral health consultants to help meet your patients' needs. Having this information will help me to better serve your needs. When would it be a good time for me to pick this up from you?

Letting providers know that what you are asking them to do is geared directly toward helping them is likely to increase the chances that they will complete the survey. In addition, knowing that you will be coming back when they say they will be finished will increase the chances that they will complete the survey and will give you the opportunity to reengage with them if it is not complete. Responding to the clinic's priorities will likely elicit enthusiasm for the behavioral health addition to the team, and your practice will grow more rapidly than if you first try to market your own specialty areas or interests.

Be a Team Member

Functioning well as a team requires each member to know his or her role and perform well in that role. Flexible collaboration, knowing your target audience, and succinct and timely feedback are keys to being a successful team member.

Collaboration.   Collaboration with medical colleagues in meeting the needs of their patients is key to a successful integrated primary care practice. It is essential for behavioral health providers to keep their scope of care as broad as possible within the limits of their training and experience. Accept all referrals and do your best to find ways to assist anyone who may need your help, including the following:

- patients with potential mental health diagnoses;
- patients needing help with health-related behavior change (e.g., tobacco cessation, increasing exercise, diet changes);
- patients with stress or coping difficulties;
- grieving or dying patients;
- family members of patients with illnesses or disabilities;
- patients with medical adherence difficulties; and
- patients with whom physician colleagues are frustrated, such as individuals who excessively or needlessly use health care resources (see chap. 16), who demonstrate personality disorders, or for whom there is no significant benefit derived from repeatedly seeing a physician.

The more of a generalist you are, the more of a team player you will be. A marketing brochure for the PCPs that outlines a full range of services you can provide can help establish you in this vein. Figure 1.2 is a sample brochure. When presenting this brochure, it may be useful to introduce it as follows:

> I was wondering if there was a time today or later this week when I could speak with you for about 2 minutes to go

over the types of patients and problems I might be able to help you manage.

Physicians as your primary customer.   Another way to establish yourself as a team player is to view the referring PCPs as your primary customers. This involves focusing on the PCP's reason for referring the patient before addressing other problems the patient may present. It also involves providing feedback to PCPs in a way that is most helpful to them. Primary care behavioral health providers must take care that their services are consistent and supportive of the health care being provided by the PCP; that is, you and the PCP should be working toward the same goals in collaboration with the patient.

Be diligent both in ensuring you know what the PCP's reason is for referring the patient and in responding back specifically about the referral problem. Other concerns may be identified during a behavioral health assessment that may need to be addressed in treatment; however, the provider's referral question must not be overshadowed. For example, a PCP may refer a woman to you to learn behavioral strategies for improving sleep. During the evaluation, you learn that significant marital distress is the patient's primary concern; this you believe is a contributing factor to the sleep difficulties. A treatment plan centered on resolving marital issues is developed and implemented. However, the education on behavioral sleep strategies requested by the physician is never delivered.

In this example, you and the PCP are working toward somewhat different goals. Although it is appropriate and ethically necessary to offer or facilitate services that address identified problem areas, it is also important to address the primary reason for referral. In this example, you might simply have added as part of the treatment plan an educational component on behavioral strategies for sleep, so that the patient can benefit from what both the PCP determined was needed and what you assessed as an additional problem area. This would represent better collaboration. Of course, there may be times when you believe the intervention requested by the PCP is inappropriate; in those instances, you should discuss your opinions and recommendations with the referring PCP. Never ignore or neglect the referring issue or request. An easy to use, yet sufficiently detailed, referral form can help facilitate communication about what the referring provider is requesting. An example is provided in Figure 1.3.

Assessment and intervention feedback.   Providing feedback to the PCP is the other key factor to working as a team. In a busy practice, this can often be neglected. However, feedback is the foundation for reaping the benefits of integrating behavioral health services into primary care. Take time to find out what PCPs find helpful when you give them feedback on a patient: How much detail do they want? Do they prefer written (clinical notes) or verbal feedback? Do they want it immediately following the patient visit or do they prefer feedback about all patients together at the end of the day?

At minimum, your feedback should include significant findings, impressions, and recommendations, and this feedback should be provided on the same day the patient is seen. It is best to keep feedback focused on the PCP's referral question and avoid unnecessary discussion of extraneous issues. Target your verbal feedback to be 60 seconds or less. If the PCP wants more information, he or she will ask. For example,

> I saw Mrs. Bennet today. Is now a good time to give you some feedback, or would another time work better? Her sleeping problems were kicked off by marital distress. She is engaging in sleep behaviors that are making her sleep worse, such as getting into bed when not sleepy, staying in bed awake for several hours, thinking about the future of her marriage, and taking naps when she comes home from work. We set a plan to change sleep behaviors that includes getting into bed only when sleepy, getting out of bed if not asleep in 15 minutes, thinking about her marriage in her living room, not her bedroom, and stopping naps. I also taught her the basics of assertive communication. She is following up with me in

2 weeks to reassess her sleep problems. When you see her again, I'd encourage you to ask her if she is getting into bed only when sleepy and getting out of bed if not asleep in 15 minutes. If not, you might encourage her to do so if she wants her sleep to improve.

Build Key Relationships
Few factors will contribute to success of an integrated behavioral health service as much as the relationships you build with the primary care team members. Establishing collegiality with administrative staff, technicians, nurses, and PCPs will make your work easier and ensure the best patient care possible. You can take several steps to promote good working relationships as you establish your primary care service.

Get support from informal leaders.   Determine who within the clinic are the informal leaders; that is, those to whom others look to shape opinion, those who have a track-record of making changes happen, and those who people come to with organizational issues and problems. These people may or may not be those in formal leadership positions. Talk with them about what you can offer patients and how your services can help them to perform their roles better and more easily. Gaining acceptance from these individuals may determine whether your practice is accepted within the primary care clinic.

Take time to get to know all support personnel within the clinic, including technicians, reception staff, billing personnel, and housekeepers. Learn their names, their history with the clinic; discuss their roles and the challenges they face. These relationships will establish goodwill and may be essential should you need their assistance in the future.

Ask the PCPs whether you can sit in on their appointments for a day. This will ensure you know each provider and they know you. It will help you better understand how they operate and can serve as a crash course in the primary care culture. In addition, you will have the opportunity to point out areas in which a referral to you would benefit patients, thus increasing the range of referrals to your practice. Finally, take steps to make yourself part of the clinic by attending formal and informal gatherings along with the other providers, including lunches hosted by pharmaceutical companies, holiday parties, and provider meetings. This will help establish you as part of the clinic team and not just a visiting provider.

Market your services. A new primary care behavioral health service will not just happen. It will require persistent marketing to PCPs and frequent reminders that you are available to assist their patients in ways that can both improve care and make their jobs easier. A variety of marketing strategies are recommended as follows to keep your services in the minds of colleagues.

Problem of the week. First, consider distributing a "Problem of the Week" flyer to all clinical staff highlighting a specific clinical condition you are seeking referrals for and what services you offer. Examples would be flyers on obesity, smoking cessation, stress management, medication compliance, depression, worry control, panic control, physical inactivity, or motivational issues. To be useful to busy primary care staff, these marketing materials must be brief; the information must be gleaned by scanning for a few seconds because longer materials are unlikely to be read. Simply state the clinical problem area and what you can you do to help in a few bulleted lines. Figure 1.4 is an example.

Daily check-ins. Second, consider conducting daily check-ins with each provider at the beginning of the day (K. Strosahl, personal communication, September 19, 2000). Ask whether any patients on the schedule might benefit from your services. Your schedule should be arranged so that some patients can be seen shortly after their scheduled medical appointments, when needed. A recommended practice is to leave every other appointment slot unscheduled to maintain availability. This practice allows for what is commonly referred to as a "warm handoff"; that is, the PCP introduces the patient he or she is seeing to the BHC at the end of a regular primary care visit. From here, the BHC can help with assessment and intervention at that

moment, avoiding delay in services and minimizing patient trips to the clinic. Again, this will likely help keep your services in the minds of the PCPs as they see their patients throughout the day.

Be Highly Available

Physicians are more likely to use a BHC who is responsive and easily accessible. Therefore, you will benefit from removing as many barriers to care as possible. Potential barriers include (a) Difficulty reaching you for consultation or referral when needed, (b) problems accessing appointments, (c) patients having to leave the clinic and return later in the day before seeing you, and (d) lack of feedback to the provider following a consultation.

BHCs can overcome these barriers by carrying a cell phone or pager and encouraging colleagues to make contact any time a question arises. Although many outpatient specialty mental health providers use a "do not disturb" sign to avoid interruptions during treatment appointments, this is not the norm in primary care settings. In primary care, knocks on the door and phone calls should be answered promptly, even during patient appointments. If you are working in primary care on a part-time basis, arrange a method for contacting you when the need arises and you are outside the clinic (e.g., cell phone, pager). It is essential to reinforce PCPs' use of your services with quick responsiveness. In addition, make yourself available during times when other PCPs are likely to be free to consult with you. These times include early morning before the first patient appointment, lunch, and the end of the business day.

Learn the Primary Care Culture

Many aspects of the primary care environment will be foreign to the traditionally trained mental health professional. Behavioral health providers typically differ from physicians on factors such as theoretical orientation, language, practice style, and expectations for assessment and treatment (Bray, 1996). Integration into primary care requires adaptation to this culture; behavioral health providers should not expect the primary care environment to adapt in response to their presence. The following suggestions are likely to help you fit in.

- Speak the same language. Use practical, no-nonsense language and avoid psychological jargon. Reading medical journals and texts can help you become more familiar with common medical terms to help communicate. Do not try to go beyond your working knowledge or you will lose credibility.

- Adopt the primary care pace. Appointment slots of 15 to 30 minutes will help ensure prompt access and will demonstrate your commitment to working as part of the primary care team. Although many behavioral health providers are unaccustomed to such brief appointments, this schedule is realistic if you are providing focused assessments and brief interventions appropriate to the primary care setting.

- Provide brief, focused interventions to a large number of the patients within the practice, rather than providing comprehensive care to a few more severe cases. For instance, avoid providing extended psychotherapy for chronic mental health conditions. This will allow you to be integrated into the routine care provided in the clinic and not be relegated to a specialist role. Patients needing extended psychotherapy or other specialty level mental health care can be referred to outpatient specialty mental health providers.

- Ensure that your feedback to providers is succinct and prompt. Comprehensive assessment reports are not the norm in the primary care setting. Verbal feedback should typically be delivered in 60 seconds or less; if more detail is needed, PCPs will ask for clarification. Written documentation can also be more abbreviated than what is typical for specialty mental health care. Mimic the writing style of the PCPs by using similar abbreviations and format. Avoid psychological jargon whenever possible.

- Make recommendations that are brief, specific, and action-oriented. Remember that PCPs may be spending as little as 5 to 7 minutes with the patient; recommendations you would like them to incorporate into their care will need to be practical within that context.

- Familiarize yourself with the organizations that are important to the PCPs. For example, family physicians may belong to the American Academy of Family Physicians (AAFP), which provides valuable resources in print and online for the entire spectrum of family medicine services. Attending a conference sponsored by such organizations can help you better understand the issues that are important to the PCPs with whom you work.

- Understand what resources the PCPs use to get information, particularly about behavioral health concerns. Physicians who focus on evidence-based care often rely on Cochrane reports, the Agency for Healthcare Research and Quality, Up-to-Date, or their organizations (e.g., AAFP, American College of Physicians) to guide their clinical practice.

The primary care culture is also one in which professionals take care of each other. PCPs consult with each other on difficult or complex cases. Personal problems—both medical and social—are discussed and advice is given. Ethical issues are discussed formally and informally. Interpersonal problems between staff members and between patients and staff are addressed. This culture is essential to creating the supportive environment in which people can successfully face the personal and professional challenges of working in health care.

A trained and experienced BHC is a valuable resource for this process and this is generally quickly recognized. In our experience, staff at all levels within the organization, from senior executives to most junior medical technician, will consult with the behavioral health provider to discuss personal problems, interpersonal conflicts, difficult patients, and personal or family mental health concerns. It can be helpful to the primary care organization if you embrace this role as caretaker of the staff. Take the time to offer whatever assistance you can. Often this simply entails listening, normalizing, and validating people's perceptions and experiences. Sometimes you will be able to give practical advice. To avoid dual relationships, it is important to keep firm boundaries on what you do in this role. Keep your role to one of support, advice, and consultation and avoid formal assessment or treatment with coworkers. If you determine that behavioral health services are indicated, you can encourage or facilitate care with a provider outside the immediate organization. In addition, ensure that coworkers have access to you without drawing excessive attention to themselves. For example, allow them to talk to you after clinic hours when fewer staff members are present, avoid putting them on your schedule as patients, or talk with them somewhere other than your treatment office so it is not apparent they are coming to you for help. Of course, it is essential that confidentiality when talking with staff members be maintained. If you can provide helpful, nonthreatening assistance to a colleague, he or she will not hesitate to send patients to you as well.

ENJOY THE JOURNEY

Working in a primary care medical setting can be a highly rewarding and positively challenging experience for a behavioral health provider. It is a setting that provides opportunities to contribute to the well-being of patients who might otherwise never use behavioral health care and to assist PCPs in delivering more effective behavioral health services.

Not all behavioral health providers are well suited for the primary care environment. This setting does not allow for time-intensive, long-term psychotherapy modalities or comprehensive psychological testing batteries. Behavioral health providers in primary care must accept working in a hierarchical system in which physicians have a higher position than nonphysicians. They must be willing and able to work as independent practitioners but also be part of a team. For those who are willing to work with these issues, however, working in the primary care environment can be fulfilling.

Primary behavioral health care is a journey, and building a solid foundation to your practice will help you thrive and enjoy this unique application of behavioral health care knowledge and skills. The material in this chapter and resources that follow can help you establish this foundation. The remainder of this volume will provide a wealth of resources for delivering high quality behavioral health care within the primary care setting.

CHAPTER 2

CONDUCTING THE INITIAL CONSULTATION APPOINTMENT

In this chapter, we detail the steps to follow in an initial consultation appointment. These include introducing the behavioral health consultant (BHC) service to the patient, identifying and clarifying the problem for which the patient was referred, conducting a functional assessment of that problem, summarizing the problem, suggesting change options, and starting the change plan. We presented the basic 5A's structure in Figure 1 of the introduction. Figure 2.1 illustrates how these steps fit into a 30-minute time frame. In this chapter, we focus on a general format for any initial consultation. The chapters in Part II suggest additional material to cover in the initial consultation specific to a particular problem area.

INTRODUCING THE BEHAVIORAL HEALTH CONSULTATION SERVICE

Patients are often unclear about what to expect when they see a BHC. Therefore, it is essential to provide the patient with information about what you do and to develop a plan early in the first encounter. In our experience, patients who do not have this information often have more difficulty answering questions, are more likely to believe you are going to provide a service you cannot provide (e.g., specialty mental health services), and are more likely to feel uncertain about how you are going to help them. Start your appointment by making the following clear to the patient:

- your profession and training,
- your role in the clinic,
- the amount of time you will be spending with him or her during the appointment,

- who will have access to the information he or she discusses, and
- what you are going to do to try to help him or her.

To assist with this process, we suggest that you provide patients with an information sheet that lists all the information you tell them. Figure 2.2 is an example of an information sheet. You might say the following:

> I'd like to begin by explaining who I am and what I do in the clinic. I'm a (psychologist, social worker, licensed professional counselor, etc.) and I work with primary care providers in situations where good health care involves paying attention to physical health, habits, behaviors, emotional health, and how these might interact with each other. This pamphlet describes my services in more detail, and you may want to read it over after our appointment today.
>
> Your provider has asked me to consult with you today. My job is to help you and your provider to better address the problems that have come up for you. To help the two of you do this, I'm going to spend about 30 minutes with you in a consultation appointment. During this time, I'd like to get a snapshot of your life and determine what's working well and what's not working so well. I'll take the information that you give me, and together you and I will

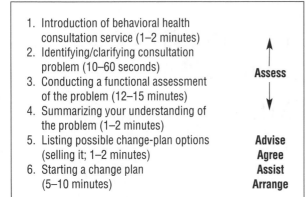

1. Introduction of behavioral health consultation service (1–2 minutes)
2. Identifying/clarifying consultation problem (10–60 seconds)
3. Conducting a functional assessment of the problem (12–15 minutes)
4. Summarizing your understanding of the problem (1–2 minutes)
5. Listing possible change-plan options (selling it; 1–2 minutes)
6. Starting a change plan (5–10 minutes)

Assess

Advise
Agree
Assist
Arrange

FIGURE 2.1. Structure for the initial consultation appointment linked with the 5A's.

come up with a plan to help you better manage what's going on.

The plan might include things you try on your own, such as reading some self-help material or practicing various skills. Or, we may decide to have you come back for follow-up appointments to help monitor your progress or to help you learn additional skills. We might also decide that you would benefit from seeing a more intensive specialty service. If that were the case, I would help your provider arrange that referral, using the information you've given me today. I'm going to write a note that will go into your medical record and I'm going to give your provider some feedback on the plan we come up with today. Do you have any questions about any of this before we begin?

If patients have questions, spend the time needed to make sure they understand the purposes of this service. It is important to allow at least a brief time for patients to ask any questions they have about your role before you start, as this will help prevent misunderstanding and confusion later on.

IDENTIFYING AND CLARIFYING THE CONSULTATION PROBLEM

After you have verbally introduced the BHC service, you might say something such as the follow-ing: "[Medical provider's name] would like me to assist the two of you in better managing or targeting [referral reason]. Is that what you see as the main problem or is it something different?" If he or she says "yes" and agrees with the main problem focus for the appointment, then begin the functional assessment by saying something such as, "OK, then I'd like to ask you several questions about [referral reason] to get a better understanding of what's involved." Then begin the functional assessment. If the answer is "no," then ask the patient what he or she sees as the main problem. This is important because primary care providers (PCPs) sometimes misunderstand what the patient considers the main problem, and sometimes the PCP and patient disagree about the main problem. However, if you spend time assessing a problem the patient is not concerned about, you are likely to have an unproductive appointment.

CONDUCTING A FUNCTIONAL ASSESSMENT OF THE PROBLEM

After the introduction, the primary focus is information gathering. A common mistake made by behavioral health and medical providers when initially gathering information is the overuse of ambiguous and open-ended questions. Although open-ended questions are certainly useful in specialty mental health care settings, time limitations make this strategy impractical as a primary way to gather information in primary care. Open-ended or ambiguous questions may elicit lengthy or ambiguous answers that may not provide much useful information. As such, BHCs may find themselves at the end of a 30-minute appointment without having obtained sufficient information from which to make recommendations or start an intervention.

Focused questions that are closed-ended or menu-driven (e.g., providing patients with several choices to pick when answering) allow the BHC to gather information needed to identify the primary problem, contributing factors, and make a diagnosis, if necessary, in a limited time frame. However, we do recommend the use of open-ended questions once you think you have collected all the information you need to understand the patient's problem. For

---

Patient Behavioral Health Consultation Information Handout

WHAT IS THE BEHAVIORAL HEALTH CONSULTATION SERVICE?

The Behavioral Health Consultation Service offers assistance when habits, behaviors, stress, worry, or emotional concerns about physical or other life problems are interfering with a person's daily life and/or overall health. The behavioral health consultant (BHC) works with your primary care provider (PCP) to evaluate the mind–body–behavior connection and provide brief, solution-focused interventions.

The BHC has specialty training in the behavioral management of health problems. Together, the BHC and your PCP can consider the physical, behavioral, and emotional aspects of your health concern and help determine a course of action that will work best for you.

What Kind of Health Concerns Do You See?

The BHC can help you reduce symptoms associated with various chronic medical conditions, or help you cope better with these conditions. A few of these are: **Headaches, Sleep, High Blood Pressure, Asthma, Diabetes, Obesity, Chronic Pain, and Irritable Bowel Syndrome.**

The BHC can help you and your PCP develop behavioral change plans for smoking cessation, weight loss, alcohol use, exercise or other lifestyle modifications. The BHC can also help you and your PCP develop skills to effectively manage emotional or behavioral difficulties such as: **Anger, Anxiety, Bereavement, Depression, and Stress.**

Who Is Eligible to Receive These Services?

The service is available to all patients within the Family Health Center as a part of good overall health care.

What Should I Expect When I See the Behavioral Health Consultant?

You can expect the BHC to ask you specific questions about your physical symptoms, the emotional concerns you are experiencing, your behaviors, and how all of these might be related. You can expect your appointments to last approximately 30 minutes and for the BHC to provide brief solution-focused assessment and treatment. You can also expect to be seen in this clinic and for the BHC to have a close working relationship with your PCP. Remember, you and your PCP remain in charge of your health care; the BHC's primary job is to help you and your PCP develop and implement the best integrated health care plan for YOU!

How is This Service Different From Mental Health Services?

The services provided by the BHC are simply another part of your overall health care and are not specialty mental health care. Documentation of your appointment and recommendations from the BHC will be written in your medical record. A separate mental health record will not be kept when you see the BHC.

Communications with your BHC may not be entirely confidential. Your BHC will make every effort to protect your privacy. However, like all providers, they may have to report information regarding child or spouse abuse, or share information regarding those at risk to harm themselves or others.

The BHC does not provide traditional psychotherapy. If you request, or the BHC thinks you would benefit from specialty mental health services, the BHC will recommend that you and your PCP consider those services.

How Do I Schedule a Behavioral Health Consultant Appointment?

Discuss with your PCP the desire to access this service. If you and your provider agree this service would be helpful, call the Family Health Center at XXX-XXX-XXXX to schedule a BHC appointment.

FIGURE 2.2. Patient behavioral health consultation information handout.

instance, you might say, "Is there anything I haven't asked about that you think is important for me to know?" As time allows, you may also choose to ask the following: "Take me through what a typical day (workday, if he or she works) looks like for you?" and "What does your non-workday look like?" Questions such as these can yield information you might not get by asking closed-ended or menu-driven questions, and sometimes that information can be valuable for understanding the problem, factors related to that problem, and intervention planning.

Another common mistake involves the frequent use of empathic or reflective statements and restatement of what the patient has just said in a manner consistent with what is done in a traditional specialty mental health service. This is typically not necessary and can be an inefficient use of time. Patients will know you are listening by eye contact, head nods, and brief verbalizations (e.g., "uh huh"). Patients will also know you have understood them when they hear the summary statement you will give once you have finished your functional assessment of the problem.

General areas to assess that can elicit more information on the primary referral problem include the nature of the referral problem, duration of problem, triggering events, frequency and intensity of the problem, factors that make the problem better or worse, functional impairment, as well as changes in sleep, interest, energy, concentration, appetite, substance use, mood, and suicidal or homicidal ideation. Examples of closed-end or menu-type questions you might ask for each category, using depression as the example, are presented in Figure 2.3. These examples demonstrate questions that are likely to get clinically rich information in a relatively short period of time; however, we are not suggesting that all of these questions should be or need to be asked of every patient. To demonstrate follow-up questions that might be asked, we have also included individual responses to some questions as examples of what a patient might say. Answers to the questions under these content areas will allow you to get a reasonable understanding of the frequency, duration, and severity of the patient's symptoms and functional impairments. Responses will also shed light on what the patient is doing or not doing that might be related to their symptoms and poor functioning.

SUMMARIZING YOUR UNDERSTANDING OF THE PROBLEM

Once you have a working understanding of the patient's symptoms and functional impairments as well as the factors adding to, perpetuating, or driving the problem, provide a summary statement of the problem, as you have understood it. This vital step provides patients with an opportunity to clarify any key information you have missed or misunderstood. A summary statement does not have to be 100% accurate to be effective; minor clarification by a patient is likely to help increase rapport and increase his or her confidence that you have an accurate understanding of their problems. In addition, a summary provides a cue to patients that you are moving on to the next stage of the appointment. This type of cue is important for effective time management. Skipping the summary can be problematic. First, patients may not be sure you completely understand the problem. Second, they may think you are still in the interview and information-gathering stage and continue to try to give you information. It is helpful to communicate directly to patients that you are preparing to switch away from the information-gathering mode. For example, you might state the following:

> Let me stop here. I'd like to summarize my understanding of what you've told me to make sure I have it right. If I don't have it right or I've missed something important, I want you to tell me what I've missed. I have some specific suggestions I'd like to review with you in a moment that are based on my understanding of what you've told me. So, it is important that I have it right or my recommendation may be off target.

Once you have finished your summary, ask the patient whether it was right or whether there is something that you missed. This invites the patient to correct misperceptions and add additional information that you may have missed.

LISTING POSSIBLE CHANGE PLAN OPTIONS

Once you are confident you have a good understanding of the problem, shift to discussing possible goals or areas of change. You might say something such as the following:

> I have some ideas about what you might focus on and things you might do differ-

---

Functional Assessment of the Problem

Examples of closed-end or menu-type questions the behavioral health consultant (BHC) might ask in each category, using depression as the example.

1. Nature of the referral problem (the first question to ask after the introduction)
    BHC: Dr. Smith would like me to assist the two of you to better manage your depressed mood. Is depressed mood what you see as the main problem or is it something different?
    Patient: Yes, its depression.

2. Duration
    BHC: Is feeling depressed something that has been going on for the past 2 or 3 weeks or has it been longer or shorter than that?
    About how long ago was it that you first noticed you were feeling depressed?
    How many months or weeks ago did you start to notice you were getting more depressed?

3. Triggering events
    BHC: Was there anything different going on in your life or anything that happened to trigger your depressed mood or did it just seem to come out of the blue?

4. Frequency and intensity of the problem
    BHC: How many times a day, week, or month would you say you feel depressed?
    On a scale of 0 to 10, with 0 being not depressed at all and 10 being the most depressed you've ever felt in your life, what was your average level of depression over the past 2 weeks?

5. Factors associated with the problem getting better or worse
    • **Physical** (what is going on in the person's body): sleep, pain, blood pressure, blood glucose, etc.
    • **Emotional** (how they feel): sad, happy, angry, worried, anxious, depressed, frustrated, stressed, etc.
    • **Behavioral** (what do they do or not do): too much or too little activity, saying or not saying things, etc.
    • **Environmental/Social** (place, time of day, friends, family, coworkers): afternoon, when boss is there, etc.
    • **Cognitive** (thoughts): what are they thinking in association with symptoms and/or poor functioning?
       BHC: Is there anything that you do or anything that happens that helps you feel less depressed?
       Is there anything that you do or anything that happens that leads you to feel more depressed?

6. Functional impairment
    • Changes in work performance
       BHC: Have you noticed any changes in your ability to do your job as your depressed mood has gotten worse?
    • Changes in work, friend, or social relationships
       BHC: Have you noticed changes in your work relationships, as your depression has gotten worse?
       Were there any changes in friend or social relationships just before or around the time your difficulties started?
    • Changes in significant familial relationships (spouse, children, etc.)
       BHC: Were there any changes in family relationships just prior to or around the time your difficulties started?
       Since you started getting depressed, has there been an impact on your relationships with your (spouse, children, friends)?
    Patient: Yes, with my wife.
    BHC: What seems to be the biggest problem with your wife since you've been more depressed?

FIGURE 2.3.   Functional assessment of the problem. (*Continued*)

- Changes in social activities (going out with friends, church, etc.).
  BHC: Often people will decrease or stop their social activities when depressed. Has that happened to you?
  Patient: Yes.
  BHC: What have you cut back on or stopped?
  Patient: Going to church and going to dinner with my wife.
  BHC: How often did you used to go to church and go out to dinner with your wife?

- Changes in fun/recreational/relaxing/meaningful activities
  BHC: Sometimes when people get depressed they cut back or stop meaningful or enjoyable activities. Have you cut back or stopped enjoyable or meaningful activities?
  Patient: Yes.
  BHC: What have you cut back on or stopped?
  Patient: Playing with the kids.
  BHC: How often did you used to play with the kids?

- Change in exercise.
  BHC: Do you exercise now?
  Patient: No.
  BHC: Have you exercised in the past?
  Patient: Yes.
  BHC: Have you stopped since you started feeling depressed?
  Patient: Yes.
  BHC: What did you used to do and how many days a week did you do it?
  When you were exercising before, what benefits did you get from it?

7. Changes in sleep, energy, concentration, appetite
   BHC: Are you sleeping about the same, more, or less than before you started getting depressed?
   Patient: Less.
   BHC: Are you having trouble falling asleep, staying asleep, or both?
   Patient: Both.
   BHC: Over the past 2 weeks, on average, how long does it take you to fall asleep?
   Patient: 2 hours.
   BHC: Over the past 2 weeks, on average, how many times do you wake up at night?
   Patient: Three.
   BHC: About how long does it take you to fall back to sleep?
   Patient: 45 minutes.
   BHC: Have you noticed a decrease in energy?
   Has your ability to concentrate decreased?
   Have you seen any increase or decrease in your appetite or is it about the same as usual?
   Have you lost or gained any weight since you started getting depressed?

8. Caffeine use
   BHC: Do you drink caffeinated drinks?
   Patient: Yes.
   BHC: What kind: tea, coffee, soda?
   Patient: Coffee.
   BHC: How many in a typical day?
   Patient: Two.
   BHC: How many ounces in each drink?
   Patient: Twelve.

9. Alcohol use
   BHC: Do you drink alcoholic drinks?
   Patient: Yes.
   BHC: What kind: beer, wine, mixed drinks?
   Patient: Beer.

FIGURE 2.3.   *(Continued)* Functional assessment of the problem.

> *BHC:* How many in a typical day, week, or month?
> *Patient:* Three a day.
> *BHC:* How many ounces in each drink?
> *Patient:* 24.
>
> 10. Medications or supplements
>   *BHC:* Are you taking any prescribed or over-the-counter medications or supplements?
>   *Patient:* Yes.
>   *BHC:* What are you taking, how much are you taking, and what are you taking it for?
>
> 11. Mood over past 2 weeks
>   *BHC:* Over the past 2 weeks would you describe your mood as down, sad, depressed, anxious, angry, frustrated, something different, or is it a combination of things?
>   *Patient:* Sad and anxious.
>   *BHC:* How many days a week would you say you feel sad and anxious?
>   *Patient:* Six.
>   *BHC:* On a scale of 0 to 10, with 0 being not being anxious or depressed at all and 10 being the most anxious and depressed you've ever felt in your life, what would you say your average level of anxiety and depression has been over the past 2 weeks?
>   *Patient:* Five.
>
> 12. Suicide or homicide risk (These questions will likely not be asked as a routine part of your assessment but should be asked when you deem it clinically relevant, for instance in assessing depressed mood.)
>   *BHC:* Do you have thoughts of harming or killing yourself?
>   Have you ever tried to kill yourself?
>   Do you have thoughts of harming or killing anyone else?
>   Have you ever tired to harm or kill anyone?
>
> 13. Open-ended questions
>   *BHC:* Is there anything I haven't asked you about that you think is important for me to know?
>   [If time allows.] Take me through what a typical weekday is like for you from the time you get up to the time you go to bed.
>   Take me through what you typically do on the days you're not working, or on the weekend.

FIGURE 2.3. *(Continued)* Functional assessment of the problem.

ently that could decrease your symptoms and improve your functioning. I'd like to go over those in just a minute, but before I do, I'd like to know one or two things that you would like to change or that you think would make a significant difference in the quality of your life.

If the response is something outside his or her control (e.g. another person changing his or her behavior), point this out and ask the following:

So, if your mother would change her behavior, you believe you would be doing better. Unfortunately, it is very difficult to get someone else to change what he or she does or how he or she thinks. You have a lot more control over your own responses and behavior than you do over those of your mother. What about yourself might you change that could make a difference for you?

Once patients have identified what they would like to change, or if they have been unable to think of what they might change (which is most often the case in our experience), discuss one or two ideas you have for changes they might make, as follows:

There are several things I think we might do that would be helpful. I would like to tell you what those things are and how I think they might be helpful. Then you can tell me if you think you want to try one, some, or maybe none of the things I suggest. You might want to discuss these options with friends, family members, or someone else before making a decision.

Once you present the options, ask whether any of those options sound like they might be helpful. Typically, patients will think one or several of the options will be useful. Asking which option(s) they see as the easiest can be a good place to start.

If none of the options for change are of interest to the patient, it is important to address this ambivalence toward change before moving on. The principles of motivational interviewing (MI) can be helpful in this situation. Detailed information on MI strategies can be found in Miller and Rollnick (2002) and Rollnick, Mason, and Butler (1999). Chapter 3 of this volume offers additional details on MI strategies to use when patients are ambivalent about change.

Sometimes, you may find at the end of your summary that patients are functioning well, given their limitations. In this case, your primary recommendations may involve letting them know they are doing a good job of managing their difficulties, encouraging them to continue what they are doing, and discussing their prognosis or the course of symptoms to expect.

STARTING A CHANGE PLAN

Once you and the patient have mutually agreed on a change plan, briefly write the plan out. A *behavior prescription pad* can be a helpful tool for writing these recommendations (see Figure 2.4). Patients can use the written prescription as a reminder of the recommendations. In the following chapters, we present various forms and educational handouts you can use for education and treatment interventions. During this phase, you may also find yourself teaching the patient a specific skill to practice and use as part of their plan. It can be helpful to ask if the patient sees any barriers in fol-

FIGURE 2.4. Behavioral prescription pads.

lowing the change plan (e.g., money, time, friends, family members), and deal with those barriers before starting the plan. Before concluding the first appointment, you will need to determine whether a follow-up consultation appointment with you would be useful to help assess the success of the plan or to teach additional skills. We recommend that this decision be made collaboratively with the patient. If you think it would be helpful to have a follow-up appointment to reinforce the intervention, to monitor progress or to get a significant other (e.g., family member, friend) involved with the plan, you can certainly suggest it. In addition, if you did not have time to start or complete the intervention, a follow-up appointment will be needed. You might say the following:

> We can go one of two ways here. Either way is fine with me; I'd like to know what you think is best for you. We can set a follow-up appointment to help

monitor how you're doing and discuss any problems you may be having, or you can try this on your own and follow up with me or Dr. Smith as needed.

Alternatively, you might say the following:

Do you think it would be helpful to come back in two weeks to see how you are doing with this plan and add some additional skills at that time, or would it be better to try this on your own and only schedule a follow-up if things are not going as planned?

SUMMARY

Each stage of the first appointment is designed to accomplish a specific purpose. The idea of "shifting" between stages within the 30-minute consult is like shifting gears on a car as you drive down the road.

Each gear is distinct and allows you to travel a certain distance at a certain speed; you shift when you want to go another speed. The amount of time you spend in each gear may vary depending on the terrain and how fast you want to go. The same concept applies to the phases of your consultation appointment and to the unique problems and interaction styles of each patient.

We have made a number of recommendations in this chapter for conducting the 30-minute initial consultation. We expect that you will adapt the steps of this plan to your unique setting and style. In chapter 3, we describe the interventions that we have found to be most helpful to BHCs working in the fast-paced world of primary care. The following chapters will conceptually flow from the model we have presented, with an emphasis on additional assessment questions, practice strategies, and specific interventions developed on the basis of evidence-based care and our own field experience.

COMMON BEHAVIORAL AND COGNITIVE INTERVENTIONS IN PRIMARY CARE: MOVING OUT OF THE SPECIALTY MENTAL HEALTH CLINIC

The window of opportunity for intervening in primary care settings is much narrower than that in specialty mental health clinics. In specialty mental health, providers often have the luxury of over a dozen 50-minute sessions. In primary care, interventions must be selected that will have the desired effect in one to four 30-minute appointments in a typical case.

In this chapter, we describe nine such interventions that we consider the behavioral health consultant's (BHC's) basic toolkit for practicing in primary care. These interventions were selected on the basis of empirical evidence and their compatibility with a self-management model of care. With regard to empirical support, we looked for interventions that have been tested in multiple well-designed studies, have been found to be effective, and are of low risk to patients. The limited research specific to integrated behavioral health care in the primary care setting has required us to generalize and adapt such interventions to the fast-paced setting of primary care.

In terms of the self-management model of care, we have selected those skill-based interventions that patients can apply and practice outside of the office setting. The time the patient spends with the BHC is viewed as a coaching appointment in which skills involved in the intervention are first taught and then refined and monitored as needed. Patients are then expected to practice the interventions on their own. Patients who cannot do this or who do not respond quickly to these focused interventions are referred to outpatient specialty mental health care.

The nine intervention strategies we describe are not the only interventions that can or should be used in primary care settings. However, we believe that these interventions provide a foundation for the BHC practice in primary care. Experience in the primary care setting will allow the BHC to adapt their clinical training and experience to fit within this fast-paced setting.

THE BHC TOOLKIT

We have found that the following nine interventions have been effective for addressing a wide variety of symptoms and functional impairments seen in primary care: (a) relaxation training, (b) goal setting, (c) cognitive disputation, (d) motivational interviewing (MI) strategies, (e) problem solving, (f) self-monitoring, (g) behavioral self-analysis, (h) stimulus control, and (i) assertive communication.

In this chapter, we first describe the intervention and how it fits into the 5A's model (i.e., assess, advise, agree, assist, arrange). Within the structure of the 5A's, we describe how to present the intervention to a patient in plain, understandable language. For several of the interventions, handouts and worksheets are included at the end of the chapter and can also be downloaded from the American Psychological Association Books Web site (http://www.apa.org/books/resources/Hunter).We do not focus on applying these interventions to specific patient problems in this chapter as this is the focus of the chapters in Part II of this volume.

Relaxation Training

Relaxation training is one of the most versatile interventions for use in the primary care setting because it can be quickly taught, is easily learned by many patients, and can have immediate effects on physiological arousal and symptoms (Boyce, Talley, & Balaam, 2002; Carroll & Seers, 1998; Engel, Rapoff, & Pressman, 1992). We believe relaxation skills are most effective when tailored to the individual.

Assess. A functional assessment of each patient's problem (see chap. 2, this volume) is essential to determine contributing factors and to assess whether relaxation training is an appropriate intervention. Once its appropriateness has been established, further assessment of several factors will provide a basis for tailoring the intervention for optimal benefit. The following are suggested assessment questions:

- What do you do to relax (e.g., napping, television, reading, conversation, hobbies)?
- How often do you engage in these activities?
- How effective are these strategies for you?
- Have you ever been trained in relaxation techniques? If so, what have you been trained to do and when? How well did the relaxation techniques work for you?
- Do you currently practice any relaxation techniques? If so, how often? When?
- What are the primary barriers for you in using relaxation strategies?
- What are the common "triggers" or things that increase stress?
- How do you think your stress response and your current problem are connected?

Advise. The findings from the assessment phase will shape what needs to be done in the advise phase. If the patient has a number of relaxation strategies that have been effective in the past but are currently being neglected, it may be sufficient to establish a connection between relaxation and the patient's concerns and advise the patient to dedicate more time to these activities. Patients who are currently engaging only in recreational relaxation activities such as reading, watching television, or engaging in hobbies, might be advised to use more focused relaxation techniques that specifically target physiological arousal.

Some patients perceive themselves as being unable to relax despite efforts with numerous techniques and approaches. It is important that these concerns are heard in a nonjudgmental manner and that advice on relaxation is presented in such a way that it will instill hope that change can occur. Relaxation should be presented as a skill that can be learned with sufficient training and practice. The following metaphor may be helpful:

> It sounds like your difficulties relaxing are similar to someone with no musical training trying to play the piano. They may sit down at a piano and try to pound out tunes although it may never sound very good. And why would it? They have never had lessons or practiced proper techniques to develop good skills. They may even feel frustrated that others have more natural musical talent and are self-taught. It's true that some people are natural musicians but that doesn't mean the rest of us can't try to learn to play the old fashioned way: with training and practice. I have worked with a lot people who, like you, don't feel very skilled at relaxation. My experience is that most people can learn to improve their ability to relax if they work at it and consistently practice the right skills. Do you think you may be expecting relaxation to come more naturally than it does and, therefore, feel you can't do it? Are you interested in developing a plan to practice and improve your relaxation skills?

Agree. If your advice is accepted, you can move toward agreeing on relaxation-oriented goals. It is essential that you and the patient reach mutually agreeable goals before moving on with the intervention. It may be tempting to rush into this step; however, a lack of acceptance from the patient will ultimately sabotage the treatment effectiveness in almost every case. If the patient does not express motivation to learn and use relaxation, go back to the assessment phase and further explore the barriers. If the patient cannot move past these obstacles, relaxation may not be the right treatment at that time and other options should be explored.

Assist. In this phase, the patient is ready to learn the behavioral skills of relaxation. Relaxation exercises fall into three primary categories: (a) breathing exercises, (b) muscle relaxation exercises, and (c) visual imagery. Patients can be taught either a single technique or multiple techniques which they can choose from or use in different situations. We recommend that the assist phase include instruction in the relaxation technique followed by practice of that technique during the appointment with the BHC coaching the patient through the exercise.

The use of a simple self-rating scale before and after the exercise can help a patient recognize acute changes that occur with relaxation and build confidence in their ability to effectively use relaxation techniques. This can be presented in the following way: "Before we start, I'd like you to rate your level of stress, anxiety, or tension on a 0 to 10 point scale. Let 10 represent high stress, anxiety, or tension; 0 means you are thoroughly and completely relaxed." At the completion of the relaxation exercise you could say: "Now rate your stress, anxiety, or tension level again using that 0–10 scale."

Verbally praise changes and indicate that the patient was able to bring about that change him or herself. Small reductions of one to two points in self-ratings can be framed as a good start and the patient reminded that skills such as relaxation improve with regular and frequent practice. If the self-rating does not decrease, or if it increases, you can emphasize that this is normal for individuals at the beginning and that sometimes when they try too hard, their symptoms can get a little worse at first; practice is required to begin seeing benefits.

BHCs should develop their own style for instructing and coaching; however, the following scripts for each technique can provide a basic structure.

Deep (diaphragmatic) breathing. See Figure 3.1 for the patient education handout.

> Let me explain to you what deep breathing is and how it might be useful. Deep breathing is using your diaphragm muscle, which is below your lungs, to take in more oxygen then you normally would. This helps turn on the relaxation part of your nervous system and can lead to decreased heart rate, blood pressure, and increased muscle relaxation. Let me show you what deep breathing

---

Deep Breathing

What Is Deep Breathing?

Deep breathing involves using your diaphragm muscle to help bring about a state of physiological relaxation. The diaphragm is a large muscle that rests across the bottom of your rib cage. When you inhale, the diaphragm muscle drops, opening up space so air can come in. When watching someone do this it looks like your stomach is filling with air. This type of breathing helps activate the part of your nervous system that controls relaxation. It can lead to decreased heart rate, blood pressure, decreased muscle tension, and overall feelings of relaxation.

Why Be Concerned With How I'm Breathing?

- To increase your awareness of the role that breathing plays in increased physical tension and in contributing to increasing your body's stress response.
- To lower your level of stress-related arousal and tension.
- To give you a method of taking calm, relaxing breaths to break the cycle of increasing arousal during stressful situations.

What Is the Best Way To Use Deep Breathing Exercises?

- Use deep breathing frequently.
- Take deep breaths at the first signs of stress, anxiety, physical tension, or other symptoms.
- Schedule time for relaxation. My scheduled time for deep breathing will be _____.

FIGURE 3.1. Deep breathing handout.

looks like. [Demonstrate by putting one hand on your chest and one hand on your stomach and take two deep breaths by pushing your stomach out as you breathe in and letting it fall as you breathe out.] Did you notice how my bottom hand went up and down and my top hand was still? This is what it might look like if you are doing it correctly. For some people both hands will go up at the same time and this can work as well. You can breathe through your mouth or nose, whatever is most comfortable for you.

Many people find this difficult when they first try but it usually starts to feel more natural with practice. As your relaxation response starts to activate, you might notice a sense of heaviness, warmth, or floating. As we're going through this exercise, you may notice sounds inside and outside of the room you haven't noticed before or thoughts popping into your mind that distract you from the relaxation. This is normal. As a way to help you focus, you can repeat the word "calm" or "relax" to yourself silently each time you breathe out. You might also notice your heart beating or muscles twitching, which is nothing to be concerned about. Some people get dizzy when they first try this because their body gets used to running on a higher level of carbon dioxide, and suddenly providing more oxygen can temporarily disrupt the body and cause dizziness. Don't be alarmed if that happens; usually that dizziness goes away. If you're getting dizzy and feel like you are going to fall out of your chair, I want you to stop and practice at another time. When that happens it is best to start with only a few deep breaths and work your way up to more as your body adapts. Do you have any questions about what deep breathing is or how it might help?

I'd like to walk you through about a 3-minute deep-breathing exercise. I'm going to look away from you as we do this so you don't feel like you're under a big magnifying glass. This usually makes it a little easier for people to do.

So go ahead and place one hand on your chest and one hand on your stomach and I will just walk you through this exercise. If you would like, you can lightly close your eyes as we go through the deep breathing. What you can do first is notice your breathing. Don't try to change it just yet, but notice the sound and feel of the air as you breathe in and the sound and the feel of the air as you breathe out. You might notice that the air is dry and cool as you inhale and a little warmer as you exhale. Remember to repeat silently to yourself the word you chose ("calm" or "relax") each time you breathe out as a way to help you focus. Continue to breathe slowly and easily at your own pace. You can start to shift the focus of your breathing so that, as you breathe in, it feels as if the air is going past your chest and filling your stomach to help hold up pants or shorts [or skirt, if appropriate] that are a little too big. As your stomach moves out, hold it there for just a moment then let all the air leave your body at once. As you let the air out, you can allow yourself to feel more comfortable and more at ease. It might be helpful to imagine, as the air is leaving your body, that you're sinking deeper into the chair, getting more comfortable, and feeling more at ease. As you continue to breathe at your own pace, you can take three more comfortable, easy breaths, and as you exhale on the last breath, you can open your eyes and get adjusted to the light in the room.

Cue-controlled relaxation. Cue-controlled relaxation is a technique for associating a specific environmental cue or cues with the relaxation response (see Figure 3.2 for a patient education handout). Thus, the cue helps the individual remember to engage in relaxation exercises, developing a daily environment that promotes relaxation and stress relief. This strategy involves selecting a cue that patients will encounter frequently throughout their day. Each time the patient encounters these cues, he or she should engage in a brief relaxation-inducing behavior such as taking two deep relaxed breaths. Examples of cues include visual stimuli (e.g., looking at their watch, placing small notes around the house or office), auditory stimuli (e.g., the phone ringing, a watch alarm at the top of each hour), or situational stimuli (e.g., getting into the car, sitting down at a desk). With repetition, the cue will become associated with the relaxation response and will begin to automatically induce relaxation.

The following script can be a foundation for providing training in this technique.

> We can take the deep breathing you just learned and start to make it a habit so you are relaxing throughout the day. We can do that with something called cue-controlled relaxation. A cue is some

kind of reminder. Cue-controlled relaxation involves using that reminder to help you remember to take two to three slow deep breaths.

> There are two kinds of cues, external and internal. External cues are things you hear, see, or do. Examples of external cues might be looking at your watch, hanging up the phone, going to the bathroom, checking e-mail, hearing a tone or alarm, or seeing something in your home or office. A good external cue is something that occurs at least once or twice an hour. Internal cues are thoughts, emotions, or physical sensations. These don't necessarily happen once or twice an hour. In fact, they may not happen with regularity at all; however, they should occur in situations in which you would benefit from relaxation. Examples might include feeling angry, feeling your heart beating rapidly, or having thoughts about your marital problems. You might pick the first thing you're aware of when you are more distressed than you would like to be.

Cue-Controlled Relaxation

Cue-controlled relaxation can be a quick and easy relaxation technique. There are two different types of cues

- *External cues.* Things you hear, see, or do. Examples might include looking at your watch, hanging up the phone, going to the bathroom, checking email, hearing a tone or alarm, or seeing something in your home or office.
- *Internal cues.* Thoughts, emotions, or physical sensations. Examples might include feeling stressed, frustrated, anxious, panicky, or having thoughts about negative events.

It is important that once you set your cue you practice relaxed breathing every time the cue occurs, so that being relaxed becomes an automatic habit.
When the cue occurs, relax by

- taking a slow deep breath,
- exhaling comfortably and easily, and
- saying a word to yourself as you exhale (e.g., "relax" or "calm").

External cue:_____
Internal cue:_____

FIGURE 3.2.   Cue-controlled relaxation handout.

The idea is to take something that is already happening in your daily life that occurs frequently and use it as reminder to take two to three slow deep breaths. By doing this, you help turn down the "volume" on any physiological stress response that might have been building up and of which you were not aware. If you use external cues throughout the day, you will help keep yourself as physiologically relaxed as possible. Likewise, if you regularly relax as soon as you are aware of specific internal cues, you will be actively working to manage some of your high-risk situations. People commonly report that doing this can help them to feel less stressed or anxious, have better concentration, have more energy, and sleep better at night. I recommend that you identify and use both external and internal cues. What can you think of that you hear, see, or do that happens once or twice an hour? What would be good internal cues for you: a thought, emotion, or physical sensation?

Progressive muscle relaxation. Progressive muscle relaxation (PMR) is another relaxation technique that is easily adapted to the primary care setting. It involves the patient progressively tensing and relaxing muscles throughout the body. It generally takes more time to use this exercise compared with diaphragmatic breathing and, therefore, may be less convenient for a patient with a consistently busy lifestyle. However, many patients report that it produces deeper relaxation. We recommend it be used as one of several techniques so that the patient has a variety of relaxation strategies to use in different settings.

PMR is typically conducted by isolating muscle groups (e.g., feet, calves, thighs, abdomen) for tensing and relaxing. The number of muscle groups used can vary. Given the time constraints of a primary care visit, we find it useful to train patients in using only four muscle groups: legs, arms, shoulder and abdomen, and face and neck. This shortens the time needed for training and for conducting the exercise. If a patient has difficulty getting relaxed

with only 4 muscle groups, you might expand this to 8 or 16 groups. The following script can be used as a foundation for coaching this exercise.

The technique I am going to help you learn is called progressive muscle relaxation. It involves tensing and relaxing muscle groups throughout your body to bring about a state of relaxation. As I ask you to tense your muscles, only tighten them enough to feel some tension— maybe a third to a half of their fully tense state. Make sure you don't strain yourself or hold your breath when you tense your muscles. The goal is to feel what the muscles feel like when they are tense so you can more fully relax them. I'll have you hold the tension for about 4 to 5 seconds and then ask you to relax. Focus on the sensations of letting go of the tension and study the feelings of the muscle being completely relaxed. We'll have you do that for about a minute before moving on to the next muscle group.

Before we begin, get into a comfortable relaxation posture: feet on the floor, legs apart, neck straight, back against your chair, teeth slightly apart, eyes gently closed, and head upright. Take a few slow, deep, comfortable breaths. Breathe in as deeply as you can, hold for a moment, and exhale. As you breathe in, concentrate on the sound and feel of the air. As you exhale completely, notice the warmth of the air and silently say the word "calm" to yourself with each breath you let out. Take a few more slow deep breaths. Be sure to exhale slowly and completely each time. Imagine your body becoming more relaxed and feeling heavier in your chair each time you exhale. [Pause.]

Now we'll begin the progressive muscle relaxation. First, we'll start with your legs. Lift your legs slightly off the ground, tense your thighs, and point your toes toward your head. Hold that position and feel the tension. Now let your legs drop to the ground and release all the tension at once. Notice the difference between the way your legs feel now when relaxed and how they felt when they were tense.

Now we will move to your arms. With your palms facing the ceiling, make a fist and raise your forearm bringing your fist as close to your shoulder as you can while at the same time pressing your arms to your sides. Feel the tension in your fingers, hands, and arms. And now relax. As you relax you may notice your arms feel warm and heavy. Notice the difference between the relaxation and tension in your arms. Continue to breathe slowly and deeply.

While your legs and arms remain relaxed, we will now move to your shoulders and stomach. Lift both shoulders as if you were trying to touch your ears with them and at the same time suck your stomach in as if someone were pushing on it. Feel the tightness and tension across both shoulders and in your stomach muscles and hold it. And now relax. Let your shoulders fall back down and enjoy the heaviness, warmth, and relaxation in your shoulders.

Continue to breathe slowly and deeply, and scan your legs, arms, and shoulders, releasing any excess tension you notice. Focus on the sensation of relaxation in these areas. We'll now move to your face and neck. To tense your neck, press your chin to your chest or the back of your head to the back of your chair. While doing this, squint your eyes and slightly bring your back teeth together, tensing just enough to feel the muscles in your jaw. Notice the tension in your face and neck: hold it. And now relax. Let all the tension go from your face and neck.

Continue to breathe slowly and enjoy the relaxed feelings throughout your entire body. Scan your body from your head to your toes and notice what your muscles feel like. As you are doing this, take five more slow deep breaths at your own pace. After you exhale on the last breath, open your eyes.

Once patients have learned the techniques of PMR and have practiced them, introduce use of the "body scan" component as a separate relaxation technique that can be used independently of a full PMR exercise. Once they have become more aware through PMR of how tense muscles feel, they can do a body scan by drawing their attention to each muscle group and letting go of any tension there without tensing the muscle first. This is useful in stressful situations in which the patient wants to relax his or her muscles without others noticing that they are doing so.

Visual imagery. Visual imagery exercises use mental pictures to induce relaxation. By bringing to mind images that already are associated with relaxation, the patient can reduce autonomic arousal when needed or desired. Attempt to use all five senses in the imagery. The following script can be used:

Close your eyes and begin to relax. Breathe deeply and slowly and let your entire body feel relaxed and at ease. Now, imagine yourself at the back of a movie theatre. Picture a scene or a place that you associate with feeling relaxed and calm and imagine it on the screen at the front of the theatre. It can be a real place that you have been to or an imaginary place. Do you have a scene in your mind? Now imagine yourself moving closer and closer to the screen and as you get closer, the picture becomes clearer and more vivid, almost as if you're in the image. Imagine that there are three steps right in front of the screen. Walk up the first, then the second, and now the third step. You are right in front of the screen and can see the image with perfect clarity. Now walk through the screen and put yourself in that image, not as if you were outside looking in, but actually in that place. [Pause.] Now look around you. Be aware of all the details of what you see. Notice the colors of everything around you, notice how vivid those colors are and areas of light and darkness. You might notice the various shades or textures and the intensity, softness, or brightness of the light. [Pause.] Be aware of the sounds you hear or don't hear in this place. Are the sounds close or far, loud or soft? [Pause.] Become aware of the smells. [Pause.] Notice the things that you can feel and the temperature of the air. [Pause.] Enjoy the sensation of being in this place where you can feel very, very relaxed. You can use any distracting, stressful, or anxious thoughts as reminders to easily travel back to this image and relax yourself. This can be your relaxation place and you can come here whenever you wish.

Encourage the patient to practice visual imagery daily to build the skills for relaxation and to manage daily stress. Advise the patient to use the same image every time so that it becomes a familiar, comfortable place that is associated with relaxation.

Following the practice of these relaxation techniques during the appointment, it is important to explore the patient's experience while doing the exercise and attempt to identify barriers or problems. Assist the patient in problem solving around these issues. For example, if he or she did not really try the exercise, explore that hesitancy and provide further education on the rationale for using relaxation. If they did not understand the technique, provide further training. Some patients will experience anxiety related to "letting go" or fearing they will be out of control if they release tension. Further exploration and questioning of thoughts contributing to this anxiety may be necessary before the patient is ready to use a relaxation technique. These patients may also benefit from progressive exposure to relaxation to allow them to get used to the sensations of a more relaxed state. This can be accomplished with various relaxation strategies that produce progressively deeper relaxation states. You might start with coaching them in a relaxation

posture. Once the patient is comfortable with that posture, teach him or her to take a few deep breaths. When the patient can tolerate that state, progress to deeper relaxation using muscle relaxation techniques or visual imagery. Some people will also not allow themselves to relax because they perceive the techniques to be a form of hypnosis or to be inconsistent with their religious or moral beliefs. These perceptions can be explored and misinformation (i.e., that relaxation will put them in a hypnotic trance) corrected. Religious and cultural beliefs should be respected and understood. It may be necessary to find alternative strategies for treatment if the patient has concerns based on his or her faith or culture.

Arrange.   Once an individual has learned relaxation techniques, discuss potential times during the patient's daily routine in which relaxation can be scheduled. Encourage the patient to dedicate him- or herself to relaxing during this scheduled time. We also advise arranging a follow-up appointment after 1 to 2 weeks. The purpose of this follow-up is to assess the effectiveness of relaxation on symptoms, identify problems associated with incorporating relaxation practice into the patient's lifestyle and schedule, and reinforce changes made. We highly recommend repeated coaching of the techniques in subsequent appointments to enhance their skills.

Goal Setting

Patients often come to primary care with a complaint or concern; however, they often do not have a clear idea of how to address that problem. Others can articulate what changes they want but do not have appropriate and achievable goals relevant to those changes. In both of these situations, patients can benefit from focused assistance with goal setting to help attain improved health and well-being (Kolb & Boyatzis, 1970; Lapierre, Dubeú, Bouffard, & Alain, 2007; Ziegelmann, Luszczynska, Lippke, & Schwarzer, 2007).

Assess.   The assessment phase of goal setting involves identifying what the patient would like to change in his or her life. Questions for the assessment phase might include:

■ What will it take for you to look back one month from now and say, "I'm glad I went to see that psychologist"? In other words, what will have to change for you to feel this visit or series of visits was a success?

- If you were to change one thing in your life, and only one thing, what would it be?
- List five things you would like see changed in your life. Rank order them from most important to least important.

Advise. Once general goals are identified, you can advise that patient on his or her goals. Consider the following:

- Are the goals well-defined? Nonspecific goals are difficult to achieve. Patients can be encouraged to make general goals more specific to increase chance of success. For example, if the goal is "to be a better husband," advise him to specify behaviors he wants to engage in and make those his goals (e.g., criticize less, help bathe the children every evening, ask his wife about her day and spend time listening). A goal to "eat better" can be defined as "eat five servings of fruits and vegetables daily" or "eat dessert only one day per week."
- Are the goals realistic and achievable? Those with unrealistic goals are setting themselves up for failure. Advise them to reframe the goals in realistic and achievable terms. For example, a goal to eliminate a 10-year chronic pain problem may be unrealistic, whereas a goal to reduce the number of pain-related sick days away from work might be more achievable. A goal to eliminate life-long public speaking anxiety may be unrealistic, whereas managing anxiety enough to give a sufficient and successful presentation may be reasonable.
- Are the goals within the patient's realm of control or influence? Goals that require someone or something besides the patient to change may be unrealistic. Examples of goals outside the patient's control may be presented as: "I want my boss to stop yelling at me" or "My mother is always telling me what to do; I'm a grown woman and she needs to let me live my own life."
- Advising the patient to refocus on goals that are within his or her control can help. In the first example, the patient might set a goal to be less upset when the boss yells or to find another job.

In the second example, the patient might set a goal to be more assertive with her mother.

- Can the goals be broken down into subgoals that are more easily accomplished? Patients are most likely to succeed with small goals that have a high chance of success. If large goals can be broken down into small, achievable subgoals, the individual will likely be rewarded by short-term success and continue making progress toward the larger goal. For example, a goal to lose 50 pounds might best be broken down into subgoals of losing 5 pounds per month.
- Are the goals personally important to the patient or are there other factors driving the goal? Patients who do not have sufficient intrinsic motivation to make a change are not likely to succeed. Examples of this include individuals who try to stop smoking to please a spouse or exercise more to satisfy a physician. These motives are not bad; however, they are likely to be insufficient to bring about success if the change is not also personally meaningful. Advice might include having the patient examine his or her own priorities and values related to the change.
- Are there more important goals that need to be addressed first? A patient may seek help from a behavioral health provider for a worthwhile goal; however, there may be other issues that should take priority. Safety issues such as domestic violence, suicide risk, or adherence to life-saving medical treatment regimens may need to take precedence over other goals.

Agree, assist, and arrange. Once these issues are addressed, you and the patient should *agree* on a goal or set of goals. We recommend these be written down in specific behavioral terms with target dates and strategies for reaching them. This will ensure that both parties are in clear agreement about what they are working toward. The BHC can *assist* the patient in defining these goals, establishing subgoals, and determining realistic time frames. It is important, however, that the patient has a sense of ownership of the goals. At this point, you are ready to *arrange* the treatment plan for working on these goals.

Cognitive Disputation

Cognitive therapy can be a lengthy and complex endeavor unsuited to the primary care setting. At the same time, we believe there are cognitive disputation skills that are relatively easy for BHCs to learn and apply in primary care. Cognitive disputation is adaptable to the brief interventions conducted in this environment, and there is empirical evidence for the effectiveness of cognitive therapy for problems commonly presenting in primary care (Dobson, 1989; McCoy & Nathan, 2007). This section, therefore, is intended to help those who have cognitive therapy skills adapt those skills to primary care (see Figure 3.3 for patient education handout).

Assess. An assessment of a presenting problem should include exploration of contributing factors from a variety of sources. These include physiological, emotional, cognitive, behavioral, spiritual, social, and environmental components as well as the interaction between these elements. The cognitive component includes the thoughts and beliefs the patient holds that contribute to their physiological stress reaction, emotional distress, maladaptive or unhealthy behaviors, interpersonal conflict, problematic choices, and so forth. BHCs should attempt to identify these thoughts or beliefs as part of the assessment process.

A simple structure for assessing relevant cognitions in a brief primary care assessment is to listen for and explore three cognitive areas: (a) predictions, (b) expectations, and (c) evaluations.

Predictions.

- What negative events or circumstances does the patient anticipate or worry about?
- How convinced is the patient that their prediction will occur?
- Are there facts to support the prediction?
- What is the patient's belief about his or her ability to tolerate or cope with the predicted event?

Expectations.

- How does the current situation conflict with what the patient believes should be happening?
- How rigid or flexible are the patient's expectations about others' behavior or his or her own behavior?

Evaluations.

- Is the patient using emotionally loaded or exaggerated language in evaluations of situations or people that may be contributing to the distress (e.g., *disaster, terrible, horrible, awful, unbelievable, unbearable, miserable, intolerable*)?

Advise. Once the cognitive distortions or unhelpful thinking patterns that are contributing to the patient's problem are identified, the patient may benefit from evaluating the role these thoughts may play in his or her problem. Recommend that he or she focus on these thoughts and beliefs as part of the treatment plan.

Agree. Your sense of the patient's receptivity in the advise phase can help you determine where to go with this next phase. Those who are receptive to the potential role of their thought processes in their problems and who express a willingness to engage in this aspect of treatment are most likely to benefit from a primary care level of intervention. We recommend that those with little understanding or receptivity for the role their thoughts play in their current problems may be better suited for traditional psychotherapy, where more time can be dedicated to establishing rapport, overcoming barriers to change, and addressing issues more pressing for the patient. However, those who express eagerness or openness to learn more, might be better suited to a brief cognitive disputation intervention in primary care, and an agreement can be established for this plan. Alternatively, focusing on concrete behavioral interventions may be the best option.

Assist. We suggest a stepped approach when helping people learn to question their thoughts. In our experience, Step 1 is a basic way to help people learn to notice and question their thinking, and, frequently, we will start here. Step 2 is often used when step one fails to achieve the objective for which it is being used. It is also used when the patient might benefit from a more specific, directed way of questioning their thinking.

Step 1: Basic. The goal of this step is to help patients learn to respond to situations in ways consistent with their values instead of reacting to their

---

How to Question Stressful, Angry, Anxious, or Depressed Thinking

1. Am I upsetting myself unnecessarily? How can I see this another way?
2. Is my thinking working for or against me? How could I view this in a less upsetting way?
3. What am I demanding must happen? What do I want or prefer, rather than need?
4. Am I making something too terrible? Is that awful? What would be so terrible about that?
5. Am I labeling a person? What is the action that I don't like?
6. What is untrue about my thoughts? How can I stick to the facts?
7. Am I using extreme, black-and-white language? What words might be more accurate?
8. Am I fortune-telling or mind-reading in a way that gets me upset or unhappy? What are the odds or chances that it will really turn out the way I'm thinking or imagining?
9. What are my options in this situation? How would I like to respond?
10. What are more moderate, helpful, or realistic statements to replace the upsetting ones?
11. Have I had any experiences that show that this thought might not be completely true?
12. If my best friend or someone I loved had this thought, what would I tell them?
13. If someone I cared about knew I was thinking this thought, what would they say to me?
14. Are there strengths in me or positives in the situation that I am ignoring?
15. When I am not feeling this way, do I think about this situation any differently? How?
16. Have I been in this type of situation before? What happened? What have I learned from prior experiences that could help me now?
17. Five years from now, if I look back on this situation, will I look at it any differently? Will I focus on any different part of my experience?
18. Am I blaming myself for something over which I do not have complete control?
19. Thinking Mistakes That Create Stress, Anger, Depression, Anxiety, and Worry

All-or-nothing thinking. You see things in black-and-white categories. It is either one thing or another; there is no room for anything in between. "I'm 100% healthy or I must have a fatal disease."

Jumping to conclusions. You make a negative interpretation even though there are no definite facts that convincingly support your conclusion. "My husband is late because he is in a car accident and is injured on the side of the road."

Fortune-telling. You anticipate things will turn out badly, convinced the prediction is a fact. "Not getting this job will cause us to lose the house."

Should statements. "Musts" and "oughts" are also offenders. Emotional consequences can include anxiety and anger. "I should be able to handle this."

Overgeneralization. Assuming one event is actually a pattern. "My hand is a little shaky today, I must have Parkinson's Disease."

Disqualifying the positive. Filtering out or rejecting positive experiences to maintain negative beliefs. Upon hearing that your spouse has checked all the doors and windows and they are all locked you think, "But someone could cut out a piece of glass and open the window."

Catastrophizing. Predicting the worst possible outcome imaginable. "Terrible," "awful," "horrible," "worst ever" might be key words. "If I can't get my heart to stop pounding I'm going to die."

Superstitious thinking. The thought that something you do prevents something awful from happening. "Giving my spouse a hug and telling her to be careful before going to work will prevent her from getting in a wreck. I do it every morning and she hasn't gotten in a wreck yet."

Emotional reasoning. The belief that because you feel a certain way means that the assumptions and associations you have with that feeling are true. "The fear, doom, and constant anxiety must mean something is seriously wrong with me."

FIGURE 3.3.   How to question stressful, angry, anxious, or depressed thinking handout. (*Continued*)

Activating event What happened?	Consequences How did I get myself to respond?	Thoughts/ beliefs What am I telling myself? What thinking mistake am I making?	Evidence for thoughts, beliefs/ self-talk	Evidence against thoughts, beliefs/ self-talk	What different thoughts can I have based on the evidence for and against my original way of thinking?	How did or might my responses change with my new way of thinking?
	Physically (What are my body responses?)					Physically (What are my body responses?)
	Emotionally (How do I feel?)					Emotionally (How do I feel?)
	Behaviorally (What did I do?)					Behaviorally (What did I do?)

Table title: Disputing or Challenging Thoughts or Beliefs

FIGURE 3.3.   *(Continued)* How to question stressful, angry, anxious, and depressed thinking handout.

initial thoughts. Patients can identify these thoughts that are not helpful and change them or use their value system (e.g., being friendly) to help them think and respond in a useful manner even if they are unable to change or alter the initial way of thinking.

The following script is one example of how to teach patients to examine and question unhelpful thinking in the primary care setting. The idea is to let them know they can manage distress differently by questioning how their thoughts are working or not working for them.

Often when people get stressed, anxious, or depressed, their minds will tell them all kinds of things that can make them more distressed than they would like to be. You can't stop your mind

from talking to you, that's its job; however, you can improve your skills for recognizing what your mind is telling you and step back from those thoughts to ask yourself how useful they are. The idea here is to increase your ability to choose how you want to respond to situations instead of just reacting automatically. Questioning your thoughts gives you the opportunity to respond in a manner consistent with your values and with how you want to represent yourself to others. This can allow you to turn the volume down on any distressing responses you might be having; it's not that you will think happy or positive thoughts that will make everything better. It is beneficial, however, to be able to look at your initial thinking and determine if it is helpful, useful, and/or accurate and ask yourself how you would need to think differently to change how you feel.

Questioning your thoughts is a skill that you can learn and get better at with practice. Look at this list of 18 groups of questions [see Figure 3.3] and when you come to one that really jumps off the page as something that would be good to ask or tell yourself, tell me what it is.

Once the patient finds a question or statement he or she thinks might work, say: "If you were to ask or tell yourself that, how do you think it would be helpful? What would it allow you to do?" Typically, patients say it would allow them to look at the situation in a different less extreme way.

So by asking or telling yourself that, it can interrupt how you typically think and react to situations, help you look at the big picture, decide how you want to respond instead of react, and you can start to change your thinking so it works for you instead of against you.

Step 2: Advanced. This component, which is more like traditional cognitive therapy, is geared toward helping the patient identify faulty ways of thinking. It can help patients learn how their thoughts affect them physically, emotionally, and behaviorally and how they can develop more accurate, evidence-based ways of thinking that can change physical, emotional, and behavioral responses. The patient handouts in Figure 3.3 are recommended tools for introducing cognitive therapy concepts to patients in an educational format and for getting them started recognizing and disputing dysfunctional thoughts. These include suggested questions for identifying cognitive distortions, descriptions of common patterns of unhealthy thinking, and a cognition monitoring form. In addition, there are many books (e.g., Beck, 2005; Leahy, 2003) describing variants of cognitive therapy, with different forms, strategies, and procedures. We suggest you consider using cognitive disputation, including identifying thinking mistakes and evaluating evidence for and

against beliefs. In our experience, these strategies can be effectively delivered in 30-minute appointments. Cognitive disputation helps patients distance themselves from their thinking and develop skills to respond instead of reacting to their initial thoughts.

Arrange.   Following the presentation and discussion of these questions or statements, a follow-up appointment should be arranged to determine whether additional help with questioning unhelpful thoughts is needed, and if so, whether further learning and practice is sufficient or a referral for traditional cognitive therapy is indicated.

Enhancing Motivation to Change and Adhere to Treatment Regimens: Motivational Interviewing Strategies, Problem Solving, Self-Monitoring, and Behavioral Self-Analysis

Poor adherence to medical treatments or lifestyle change recommendations is often attributed to negative characteristics of the individual; he or she is seen as lazy, stubborn, unmotivated, unconcerned for his or her own health, and so forth. Many times, however, there are contingencies operating independently of personality characteristics and, fortunately, many of these are modifiable. As such, BHCs can play an important role in identifying factors contributing to inadequate follow-through on recommended changes and work with individuals to improve confidence in making behavioral changes, stressing the importance of those changes and related medical outcomes (DiMatteo, Giordani, Lepper, & Croghan, 2002).

We have found that four interventions are particularly useful in this situation: (a) MI strategies, (b) problem solving, (c) self-monitoring, and (d) behavioral self-analysis. First, we discuss the factors that often contribute to medical adherence and suggest questions to ask to help determine which factors are relevant to a particular patient. Following this, we describe how each of the four interventions can help the patient follow through with treatment recommendations.

Assess.   The reasons for nonadherence can be numerous. Gatchel and Oordt (2003) identified some of these, including treatment complexity, communication issues, patient understanding, treatment coordination issues, patient beliefs, psychosocial factors, and treatment side effects. In addition, patients are sometimes not motivated to adhere to their treatment regimens because they do not believe the treatment will help, they are not confident that they can successfully follow the medical advice, or they feel that the health problem is not a high priority for them. The following questions can help to assess factors that may be affecting individual follow-through on change or adherence to treatment recommendations.

Complexity of the patient's treatment regimen.
- Is the treatment easy, medium, or hard for you to carry out?
- What are some of the challenges it poses for you?
- Do you ever get confused or mixed up about what you are supposed to do?
- What do you do to help keep it straight?

Communication between primary care providers (PCPs) and patients.
- How is your relationship with your doctor?
- Are there things he or she says that you don't understand?
- Do you feel like he or she listens to your concerns?
- Are you getting answers to your questions?
- Do you feel you have input into the medical decisions that are being made?

Patient's understanding of the treatment and its relationship to the medical problem.
- Tell me what your doctor wants you to do and be specific.
- How often are you supposed to take your medication? How much? At what time of day?
- What is your medication supposed to do for you?
- Why does your doctor want you to change your habits (e.g., eating, exercise, smoking, drinking, sleeping)?
- Why do you think your doctor wants you to see a psychologist or social worker or behaviorist?

Coordination of how and when treatment is administered.
- Are you able to get medical appointments at times that are convenient for you?

- Are your work and family obligations flexible with regard to following your treatment regimen?

Inaccurate beliefs and unrealistic expectations about treatment.
- What do you anticipate will be the worst part of following your treatment?
- What do you worry about regarding the treatment?
- Do you know anyone who has used this treatment before? What did they say?
- What do you think the result of this treatment will be?

Psychosocial factors that serve as barriers to effective disease management.
- Are there any cultural or religious issues that are relevant to what your doctor has recommended?
- Does the medication or treatment cause a financial strain?
- How does your family feel about your health problems and the recommended treatment?
- How do your family members and friends help you to (e.g., eat better, exercise, drink less, avoid tobacco use)? What do they do that is not helpful?
- Are there any ways in which your medical treatment interferes with your work? Are there ways that people at work support you? What do they do that is not helpful?
- How do you think this treatment or lifestyle change will affect your social life or intimate relationships?

Medication side effects.
- What side effects do you experience from your medications or treatments?
- On a scale from 0 to 10, how bad are the side effects, with 0 being no side effects and 10 being severe side effects?
- Do the side effects make it hard for you to take the medicines?

Motivational factors.
- How satisfied are you with your health right now?
- How important is it to you to manage your health problem better?
- How confident are you that you do something that will improve your health?

- How confident are you that what your doctor recommended will help bring about the change you desire?
- Is there something going on in your life right now that is more important to you than your health, something you are more focused on?

Advise. Once you have identified factors that may be interfering with treatment adherence or lifestyle change, summarize these with the patient. Discuss how difficult it would be for anyone to adhere to a doctor's recommendation when there are significant barriers. Advise the patient that you are willing to work with him or her on managing or overcoming these difficulties.

Agree. Attempt to reach an agreement about which factors you will work on together. In discussing this, you might consider which factors are most important to the patient, which are within the patient's control, and which will mostly likely result in improved adherence.

Assist. Four strategies are reviewed here for assisting patients with treatment adherence within a primary care visit. Again, these are (a) MI strategies, (b) problem-solving, (c) self-monitoring, and (d) behavioral self-analysis.

Motivational interviewing Strategies. MI strategies help people recognize problems and resolve ambivalence toward health behavior change (Miller & Rollnick, 2002). Through MI, the behavioral health provider or PCP attempts to elicit self-motivational statements that reflect an underlying desire of the patient to change. MI strategies are neither coercive nor confrontational; rather, strategies involve open-ended questions, reflective listening, affirmation, and summarizing to help the patient evaluate the pros and cons of change. When signs of resistance to change are observed, the skilled motivational interviewer attempts to accept the resistance rather than confronting it head-on. The scope of this volume does not permit a thorough overview of MI strategies; interested readers should consult Miller and Rollnick (2002) for further information and evidence supporting this approach. Although MI, in its full form, is not typically a good fit for the brief appointments in primary care, various strategies from MI can be useful

for helping patients address intrapersonal obstacles to medical adherence and lifestyle change (Rollnick, Mason, & Butler, 1999). Three useful MI strategies to enhance motivation are examining readiness to change, importance of change, and self-efficacy of change (the confidence a patient has that he or she can change), and the pros and cons of change.

Patients must be ready to change before they will put the time and effort into altering how they think or what they do. Assessing readiness can give you information that can help improve readiness or motivation to change. One way to assess readiness is with the use of a simple readiness to change ruler (see Figure 3.4), following up with questions such as the following: "A rating of 0 would indicate you are not at all ready to change. A rating of 10 would suggest you are completely ready to change. You rated yourself as a 5. Why are you at a 5 and not a lower number?"

> Right now, you are at a 5. What would have to happen or change for the number to be higher?

In their responses, patients may articulate strengths of which they had been previously unaware or identify barriers they had not discussed before. You can then build on those strengths and help eliminate barriers to increase motivation to change. In addition to being ready to change, patients also need to see the change as important and have confidence that they can do what is necessary to attain the objectives. Assessing importance and confidence (see Figure 3.4) and engaging in additional assessment of these areas when rated as low can help decrease ambivalence about changing. Follow-up questions such as the following might be asked:

> What would have to happen or change for this to be more important? What keeps you from moving up to a higher number on the importance scale?

It can be helpful for some patients to discuss or view the specific pros and cons of making a change. You can do this verbally or using, for example, the cost–benefit analysis table in Figure 3.4. It has frequently been our experience that patients who are ambivalent about making changes experience decreases in ambivalence after expressly listing the benefits and costs of change. The patients, rather

---

Strategies to Improve Motivation to Change

Readiness to Change Ruler

At this moment, what number best reflects how ready you are to _____?

0	1	2	3	4	5	6	7	8	9	1 0

Not ready   *Unsure*   *Ready*

Importance and Confidence in Change

How important is it that you _____?

0——1——2——3——4——5——6——7——8——9——10

Not at all   *Most important*

How confident are you that you can _____?

0——1——2——3——4——5——6——7——8——9——10

Not at all   *Very confident*

Decisional Balance

Benefits of changing	Costs of changing

FIGURE 3.4. Strategies to improve motivation to change handout.

than the BHC, make the argument for why it would be in their best interest to change. However, if the costs outnumber the benefits of change, it could be that change is not in the best interest of the patient at the time. This exercise can also give you the opportunity to review possible benefits of change that the patient was not aware existed.

Problem solving. Often, patients understand the factors that interfere with medical adherence but have poor problem-solving skills. Therefore, they are unable to address these factors in a productive way. Teaching a simple problem-solving strategy and working together can help patients address target problems as well as equip them with a skill that can help them in other aspects of their lives. A seven step problem-solving model is recommended for the primary care setting: (a) Specifically define the problem; (b) brainstorm possible solutions without being critical; (c) critically evaluate each possible solution, discarding those that are clearly unreasonable or impossible using a listing of pros and cons to help evaluate them; (d) select the best option; (e) implement the chosen solution; (f) assess the outcome—likely in a follow-up visit; (g) if the outcome is favorable, fine-tune the solution as needed and continue to monitor the patient. If the outcome is unfavorable, return to step (d). The patient handout in Figure 3.5 can be used to guide the progression through these steps either during an appointment (or multiple appointments, if necessary) or as a homework assignment.

Self-monitoring. Self-monitoring can help patients track their progress toward a goal, stay focused on the target of change, and facilitate naturally occurring rewards as they see tangible evidence of positive change. Methods for self-monitoring will vary depending on what is being monitored; however, it is generally helpful to keep monitoring simple and brief. The following are useful strategies:

- Mark on a calendar each day that the target behavior is accomplished. This is useful for behaviors that are to occur daily (e.g., exercises, physical therapy, taking medicines).
- Keep a tally. Tallies can be successfully used both for increasing behaviors that occur several times per day (e.g., serving of fruits and vegetables, glasses of water) or decreasing behaviors that occur several times per day (e.g., cigarettes smoked).
- Chart the behavior on a graph. Graphing can be particularly useful when working with behaviors you want to change in a slowly progressing manner (e.g., minutes of walking for chronic back pain patients).

Problem-Solving Worksheet

1. Write out the problem: _____
2. Brainstorm all possible solutions. Write down anything you can think of. The goal is to get your mind flowing with ideas: _____
3. Critically evaluate your ideas.

   - Cross out any that are clearly unrealistic, outside your control or impossible.

   - Of those that remain, circle the top three. Write the top three below, in any order:

   _____   _____   _____

   - For each one list all the possible pros and cons.

   Pros:_____   Pros:_____   Pros:_____

   _____   _____   _____

   Cons:_____   Cons:_____   Cons:_____

   _____   _____   _____

4. On the basis of your pros and cons, select one that you feel has the best chances of working. Implement the chosen solution. Define how you will know if the solution is working:

   _____

   Assess the outcome on the following scale:

No improvement	Little improvement	Some improvement	A lot of improvement	Total improvement

   If the outcome is favorable, fine tune the solution as needed and continue to monitor it; if the outcome is unfavorable, return to Step 4.

FIGURE 3.5.   Problem-solving worksheet.

Behavioral self-analysis. Behavioral self-analysis is a model for teaching patients to analyze an event or activity that immediately precedes a behavior (antecedents) and immediately follows a behavior (consequences) to optimize success at managing their health and disease. The following script, which uses diabetes management as an example, can easily be applied within a primary care visit.

> I would like to introduce you to a helpful strategy that can assist you in changing health-related behavior. I call it the ABC model. The A stands for antecedents. These events or activities come before the behavior. B stands for the behavior itself. C stands for consequences, which includes what happens after the behavior and either increases or decreases the likelihood that you will engage in that behavior again. The concept is one I'm sure you are familiar with, as we use it in a lot of everyday events. For example, if you wanted to learn a new skill, such as driving a car for the first time, there are some things you might want to do before getting behind the wheel that would increase your chances of success. These would be the antecedents. Using the example of driving a car, what are some antecedents?
>
> **Instruction.** Learning how to turn the car on, how to work the controls, what the rules of the road are, what strategies help others to be successful, and what pitfalls to be cautious of.
>
> **Practice.** Driving around an empty parking lot, then moving to residential streets, then busier streets. Have an advanced driver or instructor in the car with you to coach you. Repeatedly practice the more difficult aspects, such as parallel parking, until you develop the skill.
>
> **Define the goal and determine the best route.** Decide where you are going and map out the route.

> **Identify potential problems.** What are some of the hazards that could interfere with success? How is the weather? What are the road conditions? Is the car well maintained?
>
> Now let's think about what's happening while you are driving. What are some important things to do (e.g., stay focused; avoid distractions, such as eating, listening to music, or talking; don't get discouraged if you make a mistake; apply the skills you have learned and practiced; assess how you are doing and make adjustments when necessary; take safety precautions, such as wearing a seatbelt). Once you have completed the driving, what are some of the consequences that will make it likely that you will drive again (e.g., arriving safely at your destination, pride in learning a new skill, freedom to get around easier)? By analyzing the ABCs of any new skill, you can increase your chances of success.
>
> Now that you have the idea, let's apply this to learning to manage your diabetes. What are some of the antecedents (events or activities) you may want to pay attention to for developing the skill of managing diabetes?
>
> **Instruction.** What is diabetes? How can medical science help control the disease and optimize quality of life? What skills do you need to learn? What lifestyle behaviors do you need to change? How can your family help? What equipment is available? What books or education programs are available? How often do you need to visit the doctor?
>
> **Practice.** Practice testing blood sugars, insulin injections, checking feet, and investigating new diets and exercise plans. Use a diabetes educator to help coach you. Keep working at those aspects that are difficult for you until you become good at it.
>
> **Define the goal and determine the best route.** Set behavioral goals for diet,

exercise, weight loss, medication use, and doctor visits. Establish reasonable subgoals and target dates, taking small, achievable steps.

Identify potential problems. What are some of the hazards that could interfere with success? Is there anyone in your life who will work against you achieving success, even unintentionally? How is your motivation and attitude; are they working for you or against you? Do you believe you can make healthy changes in your life? Are you getting depressed?

Now, what are some of the important factors in making lifestyle changes? Many are the same as when talking about driving: (a) stay mentally focused; (b) avoid distractions; (c) don't get discouraged if you make a mistake; (d) apply the skills you have learned; (e) assess how you are doing and make adjustments when necessary; and (f) take safety precautions, such as not keeping high fat foods readily available at home. When you do well, what are some of the consequences that will increase the likelihood that you will continue to make those changes? Again, there are parallels to our driving example: (a) arriving safely at your destination is the same as achieving better health and quality of life, (b) pride in learning a new skill is similar to gaining a sense that you are in control of your diabetes, and (c) freedom to get around more easily is like maintaining high levels of functioning and not letting diabetes limit your potential.

Now that we have identified some of the ABCs related to managing your diabetes, would you be willing to come back to work on some of these things together with me with the goal of helping you to be more successful?

Arrange. Once the barriers to adherence have been addressed, it is often helpful to arrange follow-up

care to monitor progress. One helpful strategy is to schedule the patient to see the BHC as part of medical follow-up visits.

Stimulus Control

Another useful strategy for helping patients change health-related behavior involves the behavioral principle of stimulus control (Dunkel & Glaros, 1978; Jacobson, 1978). Similar to the ABC model just discussed, stimulus control involves collaborating with the patient to identify stimuli that naturally precede a target behavior and then taking steps to alter these stimuli to bring about a desired result. Stimuli can be environmental, interpersonal, emotional, behavioral, or cognitive. Stimulus control strategies can help to increase desirable behaviors, such as increasing exercise and to decrease undesirable behaviors, such as eating too many unhealthy snacks.

Assess. The following script is a suggested way of using stimulus control in a primary care visit. The example uses eating unhealthy snack foods as a target behavior.

> Behaviors such as eating unhealthy snack foods do not happen without a variety of things occurring before you eat the unhealthy snack. There are a number of factors that can come before your eating behaviors; in fact, over time, these factors become associated with eating. In other words, they start to become triggers for eating. Triggers can be things you see, hear, smell, feel, or do. What triggers for eating junk food have you recognized in yourself?

Have the patient list factors. Categorize them as follows: (a) behaviors (e.g., watching television), (b) emotions (e.g., anger), (c) thoughts (e.g., "I'm hungry"), (d) other people (e.g., family not home), and (e) environmental (e.g., sitting at my desk at work).

> This is a good start. It's good that you are aware of many of the factors that are triggering your eating. As you can see, I've organized your triggers into the different categories you listed.

There may also be some of which you are not aware. The more triggers of which you are aware, the greater are the chances of being successful at managing your eating.

I would like to suggest that, over the next week, you monitor your eating outside of meals. For this week, don't try to make any changes, just monitor your eating. This form (see Monitoring Behavioral Triggers handout in Figure 3.6) can be used to help you recognize additional triggers. Every time you eat something or get the urge to eat something, apart from mealtime, log it on the form. Let's meet in one week and we'll review what you've observed.

At the next appointment you could say, "Let's look at your eating log. What did you observe were the most important or most frequently occurring triggers for you? Were there any that you hadn't recognized before?"

Advise and agree

It looks like you have done a good job recognizing some of the triggers related to your consumption of snack foods. I suggest we work together on trying to control these. Is that something you would be willing to do? Let's list the factors you identified on this worksheet (see Figure 3.6). Now, which of these triggers are within your ability to control and which do you feel are outside your control?

Monitoring Behavioral Triggers

Date	Behavior	What was I doing?	How was I feeling?	What was I thinking?	What were others around me doing?	Time of day/ Location/Other environmental factors

Controllling Trigger Worksheet

Trigger	Level of Control			Plan
	Lots	Some	None	

Stimulus Control Plan

Trigger	Level of Control			Plan
	Lots	Some	None	

FIGURE 3.6. Monitoring behavioral triggers handout.

Check off in the corresponding column those that the patient has direct control over, those he or she can learn to control better, and those outside his or her control.

Assist and arrange. "Now let's come up with a plan for avoiding some of these triggers so that we can help you control your eating." Discuss each of the triggers and steps that can be taken to control them. List each idea that the patient is willing to start under the Plan column. Examples are provided in Figure 3.7. After using the worksheet to develop a stimulus control plan, arrange follow-up care to monitor and assist efforts to change the target behaviors.

Assertive Communication

Assertive communication training is often used as an important component of comprehensive treatment packages for problems such as eating disorders (Shiina et al., 2005), anxiety (Wehr & Kaufman, 1987), chronic pain (Merlijn et al., 2005), depression (Ball, Kearney, Wilhelm, Dewhurst-Savellis, & Barton, 2000), and partner-

relationship difficulties (Gordon & Waldo, 1984). Poor communication with others is not frequently identified as the presenting problem. However, in our experience, passive and aggressive communication problems can exacerbate symptoms and impede functioning and goal attainment. As such, being able to teach the patient assertive communication skills can be an important part of your practice.

Assess. As part of a standard first assessment, asking the following questions can help you determine whether communication is a problem that deserves further inquiry: "Do you find that you sometimes have difficulty communicating what you think or how you feel? Do you feel that others do not respond to you in a manner that you would like them to?" If the answer to this question is "No," then you might move on to other functional assessment questions. If the answer is "Yes," you might follow with questions such as these, to further clarify and determine whether assertive communications skills training might be helpful.

	Level of Control			
Trigger	**Lots**	**Some**	**None**	**Plan**
Watching TV	X			Not willing to give up watching TV. Make a commitment to eat only while sitting at the kitchen table.
Anger		X		Avoid the kitchen when feeling angry. Take an anger management class or read a book on the topic.
Thinking, "I'm hungry"		X		Rethink with realistic thinking: "I'm not hungry; I just ate dinner an hour ago. I have an urge to eat but it is not physiological hunger."
Family not home			X	Can't avoid being home alone, however, access to snack foods can be controlled. Avoid going in the kitchen when family is not home. Don't buy unhealthy food.
Sitting at my desk at work			X	Avoid access to snack foods at work. Don't carry small change so vending machines and snack cupboards are not convenient.

Stimulus Control Plan (Sample: Control unhealthy eating behvior)

FIGURE 3.7.   Stimulus control plan handout.

- With what people, or in what situations, do you have these communication difficulties?
- Is this communication difficulty something new or has it happened with other people or in other situations during your life?
- What thoughts do you have when you are in these situations?
- What makes the communication better? What makes it worse?
- Do you notice any physical changes when you are in these situations?

Advise and agree

It sounds like there are times when you do not communicate as effectively as you would like to. You find that you get nervous in these situations and your words do not come out the way you would like them to. You feel humiliated, which leads you to not want to say things in future situations, but you feel angry and frustrated by not saying anything because people take advantage of your generosity. One of the things we can do is to help you learn to communicate more effectively so that you can improve the chances that situations such as this can turn out differently. Is learning how to communicate more effectively something you are interested in doing?

This is a handout (see Figure 3.8) I would like you to review between now and our follow-up appointment. When you come back, I'll teach you some assertiveness skills and we'll review this handout to make sure you understand it, and then we'll set a specific plan for you to improve.

Assist. The primary goal is to help the patient learn the difference between passive, assertive, and aggressive communication and how to speak assertively when needed. You can use the handout in Figure 3.8 to assist with this. We use the Honest, Appropriate, Respectful, Direct (HARD) acronym to help the individual assess their communication style in any situation. We also teach the XYZ* formula in Figure 3.8 as

a format for practicing direct communication that may be more healthy and effective in meeting their needs. The XYZ* Formula is a way for the patient to assertively express thoughts by putting the appropriate words in the XYZ* positions. We recommend the following to help the patient learn effective assertive communication.

- Review the HARD acronym handout, explaining differences in communication styles.
- Demonstrate with your own example the differences between speaking passively, assertively, and aggressively. Change voice tone, affect, body posture, and eye contact appropriately.
- After you have demonstrated each, ask the patient which was the easiest to listen to.
- Highlight the point that if the words do not match what the listener sees (nonverbal communication), the listener may pay more attention to what they see than to what they hear.
- Develop appropriate statements for situations and demonstrate how those might be verbalized using the XYZ* Formula.
- Set a plan for the patient to practice the statements at home in front of a mirror.
- You might also recommend that the patient obtain a self-help book on assertive communication (e.g., Alberti & Emmons, 2001) for further information and skill development.

Arrange. We recommend having patients return for a follow-up consult to demonstrate their practiced skill through role play. This allows you to provide additional feedback and modeling as necessary. At this point, you may also set a specific plan to use the skill. You may decide not to schedule any follow-up consults at this point, or you may recommend additional follow-ups as necessary if the patient's communications skills plans are not as effective as predicted.

SUMMARY

The cognitive and behavioral skills discussed in this chapter are applicable to a broad range of medical and behavioral health concerns. We

---

Assertive Communication

Assertiveness Is Simple but Hard

NonAssertive	Assertive	Aggressive
(Passive)	(Tactful)	(Rude)
☹ ✎ **H** onest	✓ **H** onest	✓ **H** onest
✓ **A** ppropriate	✓ **A** ppropriate	☹ **A** ppropriate
✓ **R** espectful	✓ **R** espectful	☹ **R** espectful
☹ **D** irect	✓ **D** irect	✓ **D** irect

Assertiveness involves respecting your rights and the rights of others.

Important Facts About Assertiveness

- Use "I" or "me" statements such as "When you do _____, I feel _____."
- Voice tone, eye contact, and body posture are important parts of assertive communication.
- Use a steady and calm voice, stand or sit up straight, look the other person in the eyes without glaring.
- Feelings are usually only one word (e.g. angry, anxious, happy, sad, hurt, frustrated, joyful)
- Remember, assertiveness doesn't guarantee that you will get what you want or that the other person will understand your concerns or be happy with what you said. It does improve the chances that the other person will understand what you want or how you feel and thus improve your chances of communicating effectively.

Four Essential Steps to Assertive Communication

1. Tell the person what you think about their behavior without accusing them.
2. Tell them how you feel when they behave a certain way.
3. Tell them how their behavior affects you and your relationship with them.
4. Tell them what you would prefer them to do instead.

XYZ* Formula for Effective Communication

The goal of the XYZ* formula is to express the way you feel (internal world) in response to other's behavior (external world) in specific situations. You are the only person who has access to your feelings. Others have no access to your internal world. The only way they will know what you are feeling is if you tell them. Similarly, you only have access to other people's external world. It is very easy to make a mistake when trying to guess what others are feeling or intending.

I feel *X*	when you do *Y*	in situation *Z*	and I would like *
I feel angry	when you leave your socks and underwear on the bedroom floor	after work	and I would like you to put them in the hamper.
I felt insignificant	when you left me with an empty gas tank	yesterday	and I would like you to leave the car with at least 1/4 tank of gas.
I feel angry	when you don't call me	if you are staying late at work	and I would like you to call as soon as you know you will be late.
I feel loved	when you kiss me	when you get home	and I would like you to do that everyday.

FIGURE 3.8.   Assertive communication handout.

reviewed strategies and suggested methods of application that we have found to be suitable for the demands and limitations of the primary care environment. The chapters in Part II that address specific patient problems will often refer to these interventions, and many of the scripts in this chapter can be easily modified to address these problems.

CHAPTER 4

CULTURAL COMPETENCE

Culture has been defined as a complex interwoven pattern of learned behaviors and beliefs shared among groups. Culture includes ways of thinking, communicating, interacting, and views on roles, relationships, customs, and values (Betancourt, Green, & Carrillo, 2002). The looking glass through which information is filtered, culture determines how an individual sees and makes sense of the world (Gregg & Saha, 2006; Núñez, 2000). As one might expect, doctors and patients may see health care and disease in different ways when interpreting the world through different sets of values and guidelines, opening the door for miscommunication. In fact, there is a growing body of evidence showing that race, ethnicity, socioeconomic status, and factors such as limited English proficiency have a negative impact on health and clinical care, producing health disparities throughout the U.S. health care system (Agency for Healthcare Research and Quality [AHRQ], 2006; Betancourt, 2006). These disparities are consistent, found across a range of medical conditions and types of services, are correlated with worse health outcomes, and are independent of education, income, and insurance status (Institute of Medicine [IOM], 2002b). These disparities exist for the largest minority groups in the U.S. including "Black", "Asian", and "Hispanic" groups in comparison to "White" groups (AHRQ, 2006).

Improving cultural competence in the provision of health care services has received increasing attention as a potential means of decreasing these disparities (Betancourt, Green, Carrillo, & Ananeh-Firempong, 2003; Eiser & Ellis, 2007; Hays, 2008). In the past, efforts to improve cultural competence have been geared toward teaching providers about the beliefs, attitudes, values, and behaviors of various groups, in addition to the key things to do and avoid for effective practice with individuals from a specific culture (Betancourt, 2006; Hays, 2008). Learning about the values, customs, and norms of the cultural groups you work with can be helpful, but applying a one-size-fits-all approach to an ethnic group can lead to stereotyping and oversimplification of a complex, multidimensional construct that is continually being altered by social and economic influences (Betancourt, 2004, 2006; Gregg & Saha, 2006; Hays, 2008). As such, culturally competent health care has evolved as a multilevel construct to include organizational factors (e.g., diversity among leadership of health care organizations), structural factors (e.g., linguistically appropriate education materials), and clinical factors (e.g., interactions between the health care provider and the individual; Betancourt et al., 2003).

According to Betancourt et al. (2003), culturally competent health care involves the following:

> Understanding the importance of social and cultural influences on patients' health beliefs and behaviors; considering how these factors interact at multiple levels of the health care system (e.g., at the level of structural processes of care or clinical decision-making) and, finally, devising interventions that take these issues into account to assure quality health care delivery to diverse patient populations. (p. 297)

Culturally competent care at the provider and patient level has evolved from making assumptions about individuals on the basis of their background or race to include principles of patient-centered care that involves empathy, responsiveness, and compassion regarding the values, needs, and preferences of the individual (Betancourt et al., 2003b; Paasche-Orlow, 2004). Patient-centered care takes into account an individual's cultural traditions, preferences, values, lifestyle, and family situation. It also includes the patient and significant others in making shared clinical decisions and providing them with the support and tools needed for good care (Institute for Healthcare Improvement, 2007).

Culturally competent patient-centered care is important for multiple reasons. The United States is becoming increasingly diverse, and providers are likely to have increased contact with individuals holding a range of beliefs and values. These beliefs and values may influence how patients report symptoms, when they seek health services, their expectations for care, and how they adhere to recommendations (Betancourt, 2006). Being able to effectively assess a medical concern and communicate the findings in an understandable, culturally appropriate manner is important and has been associated with improved patient adherence to treatment, improved health outcomes, and greater satisfaction with care (M. Stewart et al., 1999). Furthermore, organizations such as the IOM (2002a) and the American College of Physicians (2004) have advocated the importance of cultural competence and patient-centered care as a way to decrease health disparities through improved communication.

CULTURAL COMPETENCE AND BEHAVIORAL HEALTH CONSULTATION

In specialty mental health clinics, providers commonly work collaboratively with individuals, recognizing social and cultural differences, assessing and being sensitive to the individuals' unique world perspective and what they want from treatment. If you have not had this training, or if you need to refresh your skills, it might be valuable to do a self-assessment of your current cultural competence. A cultural competence self-assessment and provider cultural self-assessment can be found at the American Academy of Family Physicians' Web

site (http://www.aafp.org/fpm/20001000/58cult.html) and Hays (2008) respectively. Most graduate school programs incorporate some type of culturally oriented training regarding assessment and intervention. Models and recommendations for culturally informed functional assessments for specialty mental health care have been proposed (e.g., Aklin & Turner, 2006; Hays, 2008; Okazaki & Tanaka-Matsumi, 2006; Tanaka-Matsumi, Seiden, & Lam, 1996). The model component of Okazaki and Tanaka-Matsumi and Tanaka-Matsumi, Seiden, and Lam are particularly amenable to primary care. These are discussed and adaptations for the primary care setting are suggested.

Similar to Betancourt (2006), we believe it is important to have a framework that allows a patient-centered, culturally competent approach for effective communication and care for any individual, regardless of cultural background. To assist with this, we describe five areas that are likely important to attend to across cultures to minimize misunderstandings. We also provide a focused description of the model that includes the Explanatory model of health and illness, Social and environmental factors affecting adherence, Fears and concerns about medication and side effects, Treatment understanding model of culturally competent practice (ESFT; Betancourt, 2006; Carrillo, Green, & Betancourt, 1999), which is geared for physician use and cited as enhancing provider–patient communication, satisfaction, and adherence (Stanton, 1987). We also discuss the *Culturally Informed Functional Assessment interview* (CIFA) model of culturally competent assessment (Tanaka-Matsumi et al., 1996), which was developed for mental health providers. The CIFA model has been found to facilitate the interview process, build rapport, and increase the likelihood of obtaining accurate knowledge of the individual's cultural definition of the problem, cultural norms, and culturally appropriate change and intervention strategies (see Okazaki & Tanaka-Matsumi, 2006). In addition to these models, there are resources available on the Internet (e.g., http://erc.msh.org/mainpage.cfm?file=1.0.htm &module=provider&language=English and http://search.aafp.org/search?q=cultural+competence&x=0&y=0&site=a&client=aafp&proxystylesheet=aafp&filter=0&output=xml_no_dtd&getfields=*

&hl=en&lr=lan_en) that can be helpful for learning about cultural considerations for medical care. We provide a series of suggestions toward the end of the chapter based on a merging of these two models designed for the behavioral health consultant (BHC) and geared toward enhancing communication and providing a patient-centered approach to assessment and intervention.

CROSS-CULTURAL AREAS OF MISUNDERSTANDING

Betancourt (2006) and Carrillo et al. (1999) have described several areas in which cultural misunderstandings can occur. If not attended to, these misunderstandings have the potential to result in a range of negative outcomes. Greater attention should be paid to these areas when interacting with individuals from a cultural background different from your own. It would be impossible to provide a detailed list of what to do within each category. However, if you regularly see individuals that vary significantly from your own cultural background, consider educating yourself about the cultural factors falling under these topic areas as a way to maximize effective communication during a 30-minute appointment.

Communication Style
Communication style includes both verbal and nonverbal communication and comprises personal space, eye contact, and touch. As an example, Hispanic Americans may be more likely than their White counterparts to communicate in less assertive and more covert ways, using subtle remarks or humor so the listener can retain their sense of dignity (Falicov, 2001). When providing care for patients in this culture, not attending to this trait and speaking to the patient in a direct assertive manner may offend the patient and, as a result, he or she may not follow recommendations or return for care.

Mistrust
There are a variety of reasons behavioral health and medical providers are not trusted. These include events in history, myths or folklore, misperceptions about the medical profession handed down through cultural groups or families, and negative individual medical experiences that are generalized to all medical personnel. As an example, African Americans, because of historically poor quality and quantity of medical care, medically related discrimination, and negative clinical experiences, may carry more mistrust of medical providers and the system than their White counterparts (Eiser & Ellis, 2007). Thus, providing optimal care for patients who are African American may include the involvement of additional health care personnel of various ethnicities and demonstrations of emotional support, including expressed empathy and understanding of the current situation and the patient's fears and concerns (Eiser & Ellis, 2007).

Decision Making
Many Americans place a value and importance on being free to make personal decisions independently. At the same time, there can be great variability within and between cultures, and individuals may want to include or consult with family members or others from their cultural tradition during or before making decisions to follow a treatment plan. For example, in some cultures it may be expected that a woman will consult and get approval from her husband, father, or other elders in the community before making decisions about health care changes. In other cultures, individuals may prefer to consult religious or spiritual advisors to obtain permission before medical action or change can take place. Some cultures may rely on the advice of a recognized "health expert" in the community. An example of this is the *promotora,* a Hispanic liaison between health care providers and patients, who provides education, makes referrals for service and home visits, and identifies barriers to care. The standard statements we suggest you use when providing treatment options may work well regardless of what is important to that individual's decision-making process (see chap. 2, this volume).

Spirituality, Traditions, and Customs
Spirituality, traditions, and customs can influence the way patients conceptualize the causes, symptoms, and effective treatment of their condition.

For example, current symptoms might be attributed to deviating from religious values or standards. Resolution of those symptoms may be achieved through specific cleansing or correcting actions or through actions of forgiveness or ritual ceremony with a religious leader or healer. Another example is the belief that symptoms stem from interpersonal conflict or wronging someone; the traditional or customary way to get better is to repair the conflict or right the wrong. Other traditions and customs include not discussing problems or symptoms that could be interpreted as compromising dignity, portraying weakness, or shaming the family. Asking about and being aware of how spirituality, traditions, and customs influence how the patient thinks and what he or she is willing to do or not do as well as who else needs to be part of their treatment (e.g., family, friends, spiritual leaders) are all important in developing a patient-centered approach to care that maximizes the chances of success.

Gender and Sexual Issues

Gender, gender roles, and sexuality may be important areas to understand regarding the effect of symptoms and functioning on those roles and how thoughts, behaviors, and social interactions are influenced in a positive or negative manner. Knowledge about male and female roles in a partnerships, marriage, family, and community, the effect of symptoms on those roles, and what sexual functioning means about or for the individual can be important to consider when developing an intervention that is patient-centered and focused on areas that are motivating for change on the basis of the patient's belief system. This knowledge may be important to understand what the patient's family and community is willing to do or not do to assist the patient to return to previous functioning.

THE ESFT MODEL OF CULTURALLY COMPETENT PRACTICE

The ESFT model (Betancourt, 2006) consists of the factors described in the following subsections. Under each factor are questions suggested by Betancourt that might be asked to elicit relevant information.

Explanatory Model of Health and Illness

Cultural factors may influence beliefs about what is causing the health problem or the related symptoms, what the patient's symptoms or illness means, or the meaning of treatment.

- What do you think caused your problems?
- Why do you think it started when it did?
- How does it affect you?
- What worries you most?
- What kind of treatment do you think you should receive?

Social and Environmental Factors Affecting Adherence

The patient's ability to afford and obtain medication may result from social and environmental factors that ultimately affect the patient's adherence to the medication regimen. If barriers are identified, the provider may seek less costly medication or referral for social services assistance.

- How do you get your medications?
- Are they difficult to afford?
- Do you have time to pick them up?
- How quickly do you get them?
- Do you have help getting them if you need it?

Fears and Concerns About Medication and Side Effects

Individuals may have fears about medication that could lead them to not take it or take it incorrectly.

- Are you concerned with the dosage, color, or size of the pill?
- Have you heard anything about this medication?
- Are you worried about side effects?

Treatment Understanding

To ensure that the individual understands the plan, have them repeat back to you what they are to do. Provide written or pictorial instructions.

- "Do you understand how to take the medication?"
- "Can you tell me how to take it?"

THE CIFA MODEL OF CULTURALLY COMPETENT ASSESSMENT

The components of the CIFA model (Okazaki & Tanaka-Matsumi, 2006; Tanaka-Matsumi et al., 1996) are discussed in the following subsections.

Assessment of Cultural Identity and Level of Acculturation

The goal is to examine the match or mismatch in culture between the individual and the provider. Identifying the primary language spoken by the patient and the behaviors of the individual's reference group may help assess cultural identity and level acculturation.

Assessment of the Presenting Problem

When you are evaluating the individual's problems and explanation for those problems, it is important to consider the individual's cultural norms. How similar or different the individual's behaviors and symptoms are from his or her cultural norm will influence how the type and severity of problems are judged and what treatment might be pursued.

Eliciting Conceptualization of the Problem and Possible Solutions

It is valuable to ask the individual what he or she believes is the cause of his or her problem(s) and then compare it with the family's explanation and the cultural norms of the individual.

Functional Assessment of Factors Related to Initiation and Maintenance of the Problem

Examine modifiable causal variables, motivation to change, consequences of problems for the family, and what happens to the family if the treatment is successful. Explore what the individual's reactions might be to variables in his or her environment that are consistent or inconsistent with cultural norms.

Causal Explanatory Model Comparison and Negotiation

The provider should discuss and explain the hypothesis of what is happening to the individual, compare it with the individual's hypothesis, and work with him or her to resolve discrepancies.

Development of an Acceptable Treatment Plan

When one is developing a treatment plan, it is important to negotiate and agree on a plan that includes culturally acceptable goals, target behaviors, and intervention techniques. The provider may actively involve others in the individual's life to reinforce changes. The provider may also ask about prior help-seeking, preferences for treatment, or culture specific treatment techniques or practices.

Data Gathering That Facilitates Ongoing Assessment of the Individual's Progress

It may be important to spend time discussing the acceptability and disadvantages of collecting self-monitoring or treatment outcome data.

Treatment, Duration, Course, and Expected Outcome

Individuals may come in with different preconceived ideas about the treatment and how that treatment will be delivered. Therefore, early in the development of the treatment plan, spend time discussing individual and family concerns related to transportation, scheduling, money, and confidentiality.

BRINGING IT ALL TOGETHER FOR THE INITIAL APPOINTMENT

In chapter 2, we detailed phases of the initial consultation appointment as well as potential questions and statements to effectively and efficiently gather information to treat individuals. These phases already include patient-centered care strategies that are also part of operating in a culturally competent manner. What follows is a synthesis of "Cross-Cultural Areas of Misunderstanding," and the ESFT, and CIFA models to the primary care setting. We use this synthesis as a guide to decrease miscommunication and increase patient-centered care that is culturally responsive and appropriate for all individuals. We lay out the content areas we have adapted, and the concepts that these functional areas include. We then give specific suggestions for questions and statements, including relevant areas from chapter 2 that we believe are important for providing the best patient-centered, culturally competent care within the Primary Care Behavioral Health model of integrated care.

The following is a list of content areas from "Cross-Cultural Areas of Misunderstanding," and the ESFT and CIFA models. These areas are important to focus on in the 5A's of an initial consultation.

- *Trust.* This includes "Mistrust" from "Cross-Cultural Areas of Misunderstanding."
- Faith and customs. This includes "Spirituality, Traditions, and Customs" from "Cross-Cultural Areas of Misunderstanding."
- *Culture.* This includes "Assessment of Cultural Identity and Level of Acculturation" from CIFA.
- *Thoughts and beliefs about the problem.* This includes "Explanatory Model of Health and Illness" from ESFT and "Assessment of the Presenting Problem," "Eliciting the Conceptualization of the Problem and Possible Solutions," and "Functional Assessment of Factors Related to Initiation and Maintenance of the Problem" from CIFA.
- *Provider and individual's problem conceptualization agreement.* This includes "Causal Explanatory Model Comparison and Negotiation" from CIFA.
- *Developing an action plan.* This includes "Decision Making" from "Areas of Misunderstanding" and "Development of an Acceptable Treatment Plan" from CIFA.
- *Barriers to the plan.* This includes "Social and Environmental Factors Affecting Adherence" and "Fears and Concerns About Medication and Side-Effects" from ESFT.
- *Understanding of the plan and follow-up.* This includes "Treatment Understanding" from ESFT and "Treatment Duration, Course, and Expected Outcome" from CIFA.

THE 5A'S AND PATIENT-CENTERED, CULTURALLY COMPETENT CARE

The following are specific recommendations for improving patient-centered, culturally competent care during the initial assessment. We have placed these suggestions where we believe they fit best within the 5A's framework.

Assess

Specifically assessing trust, faith and customs, cultural identity, and belief about the problem can be important in developing a plan the patient can understand and is willing to do. Examples of questions for these areas are given.

Trust. This might be addressed through the following methods. The introductory script makes it explicit who you are, what might happen in the appointment, who is going to have access to the information the patient tells you, and how that information might be used (see chap. 2, this volume). Ask whether the patient has any questions at the end of the introductory script as follows: "Do you have any questions about who I am, my role in the clinic, what we might do during this appointment, or how the information you give me might be used?" If he or she says yes, then answer the questions; if not, then you might say, "If you should have any questions at all during our appointment, please ask." This provides the individual with an initial opportunity to discuss any fears or concerns they may have. It allows you to provide accurate information and to potentially increase trust.

If during the assessment, you get the impression the individual is holding information back, you might ask something such as the following:

> I get the impression that you are not sure how the information you tell me will be used, who might have access to that information, or what might be suggested or happen to you as a result of telling me certain things. Whether this is true, or whether there is something else you are concerned or have questions about, I'd like the chance to discuss those with you before we go any further.

Faith and customs. These might be addressed in the following way:

> Before we start today, I'd be interested in knowing whether you have any reli-

gious or spiritual values, traditions, or customs that you feel are important for me to know so that I can best understand your current situation and help us to work well together.

Culture. This might be addressed in one or more of the following ways:

- What country did you grow-up in?
- How long have you been here?
- What do you see as the main differences between the medical care where you grew up and the medical care here?
- What language do you speak at home?

Thoughts and beliefs about the problem. The suggestions from chapter 2 about areas of general assessment are geared toward a patient-centered approach to assessment and identifying from the individual's perspective what the problem is and what the factors are that are influencing the problem. The following topic areas are most applicable and additional questions are listed for some of the areas to supplement the questions from chapter 2, as needed.

- *Nature of the referral problem.* "Do your friends and family see you as having problems with (specify referral problem) or do they see it differently? Besides the provider in this clinic, whom else have you asked for help with this problem?"
- *Duration.* "When do you think other important people in your life noticed your problems starting, or have they noticed?"
- *Triggering events.* "Do friends, family, or other important people in your life see the same things as causing your problems or do they see it differently?"
- *Frequency and intensity of the problem.* "How does it affect your family when things get better or worse?"
- *Factors that make the problem better or make it worse.* "Do people who are important in your life see the same things that you see making your problem better or worse or do they see it differently?"
- *Functional impairments (changes in work, relationships with family and friends).*

The Provider and Individual's Problem Conceptualization Agreement. This is included as part of the standard recommendations for the initial appointment in chapter 2 and is administered during the summary phase. During this phase, the BHC summarizes his or her understanding of the problem and asks the patient whether it is correct. If not, it allows the patient to correct the BHC or provide additional information so the BHC and the patient have the same conceptualization of the problem.

Advise and Agree

An action plan is included as part of the standard recommendations for the initial appointment in chapter 2 and is implemented during the potential change plans phase. During this phase, the BHC asks the patient what he or she thinks would need to be changed or be different to effectively treat the problem, discusses what the provider thinks might be helpful to change or do, and reviews the results that are predicted to occur from these changes.

Assist

Barriers to the plan might be addressed through one or more of the following questions:

- Is there anything you can think of that will make it difficult to follow-through with the plan that we have set?
- Are there family members or friends that might not be happy with the changes you are planning to make?
- How do you think members of your [house/ neighborhood/community/place of worship] will respond to the changes you make as part of this plan?
- Do you have any concerns, fears, worries, or questions about the plan?

Arrange

In the *Understanding of Plan and Follow-up*, it is important to determine that you and the individual have communicated well about what the plan is, what the individual is supposed to do, why it is important, and the expected results. One way to determine the patient's understanding is to ask something such as the following:

> I would like to make sure that we both have the same idea about what the plan is. Would you be willing to tell me your understanding of the plan, what are you going to do, why that is important, and what type of result you might get?

Consistent with chapter 2, determine whether the individual needs a follow-up appointment, and with whom as well as when and how the individual should follow-up.

SUMMARY

There are health care disparities driven by ethnicity, socioeconomic status, race, and ability to speak English, which are independent of an individual's education, income, and insurance status. One way of bridging this gap is to improve the cultural competence of medical providers. Moving past the one-size-fits-all approach of applying stereotyped information to everyone within an ethnic group, cultural competence seeks to improve communication and promote better health care through a patient-centered approach. Thus, paying attention to the individual's health beliefs, behaviors, preferences, lifestyle, and family situation is seen as

important not only to improve communication but also to promote health behavior change.

In the medical and behavioral health communities, greater attention, theoretical development, research, and training are increasing culturally competent assessment and intervention. We believe that the "Cross-Cultural Areas of Misunderstanding," the ESTF, and the CIFA models of cultural competent practice and assessment contain practical areas of focus for better cultural care competence and we have blended these concepts into a working framework or set of important areas for consideration. These areas may be important to include in behavioral health consultations when working with individuals who are from a different cultural background. We have offered a practical set of recommendations that include how these content areas fit within the 5A's model with suggestions for questions to efficiently and effectively gather information and improve communication and understanding of the individual's problems and concerns.

Certainly, culture is an ever-changing entity. As theory and research develop around patient-centered and culturally competent care, our practices will surely follow. We hope that this chapter and the tools within it will serve as an adaptable base and launching point for improving your own cultural competence and that you will continue to build on this framework as theory and research develop and as you develop as a BHC.

PART II

COMMON BEHAVIORAL HEALTH CONCERNS IN PRIMARY CARE

CHAPTER 5

DEPRESSION, ANXIETY, AND INSOMNIA

Behavioral health concerns such as depression, anxiety, and insomnia are prevalent in primary care and, not surprisingly, are often treated pharmacologically (Pincus et al., 1998). One of the greatest advantages of integrating behavioral health professionals into primary care systems is the potential to identify and use evidence-based behavioral and cognitive interventions with individuals who demonstrate subclinical or mild to moderate depression, anxiety, and insomnia. Obviously, each topic could constitute its own chapter or even its own book (e.g., Robinson, Wischman, & Vento, 1996). Our intent in this chapter is to provide an overview of the main areas we often target when confronting these problems in primary care.

DEPRESSION

Community surveys suggest that the lifetime prevalence rate of a major depressive disorder is 16.9% and the prevalence rate of any mood disorder is 21.4% (Kessler, Chiu, Demler, Merikangas, & Walters, 2005). The prevalence of significant depressive symptoms for those being seen in primary care settings ranges from 10% to 30% (McQuaid, Stein, Laffaye, & McCahill, 1999; Stein, Kirk, Prabhu, Grott, & Terepa, 1995). Unfortunately, primary care providers (PCPs) do not recognize depression in roughly 67% of their patients (Coyne, Schwenk, & Fechner-Bates, 1995; Nisenson, Pepper, Schwenk, & Coyne, 1998; Spitzer et al., 1995). A major depressive episode is defined in the *Diagnostic and Statistical Manual of Mental Disorders, Fourth Edition, Text Revision* (*DSM–IV–TR*; American Psychiatric Association [APA], 2000) as a depressed mood or loss of interest or pleasure for at least 2 weeks in addition to at least four other symptoms, including significant weight changes, sleep disturbance, psychomotor agitation or retardation, feelings of worthlessness or guilt, or recurrent thoughts of death or suicide. Individuals diagnosed with major depressive disorder must have had a major depressive episode, whereas individuals with fewer symptoms or those who have experienced the symptoms for shorter periods of time may be diagnosed with depressive disorder not otherwise specified (APA, 2000, pp. 381–382).

Specialty Mental Health

Although a wide variety of therapies are offered for the treatment of depressive symptoms, evidence-based reviews have suggested that the most effective psychological treatments for depression are cognitive and behavioral interventions (Management of Major Depressive Disorder Working Group, 2000; National Institute for Clinical Excellence [NICE], 2004). These treatments often involve techniques such as behavioral activation, cognitive restructuring, problem-solving, and relaxation techniques. In addition, there is evidence that brief interventions, including guided self-help (Bower, Richards, & Lovell, 2001), can be effective for reducing depressive symptoms.

Behavioral Health in Primary Care

Consistent with the NICE (2004) stepped-care model, behavioral health consultants (BHCs) play particularly important roles as collaborative partners on the primary care team for individuals demonstrating mild to severe depression. The Agency for Health Care Policy and Research Guidelines (Schulberg, Katon, Simon, & Rush, 1998) as well as other reviews (e.g., Schulberg, Raue, & Rollman, 2002) suggest that time-limited, depression-targeted psychotherapies are efficacious when used in primary care settings. Broadly defined, care management models of collaborative care (i.e., those using a care manager to assist with monitoring of medication adherence and follow-up on referral to specialty mental health) have been shown to be more effective for improving short- and long-term depression outcomes when compared to standard care (Gilbody, Bower, Fletcher, Richards, & Sutton, 2006). In a more recent review of psychosocial interventions for depression in primary care, Wolf and Hopko (2008) concluded that problem-solving therapy, interpersonal psychotherapy, and pharmacotherapy are efficacious interventions for major depression, whereas cognitive behavior and cognitive therapies are "possibly efficacious" (p. 130). However, methodological limitations (e.g., different outcome measures, deliveries of treatment) may have confounded the results. In addition, many of the reviewed studies used interventions that were more similar to co-located care (e.g., meeting 6–12 times for 50 minutes) rather than brief interventions that could be incorporated into the primary care environment by a BHC. Given the breadth of data in specialty mental health settings and the developing evidence in primary care settings, our recommendations for assessments and interventions for depressive symptoms rely heavily on cognitive and behavioral techniques.

Primary Care Adaptation

Assessing and targeting depressive symptoms in primary care requires the BHC to use focused questions and interventions. Using the 5A's provides a useful guide.

Assess.   There are several self-report measures that are both short and easily scored and therefore can be useful for screening for depressive symptoms in primary care. Sharp and Lipsky (2002) provided a broad review of depression screening measures for use in primary care. Several popular measures used

to screen for depression in primary care include the Beck Depression Inventory-Primary Care (BDI-PC; 7 items; A. T. Beck, Guth, Steer, & Ball, 1997), the Center for Epidemiologic Studies Depression Scale-Revised (CESD-R; 20 items; Eaton, Smith, Ybarra, Muntaner, & Tien, 2004), and the Patient Health Questionnaire-9 (PHQ-9: 10 items; Kroenke, Spitzer, & Williams, 2001).

The Patient Health Questionnaire-2. The Patient Health Questionnaire-2 (PHQ-2; Kroenke, Spitzer, & Williams, 2003) is a particularly short measure that uses the first two questions of the PHQ-9 to screen for depression.

> "Over the last 2 weeks, how often have you been bothered by any of the following problems:"
>
> 1. Little interest or pleasure in doing things?
> 2. Feeling down, depressed, or hopeless?

Given its length, the PHQ-2 is a particularly good screening measure with 87% sensitivity and 78% specificity for a major depressive disorder and a sensitivity of 79% and a specificity of 86% for any depressive disorder (Lowe, Kroenke, & Grafe, 2005). For older adults, the PHQ-2 also demonstrated a high sensitivity of 100% and specificity of 77% for major depressive disorders (Li, Friedman, Conwell, & Fiscella, 2007). The PHQ-9 can be retrieved from http://www.depression-primarycare. org/clinicians/toolkits/materials/forms/phq9/.

Sleep, interest, guilt, energy, concentration, appetite, psychomotor retardation or agitation mnemonic. Even relatively brief measures can be administratively difficult to administer in fast-paced primary care environments. In addition to, or instead of, the PHQ-2, we suggest that you ask about mood and then incorporate the commonly used Sleep, Interest, Guilt, Energy, Concentration, Appetite, Psychomotor agitation or retardation, Suicidal ideation (SIGECAPS) mnemonic:

■ Mood.

> How would you describe your mood? Happy? Mad? Sad? Irritable? On a scale of negative 5 to positive 5, where nega-

tive 5 is the *most depressed or worst you can imagine yourself feeling* and positive 5 is the *happiest or best your could imagine yourself feeling,* with 0 right in between where you feel neither sad nor happy, how would you rate your mood on average? Right now? At its worst? At its best?

- Sleep. "Are you sleeping more? Less? Do you wake before your alarm?"
- Interest. "Do you have less interest in activities that you used to enjoy?"
- Guilt. "Do you have increased feelings of guilt? Worthlessness?"
- Energy. "Do you have less energy to do things that you want to do?"
- Concentration. "Do you have difficulty concentrating?"
- Appetite. "Has your appetite increased? Decreased? Has your weight changed?"
- Psychomotor retardation or agitation. "Do you feel slowed down or keyed up?"
- Suicidal ideation. "Do you think about hurting or killing yourself?"

Functional assessment. As with any functional assessment, it is important to determine the onset, duration, intensity, and frequency of the symptoms. We use targeted and more closed-ended questions than would be used in specialty mental health clinics. In Figure 2.3 of chapter 2, we presented specific questions you can ask during a functional assessment of depression. As in any situation, when you are screening for depressive symptoms it is important to be mindful of medical causes of depression such as endocrine disorders (e.g., hyper- and hypothyroidism, hyper- and hypoparathyroidism), infectious diseases (e.g., HIV, hepatitis, mononucleosis), nutritional deficits (e.g., vitamin B_{12} deficiencies), diseases of the central nervous system (e.g., stroke, traumatic brain injuries), or substance use (e.g., excessive caffeine use interfering with sleep, excessive alcohol, or hypnotic use).

Positive responses to any question related to depressive symptoms may result in further follow-up questions, but this is particularly the case if there are positive responses to questions about suicidal ideation. It is beyond the scope of this chapter to discuss fully how to manage the full range of suicidal ideation. Providers should establish policies and guidelines to help them determine whether someone should be managed in primary care, referred to specialty mental health care, or hospitalized. Rudd, Joiner, and Rajab (2001) provided an excellent overview of the assessment and treatment of suicidal ideation in tertiary care settings. As the authors pointed out, it is not possible to predict suicide but only to assess suicide risk in a "reasonable, reliable, consistent, and clinically useful manner" (p. 128). According to Rudd, Joiner, and Rajab, to assess risk it is important to determine

- a patient's predisposition to suicidal behavior (e.g., history of psychiatric diagnoses, suicidal behavior, abuse). "Have you thought about killing yourself? Have you been diagnosed with depression, anxiety, or any other behavioral health problems in the past? Do you have a history of emotional, physical, or sexual abuse?"
- current precipitants of the suicidal ideation (e.g., significant stressors, chronic health problems, family problems). "What started these suicidal thoughts? Are you experiencing any significant stressors, such as relationship, financial, or health problems?"
- affective symptoms (e.g., intensity and duration of depressive, anxiety, or anger symptoms). "Have you been feeling sad, down, or depressed? How about on edge or anxious? Have you felt angry or unusually irritable? How long have you been feeling this way?"
- hopelessness. "Are you feeling hopeless, as if things won't get better?"
- components of the suicidal thinking (e.g., current frequency, intensity, and duration of thoughts; specificity; access to method; intent).

  How often do you think about killing yourself—every day, once a week, once a month? How long do the thoughts last—a few seconds, minutes, hours, days? How would you kill yourself? Do you have access to those things that you would use to kill yourself? On a scale of 0 to 10 where 0 is *not likely at all* and 10 is *very likely,* how likely is it that you will kill yourself?

- previous suicidal behavior and preparatory behaviors (e.g., frequency of previous attempts, intent, outcome, opportunities for rescue, current writing of notes, getting finances in order).

> How many times have you tried to kill yourself in the past? Did you think that you would die? Did you think that someone would find you or help you before you died? Are you doing things now to get ready to kill yourself, such as writing a note, giving away meaningful items, trying to get things in order?

- impulsivity and self-control factors (e.g., perceived control, factors that may affect impulsivity).

> Do you feel out of control? Can you control your suicidal impulses? Have there been times when you have been out of control in the past? Do you drink alcohol or use any drugs? How often are you using those substances?

- protective factors (e.g., social support, problem-solving, coping, current treatment, hopefulness). "What has kept you from killing yourself? Who can you talk to about your problems? Have you told them how you are feeling?"

Rudd et al. (2001) suggested that the severity range of suicidality includes the following:

- Nonexistent. No suicidal ideation.
- Mild. Limited suicidal ideation, with no intent, few risk factors, and the presence of protective factors.
- Moderate. Frequent suicidal ideation, potentially some plans, but without intent; good self-control, limited emotional distress, some risk factors, some protective factors.
- Severe. Suicidal ideation is frequent, intense, and enduring. The patient may not endorse intent, but has indicated some preparatory behavior and/or access to the method. Multiple risk factors, few protective factors.
- Extreme. In addition to frequent, intense, and enduring suicidal ideation, there is a plan with intent, multiple risk factors, impaired impulse control, and no protective factors.

After assessing suicide risk, evaluate whether the severity of risk seems reasonable to manage in primary care, whether the individual should be managed in a specialty mental health setting, or whether he or she needs to be taken immediately to the emergency department. Although it is obvious that you would ask about suicidal ideation among individuals demonstrating depressive symptoms, it may also be important to assess for suicidal ideation among individuals with chronic medical conditions (e.g., chronic pain, coronary artery disease, cancer pulmonary disease) because these populations may be at increased risk of suicidal ideation and behaviors (e.g., Goodwin, Kroenke, Hoven, & Spitzer, 2003).

Advise. Following the functional assessment, and depending on the data you gathered, you might use the analogy of a spiral to describe to patients how removing activities from their lives and doing less can affect their mood and increase negative thinking. In turn, their negative mood and thoughts can contribute to doing still less, and hence they spiral in a downward direction. We show how this process works on the first page of the depression handout (see Figure 5.1). To begin to move upwards on this spiral, there are varieties of things they might consider, including (a) developing a plan for change, (b) pursuing specialty mental health care, (c) taking medications (i.e., antidepressants), and (d) doing nothing (i.e., keep doing what they are doing and evaluate whether their depressive symptoms improve).

We typically suggest that the interventions we offer would be a useful place to start as part of a stepped-care approach. If a patient has been started on an antidepressant, you can help the PCP by assessing adherence to the prescribed regimen and asking whether the patient has any concerns or questions about the use of the medication. For this reason, it is important to have an understanding of the most commonly prescribed antidepressants.

We recommend and refer patients to specialty mental health care providers when patients demonstrate complex depressive symptoms that are beyond the scope of management in a primary care setting (e.g., psychotic features, prolonged and severe symptoms, multiple failed treatments with

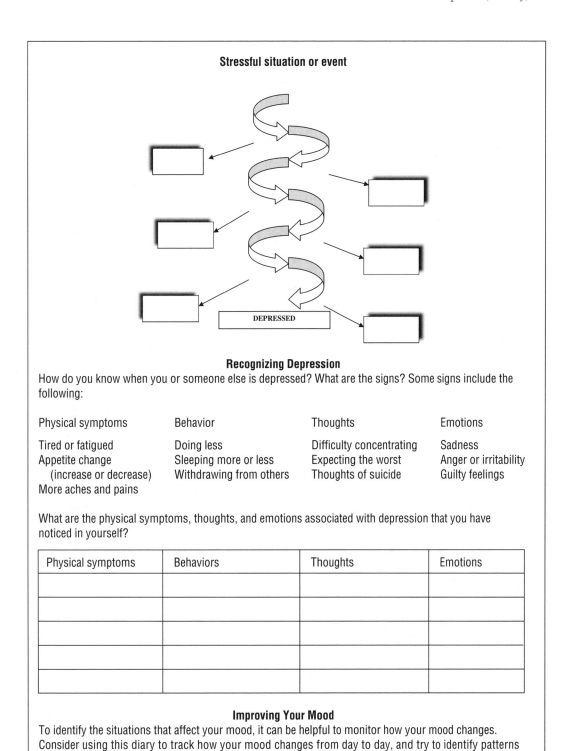

Stressful situation or event

DEPRESSED

Recognizing Depression

How do you know when you or someone else is depressed? What are the signs? Some signs include the following:

Physical symptoms	Behavior	Thoughts	Emotions
Tired or fatigued	Doing less	Difficulty concentrating	Sadness
Appetite change (increase or decrease)	Sleeping more or less	Expecting the worst	Anger or irritability
More aches and pains	Withdrawing from others	Thoughts of suicide	Guilty feelings

What are the physical symptoms, thoughts, and emotions associated with depression that you have noticed in yourself?

Physical symptoms	Behaviors	Thoughts	Emotions

Improving Your Mood

To identify the situations that affect your mood, it can be helpful to monitor how your mood changes. Consider using this diary to track how your mood changes from day to day, and try to identify patterns that occur.

FIGURE 5.1.   Depression spiral handout. (*Continued*)

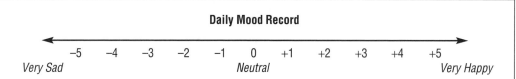

Daily Mood Record

| −5 | −4 | −3 | −2 | −1 | 0 | +1 | +2 | +3 | +4 | +5 |

Very Sad   Neutral   Very Happy

1. Using the scale above, rate your general level of sadness at the end of each day.
2. This rating is based on how you felt on average over the course of each day.
3. If you felt great, mark +5.
4. If you felt really bad (the worst you have ever felt or can imagine yourself feeling), mark −5.
5. If it was average, mark 0.

	Mon	Tues	Wed	Thurs	Fri	Sat	Sun	Average
Week 1								
Week 2								
Week 3								
Week 4								
Week 5								
Week 6								
Week 7								
Week 8								

Increasing Activities

When we perceive ourselves as overwhelmed or not feeling well, we often choose to avoid activities that we once enjoyed. However, by not spending time in those activities, we have fewer opportunities for enjoyment. One of the most important steps to help reduce depressive symptoms is to engage in potentially enjoyable or meaningful activities.

Setting Enjoyable and Meaningful Activities or Physical Activity Goals

- Is the goal realistic?
- Is a target date set for completion?
- Is the goal measurable?
- Is the goal broken down into small realistic parts?
- Once accomplished, what rewards will you use?
- Is the goal personally meaningful?
- Is a relapse plan clearly established?

An example of goal setting:

Week 1: Walk 8 minutes/day, 3 days/week   Week 6: Walk 16 minutes/day, 4 days/week
Week 2: Walk 10 minutes/day, 3 days/week   Week 7: Walk 16 minutes/day, 5 days/week
Week 3: Walk 12 minutes/day, 3 days/week   Week 8: Walk 18 minutes/day, 5 days/week
Week 4: Walk 12 minutes/day, 4 days/week   Week 9: Walk 20 minutes/day, 5 days/week
Week 5: Walk 14 minutes/day, 4 days/week   Week 10: Walk 20 minutes/day, 5 days/week

FIGURE 5.1.   *(Continued)* Depression spiral handout.

antidepressants) or when they exhibit significant suicidal thoughts (e.g., evidence of a plan or intent) that are difficult to adequately monitor in a primary care environment (e.g., weekly return appointments would be required over time).

When advising on a plan for change, describe what the option involves and how it will help target their specific problems. For instance,

> One of the things we might do is set a plan to increase the potentially enjoyable and valued activities in your life. You've noticed that as you've cut back or cut out these activities, your mood has gotten worse. The idea is, if you're not doing fun, enjoyable, and valued activities in your life, your life is not fun, enjoyable, or valuable. So this plan would be like the old Nike commercials where you "just do it." We could set a specific day, time, and plan for what you might add back into your life.

You could also say,

> Another thing we might do is help you get really good at questioning the depressive thoughts you have. Your mind will tell you things that are not true, not helpful, and inconsistent with your values. You can't stop your mind from telling you things, but you can get really good at questioning those thoughts and developing new ways of thinking that can decrease depressed mood and make it easier for you to live your life in a way that is consistent with your values.

Agree.   It is important for patients to agree to do something before you try to start an intervention, even if that something is just doing a little more than what they are currently doing. If they seem unwilling to try any of the options, then you might ask them whether they have additional ideas on how you might assist them. Another option is to have a follow-up appointment to discuss the options further. The follow-up appointment itself may start to help decrease depressed mood as a result of the increased social activities with you and others in the clinic, and thus may make it easier for the patient to choose a viable evidence-based plan.

Assist.   We use a handout such as the one in Figure 5.1 to introduce evidence-based components of cognitive and behavioral interventions, including behavioral activation, cognitive disputation, and problem-solving for intervening with depressed mood.

Behavioral activation.   Our experiences suggest that one of the easiest and most effective initial interventions is behavioral activation (Cuijpers, van Straten, & Warmerdam, 2007). The functional assessment usually identifies activities patients have decreased or stopped. We use the depression handout (see Figure 5.1) to help patients recognize the symptoms of depression, get them started with monitoring their mood, and start them on a behavioral activation plan with realistic goals. We suggest starting with a plan to add these activities back into their daily or weekly schedule. Set specific goals, including time, place, duration, and frequency (see chap. 3, this volume, for specifics on goal setting). The activities might involve little effort and represent doing just a little more than they do currently. For example you might say, "You mentioned that you used to go out with your friends once a week. Would it be realistic for you to plan an outing with your friends at least once between now and the next time we meet?" An even more simple change plan might be to say, "You indicated that you used to walk your dog in the neighborhood for 20 minutes a day. Would it be realistic for you to start to do that again?"

We use the goal setting sheets in the handout in Figure 5.1 to develop a plan for how patients will begin their behavioral activation plan. As part of behavioral activation, we encourage individuals to increase physical activity or exercise because exercise has been shown to be a valuable antidepressant interventions (Stathopoulou, Powers, Berry, Smits, & Otto, 2006). Again, it is important for the goal to be specific and realistic for the patient. For individuals who have not exercised in the past, we often start with a simple walking program, whereas for those individuals who have exercised regularly in the past, we build on what they used to do.

Cognitive disputation. In addition to behavioral activation, we discuss methods for changing the way patients think. We may use cognitive restructuring techniques or acceptance and commitment therapy (ACT) techniques (Zettle, 2004) that have been shown to be effective for improving functioning. Rather than focusing on trying to change or control negative or depressive thinking, ACT interventions use the premise that people cannot control or stop their negative thinking. Instead, ACT encourages patients to allow thoughts and emotions to happen and to focus on making changes in areas of their life that they can control. (Hayes & Strosahl, 2004; Hayes, Strosahl, & Wilson, 1999). In chapter 3 (see Figure 3.3, chap. 3, this volume), we discussed how we use two levels of cognitive disputation, which can target the negative and alarming thinking associated with depressive symptoms. Identifying thoughts that are inconsistent with how individuals want to live their life, and either changing those thoughts or living with them, can be an important component of improving functioning in individuals demonstrating depressive symptoms. We often encourage patients to write down the three or four questions that seem most applicable to them on a note card to help them remember the questions. We focus on the demands that patients place on themselves and discuss issues related to what they can and cannot control (see chap. 3, this volume, for additional information).

Problem Solving. Problem solving is another skill we discuss with patients to help them to effectively manage their depressive symptoms. Using the outline we presented in chapter 3, we take time with the patient to identify a problem they are struggling with, and then brainstorm on solutions, evaluate those solutions, help them to choose the best ones to try, and then discuss how to evaluate the outcome and decide whether they will need to try another possible solution. Often, problem solving involves engaging in an activity and can become a part of the behavioral activation plan.

Arrange. Follow-up appointments can vary greatly between individuals. Some return after the initial appointment, having successfully increased their participation in activities, exceeding their goals and appearing to demonstrate significantly improved functioning and mood. However, some individuals may return for two or three appointments and will not have changed their thinking or behaviors; you might consider recommending these individuals for specialty mental health treatment if obvious barriers cannot be overcome. For individuals demonstrating suicidal thoughts, the BHC should consider frequent appointments, or even multiple appointments in the same week to monitor whether the intensity and frequency of the thoughts change over time. Feedback should always be provided to the PCP about the plan for managing the depressive symptoms and existing suicidal thoughts.

ANXIETY DISORDERS

An estimated 20% of the patients in primary care clinics meet the criteria for one of the following: generalized anxiety disorder (GAD), panic disorder, social anxiety disorder, or posttraumatic stress disorder (PTSD; Kroenke, Spitzer, Williams, Monahan, & Löwe, 2007; Nisenson et al., 1998). One study found that patients who were eventually diagnosed with these disorders had been seen in primary and specialty care clinics an average of six times before being identified as having an anxiety disorder (Deacon, Lickel, & Abramowitz, 2008). In addition, anxiety disorders have been associated with the occurance of multiple medical problems including irritable bowel syndrome, asthma, cardiovascular disease, and chronic pain (Roy-Byrne et al., 2008). In this section, we discuss methods for managing GAD, panic disorder, and PTSD.

GENERALIZED ANXIETY DISORDER

According to *DSM–IV–TR* criteria (APA, 2000, p. 476), GAD is associated with difficult-to-control excessive anxiety and worry, with symptoms of restlessness, fatigue, difficulty concentrating, irritability, muscle tension, and/or disturbances of sleep. The source of the worry cannot involve features of other

Axis I disorders (e.g., embarrassment in public [social phobia], fear of contamination [obsessive–compulsive disorder], the patient's belief that he or she has multiple health problems [hypochondriasis]). Twelve-month prevalence rates of GAD were found to be 3.1% among a U.S. population (Kessler et al., 2005).

Specialty Mental Health

In systematic reviews of the literature, cognitive–behavioral therapy has been shown to be effective for treating GAD in the short term (Hunot, Churchill, Teixeira, & Silva de Lima, 2007). Cognitive–behavioral treatments for GAD focus on reducing physiological symptoms using relaxation training (e.g., progressive muscle relaxation), changing anxious and worried thinking, behaviorally reducing avoidance of feared situations, and improving problem-solving and time management skills (Brown, O'Leary, & Barlow, 2001).

Behavioral Health in Primary Care

Preliminary findings by Stanley et al. (2003), who implemented a treatment program for GAD among older adults in primary care, support the use of cognitive–behavioral interventions. However, Stanley's program is more similar to a co-located model of treatment (i.e., it uses eight sessions) than to an integrated model using time-limited

interventions. Some data have suggested that GAD symptoms have improved using self-help or physician-guided evidence-based interventions (van Boeijen et al., 2005).

Primary Care Adaptation

Assess. To begin screening for GAD, you can simply ask individuals, "Do you worry most days? Is it difficult to control your worry? How does worry affect your life?"

Generalized anxiety disorder-7. A screening measure such as the Generalized Anxiety Disorder-7 (GAD-7), with a cutoff score of 10, has good specificity (82%) and good sensitivity (89%) for screening for GAD (Spitzer, Kroenke, Williams, & Löwe, 2006). A slightly lower cutoff score of 8 on the GAD-7 provides a specificity of 82% and a sensitivity of 77% for identifying individuals with any anxiety disorder (Kroenke et al., 2007). The even shorter GAD-2, with a cutoff score of 3, may be a useful screening measure for identifying individuals who would benefit from additional assessments for GAD (specificity, 83%; sensitivity, 86%) and other anxiety disorders (specificity, 88%; sensitivity, 65%; Kroenke et al., 2007).

Functional assessment. We suggest using a screening mnemonic such as AND I C REST, proposed by Seitz (2005), which we present in Table 5.1, to help guide the functional assessment of worry symptoms.

TABLE 5.1

Mnemonic to Screen for Generalized Anxiety Disorder

Letter	DSM–IV–TR symptoms	Screening question
A	**A**nxious, nervous, or worried	Do you feel anxious, nervous, or worried most of the time?
N	**N**o control over worry	Is it difficult to control the worry?
D	**D**uration of 6 months	How long has worrying been a problem?
I	**I**rritability	Are you more irritable, or do you get frustrated more easily than usual?
C	**C**oncentration impairment	Do you have difficulty concentrating?
R	**R**estlessness	Are you restless, fidgety, or feel like you can't sit still?
E	**E**nergy decreased	Do you feel tired more than you used to?
S	**S**leep impairment	Do you have difficulty falling or staying asleep?
T	**T**ension in muscles	Do your muscles feel tense?

Note. From "Screening Mnemonic for Generalized Anxiety Disorder," by D. P. Seitz, 2005, *Canadian Family Physician, 51,* pp. 1340–1342. Copyright 2005 by Canadian Family Physician. Reprinted with permission.

Advise. GAD is generally treatable by cognitive and behavioral interventions, although in the primary care setting it is common to see individuals who have been prescribed anxiolytics to help manage symptoms. When physicians know that they can easily help their patients access alternative evidence-based strategies, they may be more likely to try those interventions before starting medication. Nonetheless, it is important to be familiar with the medications often prescribed for anxiety disorders. Medications that have been shown to be effective for GAD include selective serotonin reuptake inhibitors (SSRIs; e.g., paroxetine), benzodiazepines, serotonin–norepinephrine reuptake inhibitors (SNRIs; e.g., venlafaxine), and antihistamines (e.g., hydroxyzine; McIntosh et al., 2004).

When introducing cognitive and behavioral interventions, it is important to discuss what changes patients will be asked to make and how those changes will help them manage symptoms and function more effectively. For example, you might say the following:

> The interventions that I can discuss with you are skill-based, that is, they require practice to be effective. The interventions are intended to help you change the way that you think and what you do to help you become distressed less often. Research has demonstrated that these interventions help the majority of individuals who have difficulty managing their worry.

If the individual is taking an anxiolytic, you could say, "Changing your thoughts and what you do may help you reduce your need for taking medications, if that is something you and your medical provider are interested in accomplishing."

Agree. To effectively target worrying, patients must be willing to consider methods of accepting and managing their thinking. Relaxation exercises may help to reduce the physiological effects of worried thinking; however, without thinking differently about their worries, relaxation will likely not be sufficient to have an impact on the frequency, duration, and intensity of those worries. We suggest you carefully explain that the goal is not to eliminate anxiety or worry; instead, the goal is to reduce anxiety and worry to a level that does not interfere with functioning. Therefore, a key aspect of targeting worried thinking is to discuss with patients possible methods of managing their worries and eliting a willingness from patients to pursue those changes. For example, you might say the following:

> It sounds as if you spend a significant amount of your time worrying about things that you have very little control over. To reduce your worrying, we can discuss several methods, such as writing your worries down, which can help reduce the frequency, duration, and intensity of your worrying. However, these techniques won't eliminate all of your worries. Worrying is a normal part of human existence, and it would be unrealistic to totally eliminate worries. Nevertheless, the techniques that we'll discuss require practice for them to work. Are you willing to use and practice these techniques with the goal of reducing your worrying?

As part of the agree phase, you are beginning to educate patients and lead them into the assist phase.

Assist. Once a patient demonstrates a willingness to engage in an intervention for worrying, we always spend some time normalizing the behavior and educating him or her about the factors involved in worrying. We use handouts, such as the one provided in Figure 5.2, to guide patients through understanding worry, overcoming barriers associated with changing worry behavior, and interventions that can help reduce worry. We take time to discuss the effects of worry, and help them distinguish between helpful worry and anxiety, and how the intensity of worry symptoms may interfere with their functioning. We also highlight how thinking can interfere with attempts to change their responses to anxiety.

We also suggest the use of a worry log, such as the one in Figure 5.3, as an effective way to manage worry. The goal of a worry log is to decrease overall daily worry by creating a specific place and time the individual can engage in worry. The

Common Symptoms of Anxious Worry

Anxiety is a normal human emotion that is experienced by everyone at one point or another. Anxiety is an adaptive function that motivates us to correct or flee situations that may be stressful or hazardous. Because of anxiety's protective factor, the body is designed to experience this emotion. The body is also designed to counteract this response in time, once the danger is over.

These are some signs that worrying may be a problem for you:

- Worrying more often than not for at least 6 months
- Difficulty falling or staying sleep
- Worrying that interferes with some aspect of your life
- Chronic muscle tension
- Feeling restless, on edge, or "keyed up"
- Feeling irritated
- Easily fatigued
- Difficulty controlling your worries
- Difficulty concentrating, mind going blank

Is Worrying Bad?

The anxiety associated with worry can be helpful. We can be motivated by worry. If we have deadlines or goals that we want to meet, anxiety can be useful. However, once anxiety gets too extreme, our performance can begin to decline; therefore, the goal is to keep worrying and anxiety within a healthy range.

Barriers to Treatment

Sometimes the way we think can affect whether we can change our worry. The following are some examples of worried thoughts.

"My worries are perfectly justified because of all the stress in my life. Since the stress will never go away, I will never stop worrying."

No one could realistically guarantee that all the stress in your life could be removed. Nevertheless, you can change the way that you interpret and deal with the events in your life. It is a fact that some worry is justified. However, individuals experiencing difficulties with anxious worry often overestimate the amount of justifiable worry in their lives, and stand to gain from skills aimed at improving this judgment.

"Worrying about things is how I prepare. If I don't worry, how I will handle different situations beforehand? I won't be prepared when situations arise, and I'll be overwhelmed."

For those with anxiety, worrying does serve a purpose. It can serve as a form of avoidance for the worrier because of the distraction it provides. For others, worrying is a coping strategy, a form of busywork that provides the worrier with a small degree of control over the situation. You've probably had some experience with successfully handling one or two of these unexpected crises, even though you had no time to worry about it beforehand. Treatment for anxiety replaces worry with more adaptive ways of coping.

"My life is so stressful. I don't have time to relax."

When crises arise, we often sacrifice personal time to meet deadlines. For individuals with chronic anxiety who spend most of their time worrying, even small breaks for relaxation can be beneficial. Most people can find 15 minutes a day to devote to relaxation.

"I'm afraid to focus on my anxiety because I think it might be a sign that I'm going crazy."

People experiencing difficulty with anxious worry often report that it is difficult to stop worrying once they get started. This perceived loss of control is very disturbing. However, difficulty controlling anxious thoughts or feelings is different from an inability to control one's behavior or perceptions of reality. People who experience anxiety disorders do not develop the various thought disorders that people often think of when they describe "going crazy."

FIGURE 5.2.   Common symptoms of anxious worry handout.

Worry Management

The following strategies may be used to deal with your worries when you feel that they are becoming over-whelming.

1. **Worry Place and Time.** Set a 30-minute worry period that will take place at the same time and same place each day. Your worry place and time will be:

   _____

2. **Delay Worry.** If you notice you are worrying outside of your scheduled worry time, tell yourself, "I have plenty of time to focus on this later. Right now I'm just going to be in the moment and notice what I'm doing, what others are doing, the environment, and other things I see, hear, or smell."
3. **Worry Log.** Record all your worries during your worry time on the Worry Log on the following page and then take time to categorize these worries. You can choose categories that are helpful for you. You might organize them by "Big Concerns," "Medium Concerns," and "Small Concerns." Another option would be to categorize them by content area, such as "Work Concerns," "Family Concerns," "Financial Concerns," and "Relationship Concerns." Any means of categorizing can be used; however, it is important not to use too many categories; usually between three and seven work best.

   In the next column of your worry log, you can write how you will manage the problem. If the problem is something you have absolutely no control over, you might write down, "I'm not going to worry about this problem because there is nothing I can do about it right now."

Worry Log

Worrisome thought	Category	Management strategy

FIGURE 5.3. Worry management handout.

specific day and time become the cue to worry, whereas other cues to worry throughout the day become less powerful and fade as worry initiators (Borkovec, Wilkinson, Folensbee, & Lerman, 1983). We ask patients to list their worries, to categorize them, and then to think of solutions, if any exist. It can be helpful to get a baseline assessment of the amount of time and average intensity of worry before engaging in this intervention so

changes can be tracked as the patient implements worry management strategies.

As a primary worry management strategy, patients are encouraged to have a 30-minute worry period that occurs at the same place and time each day. They are asked to write out their worries during this time, identifying data to support or not support the worries. Worry outside of this period is delayed, and the individual is asked to instead focus on the present moment, on what they are doing, what others are doing, the environment, what they see, and what they hear.

In addition to methods for addressing cognitive changes, we may also teach relaxation methods (e.g., relaxed breathing) and ways to reduce alarming thinking (see chap. 3, this volume) to help lower sympathetic arousal and alarming thinking associated with worrying.

Arrange.   Often patients who adopt new patterns of thinking will quickly notice decreases in their worrying. Follow-up appointments may focus on teaching new skills or overcoming barriers associated with modifying thinking habits. For those individuals who demonstrate difficulty in making changes in their thinking or behaviors, specialty mental health may be useful for providing a more intensive treatment for worrying.

PANIC DISORDER

DSM–IV–TR (APA, 2000, p. 440) criteria for panic disorder includes recurrent panic attacks (i.e., approximately 10 minutes of intense fear or discomfort with multiple physical or cognitive symptoms, such as heart racing, sweating, nausea fear of death, fear of losing control) associated with concern about having attacks in the future, worry about the implication or consequences of the attack, or significant behavior changes caused by the attacks. Panic disorder may or may not be associated with agoraphobia (i.e., anxiety about places or situations that may be difficult or embarrassing to escape; those situations are avoided or are associated with marked distress or anxiety). Lifetime prevalence data suggest that panic disorder affects approximately 4.8% of the population; 23.5% experience isolated panic, without panic disorder (Kessler et al., 2006). Patients demonstrating panic disorder have higher rates of utilization of medical services compared with individuals with other anxiety disorders (Deacon et al., 2008).

Specialty Mental Health

Behavioral and cognitive–behavioral therapies have been found to be effective treatments for panic disorder either alone or combined with pharmacother-

apy (Furukawa, Watanabe, & Churchill, 2007). Interventions for panic disorder typically incorporate relaxation techniques, in vivo and imaginal exposure, breathing retraining, and cognitive restructuring. Similar to those of GAD, panic symptoms have been improved through the use of self-help or physician-guided, evidence-based interventions (van Boeijen et al., 2005).

Behavioral Health in Primary Care

Some data have shown that cognitive and behavioral interventions delivered by BHCs in primary care can be effective (Roy-Byrne et al., 2005). Evidence-based treatment guidelines recommend the use of cognitive and behavioral interventions, as well as SSRIs for the treatment of panic disorder in primary care (McIntosh et al., 2004).

Primary Care Adaptation

The 5A's help to guide BHCs through the process of assessing and treating panic disorder in primary care.

Assess.   To screen for panic disorder you can ask targeted questions about experiences with panic related symptoms, as follows:

- "Have you ever had an episode when you suddenly felt your heart racing, had difficulty breathing, started feeling shaky or dizzy, and/or you were worried that you might die, suffocate, or something bad would happen?"
- "How long did that episode last? How many experiences have you had like that?"
- "Are you worried that it would happen again? Did you change what you did because you were concerned about the attacks?"
- "Have you avoided places that might be difficult to get out of or might be embarrassing if you had one of these attacks?"
- "What do you do to avoid having an attack? Have you avoided driving? Going to the store? Going to social gatherings?"

The goal of the questioning is to determine whether the individual experienced a panic attack and how they changed their behavior in response to concerns about the attacks. The GAD-7 and

GAD-2 may be helpful as screening tools for panic disorder. Similarly, the Autonomic Nervous System Questionnaire (ANS) is a 5-item measure, in which positive responses to either of the first 2 items are used to identify individuals who may meet criteria for panic disorder. Although the ANS is highly sensitive (95%–100%), its low specificity (25%–59%) may result in an unacceptably high number of false positives (Stein et al., 1999).

Advise. Once our functional assessment has identified a patient with panic disorder, we discuss the various treatment options. Patients diagnosed with panic disorder commonly use medications to manage their symptoms. Medication recommendations for panic disorder include SSRIs or possibly imipramine or clomipramine; however, benzodiazepines are not recommended (McIntosh et al., 2004). We discuss with patients the importance of education and the possibility of using cognitive and behavioral techniques to manage their anxiety symptoms. We tell them that these techniques have been shown to be superior for long-term treatment of panic symptoms. This is often a good time to use some of the motivational enhancement techniques that we reviewed in chapter 3. Thus, you could say the following:

> It sounds as if you have used medications to manage the uncomfortable symptoms of your anxiety. I'm wondering whether it would be beneficial for you to learn other ways to manage this anxiety so that you didn't need to use the medication as often. We know that, over the long term, these techniques can be as, or more, effective interventions for panic symptoms. What would be the benefits of changing? What would be the risks?

Agree. As with depressive symptoms, it is necessary to assess what the patient is willing to attempt regarding change. Cognitive and behavioral interventions often involve a willingness to tolerate the uncomfortable physiological symptoms that occur with anxious thinking. Relaxation techniques can reduce the intensity of these symptoms, but the patient must be willing to think about his or her

exaggerated physiological symptoms in a different way and be willing to implement and practice a new set of skills for managing these symptoms. Review the options for treatment (e.g., continue taking medication, learn cognitive and behavioral techniques, do nothing), and ask the patient what he or she wants to pursue.

Assist. We have included a patient handout in Figure 5.4 that guides the patient through the interventions for panic disorder. In general, we educate the patient about panic, teach ways to manage their alarming thoughts, and may teach relaxation and ways to decrease behavioral avoidance.

Education. To decrease symptoms associated with panic disorder, we start by educating patients about panic attacks and discussing how these attacks are due to exaggerated sympathetic responses, which are usually helpful for managing stressful situations. It is often important to draw on the fact that the medical provider has ruled out any serious medical problems. Thus, we might say the following:

> Your doctor has ruled out any significant medical problems at this point, so we think that the physical symptoms you are experiencing are related to what we call the fight or flight response, a reflex that helps all of us to react to potentially dangerous situations. This response does everything possible to allow us to respond as quickly as possible to these situations, including increasing our heart rate, tightening our muscles, and slowing down our digestive system, so that we can fight or flee from something that is potentially dangerous. In individuals who have panic attacks, this system seems to activate for no reason, and people notice an intense unexpected physiological response. The symptoms can feel as if they are life-threatening, and all you want is for those symptoms to stop.

Changing thoughts. We then focus on discussing how thoughts and fears associated with these responses, as well as attempts to avoid panic-related

Panic Disorder Handout

What Is a Panic Attack?

Sometimes we experience a sudden and severe onset of symptoms that can be scary. These symptoms can include some or all of the following:

- Pounding heart or increased heart rate
- Sweating
- Nausea
- Trembling or shaking
- Shortness of breath
- Feeling of choking
- Chest pain

- Feeling dizzy, unsteady, lightheaded, or faint
- Feelings of unreality or being detached from yourself
- Fear of losing control or going crazy
- Fear of dying
- Numbness or tingling
- Chills or hot flashes

Although we don't fully understand why some people experience panic attacks and other people don't, we do know that these symptoms are related to a very normal response called the *fight-flight response*. This response allows our body to react quickly when we think that something is dangerous, such as being attacked or being cut off when we are driving.

How Panic Attacks Affect Our Lives

Because symptoms of a panic attack occur out of the blue, we can become worried about them, and we may begin to avoid situations that we think will result in these panic symptoms, such as crowded stores, public transportation, or driving. What situations have you avoided because of panic attacks?

_____

_____

Changing Thinking Patterns

One of the most important changes associated with decreasing panic attacks is changing how we think. The fear associated with having a panic attack may increase the likelihood of having an attack. Therefore, a willingness to experience a panic attack, knowing that the symptoms, although uncomfortable, will not harm you, is an important aspect of managing the symptoms of panic.

Thinking that increases panic	Thinking that decreases panic
I'm having a heart attack!	This is not an emergency.
I'm going to die.	This doesn't feel good, but it won't hurt me.
I can't stand this.	I can feel uncomfortable and still be OK.
I have to get out of here.	This will go away with time.
Oh no, here it comes!	I can handle this.

What are the things that you say to yourself that may increase panic symptoms?

_____

_____

What could you say to decrease panic symptoms?

_____

_____

Breathing Retraining

People who have panic attacks show some signs of hyperventilation or overbreathing. When people hyperventilate, certain blood vessels in the body become narrower, which can contribute to numbness or tingling in the hands or feet or the sensation of cold, clammy hands, and increased heart rate. You can help overcome overbreathing by learning breathing control.

FIGURE 5.4.   Panic disorder handout. *(Continued)*

Instructions for Breathing Retraining
1. Choose a comfortable quiet location.
2. Count, "One," on the first breath in, and think, "Relax," on the breath out.
3. Focus your attention on breathing and counting.
4. Maintain a normal rate and depth of breathing.
5. Expand your abdomen on the breath in and keep your chest still.
6. Continue counting up to 10 and back to 1.
7. Practice two times per day, for 10 minutes each time.

Decreasing Avoidance
Regardless of whether you can identify why you began having panic attacks or whether they seemed to come out of the blue, the places where you began having panic attacks often can become triggers themselves.

To break the cycle of avoidance, it is important to first identify the places or situations that are being avoided and then to do some "relearning." Just as the negative experience of a panic attack can result in learning to avoid certain locations, having positive, successful experiences can result in learning that the location is nothing to be afraid of.

Which item on your list of avoided locations or situations would you like to target first?
Please list this situation here: _____

Now, you can develop a hierarchy for this situation or location. A hierarchy is a list of situations that result in increasingly higher intensities of anxiety. Develop a list of situations that result in a range of anxiety intensities, that is, some result in low intensity and others result in higher intensities. Then rank order the situation from the lowest to the highest anxiety producing situations. This hierarchy will help guide you as you gradually begin to "expose" yourself to the situation or location that you have been avoiding.

FIGURE 5.4. *(Continued)* Panic disorder handout.

symptoms, can increase the intensity and frequency of these symptoms. This component, which is more like traditional cognitive therapy, is geared toward helping the patient identify faulty ways of thinking (see "Cognitive Disputation" in chap. 3, this volume, for further details). We also incorporate simple analogies used with ACT, such as the Chinese finger trap (Hayes et al., 1999, pp. 104–105), to help illustrate this point. Therefore, we might say the following:

When we experience these physical symptoms, often our first instinct is to want them to go away. Sometimes we may leave the situation, we may try to gain control of our breathing, we may try to distract ourselves, but if the symptoms don't go away, we get more worried. Sometimes our attempts to control these symptoms may make the symptoms worse. For example, have you ever played with Chinese finger cuffs? [Explain that you put one finger of each hand into each end of a woven tube-like device; when you try to quickly pull your fingers out of it, the tube holds your fingers in place.] If you try to quickly pull your fingers out of the finger cuff, the cuff gets tighter. Panic symptoms can be very similar to that finger cuff; the harder we try to control the symptoms, the "tighter" or the more intense the symptoms can become. So instead of trying to make the symptoms go away, maybe it would be possible to let the symptoms occur, and relax our fingers in the cuff, knowing that, in time, the symptoms will go away.

Relaxation training. We may teach relaxation methods, such as controlled breathing, to help manage hyperventilation or over-breathing, which is experienced by some patients with panic disorder. Such breathing strategies provide a way for the patient to cope with a panic attack when it occurs.

Decreasing behavioral avoidance with exposure. Detailed explanations for behavioral exposure treatments are explained in many publications (e.g., Richard & Lauterbach, 2007; Rosqvist, 2005). Readers should consult these or other information sources, as needed, for details about these procedures. The goals of exposure are to decrease general fear, avoidance, and safety behaviors.

Situational exposure is being in or around an object, person, or place that is harmless but produces fear. It is used to desensitize the patient to people, places, and objects the patient avoids because of fear. The goal is to test the patient's belief and to decrease anxiety associated with the avoided people, places, or objects. Have the patient complete the Situational Exposure Hierarchy in Figure 5.5 on his or her own. At a follow-up consult, discuss specifics and devise a plan to go through the hierarchy and set times for exposure.

Interoceptive exposure involves exercises that produce a physical symptom (e.g., breathing through a straw for 2 minutes to produce a rapid heartbeat and short shallow breaths). Interoceptive exposure can be done in a 30-minute appointment in much the same way as in a specialty mental health appointment. This exercise should be geared toward the feared body sensations. The goal is to help the patient learn that his or her feared prediction about what might happen is not true and to desensitize them to these sensations (see Figure 5.5 for patient handouts).

Arrange. Many individuals treated with brief interventions for panic disorder improve quickly. If significant improvement is not seen in a short period, or if there are comorbid disorders (e.g., substance abuse) that significantly complicate the treatment of the anxiety disorder, then consider a referral to specialty mental health care. If possible, the specialty mental health provider should be trained in cognitive and behavioral interventions for panic disorder, as evidence-based guidelines suggest that there is insufficient evidence to support the use of many other treatments (e.g., hypnosis, interpersonal therapy, psychoanalysis; McIntosh et al., 2004).

POSTTRAUMATIC STRESS DISORDER

The *DSM–IV–TR* (APA, 2000) diagnosis of PTSD is dependent on: (a) Exposure to a traumatic event, involving actual or threatened death, serious injury, or a threat to the physical integrity of others; (b) the reexperiencing of the event (e.g., recurrent thoughts, images, perceptions); (c) avoidance of stimuli associated with the traumatic event; and (d) persistent symptoms of arousal. The symptoms (b), (c), and (d) must last longer than 1 month. Although over half of men and women report at least one traumatic event, there is a lifetime prevalence of PTSD in 10.4% of women and 5.0% of men (Kessler, Sonnega, Bromet, Hughes, & Nelson, 1995). The traumas most commonly associated with PTSD were combat exposure for men, rape and sexual molestation for women (Kessler et al., 1995).

Specialty Mental Health

Traditionally, in outpatient mental health settings, stress inoculation training, exposure techniques, and cognitive processing therapy have been the primary modes of treatment. According to a systematic review of the literature, trauma-focused cognitive–behavioral therapies significantly reduce trauma-related symptoms (Bisson & Andrew, 2005). Most patients with PTSD, who are treated with psychotherapy recover or improve (Bradley, Greene, Russ, Dutra, & Westen, 2005). Trauma-focused cognitive–behavioral therapy has the largest empirical database supporting its use for the treatment of PTSD (NICE, 2005); however, these interventions have not been tested in the primary care environment. In primary care settings, physicians are encouraged to consider pharmacotherapy and referrals for psychotherapy to treat PTSD (Bobo, Warner, & Warner, 2007). Currently, there are no data supporting the use of brief therapies that could be implemented in primary care settings for the successful treatment of PTSD.

Adaptations for Primary Care

Although the literature does not give specifics on how to best manage PTSD in primary care, use of the 5A's can help you efficiently integrate evidence-based care in an effective manner.

Situational Exposure Hierarchy

Example: Fear of driving	Your fear: _____
List situations from least to most anxiety provoking.	List situations from least to most anxiety provoking.
1. Visualizing driving to store	1.
2. Sitting in car in the driveway, with car off	2.
3. Sitting in car in driveway, with car idling	3.
4. Driving to end of driveway and back	4.
5. Driving to end of street and back	5.
6. Driving from driveway to main street and back	6.
7. Driving car from house to store	7.

Situational Exposure Rating Form

Date	Number of times practiced	Exposure situation	Maximum anxiety (0–10)*

*0 = *no anxiety*; 10 = *severe anxiety*.

Interoceptive Exposure
Activities that can produce feared body sensations

Activity	Physical sensation
Holding breath as long as you can	Tight chest, breathlessness
Overbreathing: take short shallow breaths with chest going out for 60 seconds	Numbness, racing heart, tingling fingers
Spinning in a chair for 90 seconds	Dizziness, nausea
Breathing through a straw for 2 minutes	Increased heart rate, breathlessness
Shaking head from side-to-side for 30 seconds	Blurred vision, dizziness
Tensing all muscles while sitting in a chair for 60 seconds	Trembling, shakiness
Swallowing six times quickly	Sore, uncomfortable throat
Clear throat six times quickly	Sore, uncomfortable throat
Jog in place for 3 minutes	Racing heart, tight chest

FIGURE 5.5. Situational exposure hierarchy handout. (*Continued*)

Feared Physical Sensation Exercise

Physical activity	Feared prediction or belief about the physical sensations of the activity	Alternative or rational prediction or belief about the sensations of the activity	Physical sensations produced by the activity	How similar were the sensations to what you experience naturally? 0–10*	Anxiety in response to the sensations 0–10**

*0 = *not at all;* 10 = *severe.* **0 = *none;* 10 = *severe.*

FIGURE 5.5.   *(Continued)* Situational exposure hierarchy handout.

Assess.   The need for improved identification of PTSD in primary care has been discussed repeatedly (e.g., NICE, 2005; Wilson, 2007). Particularly with individuals who demonstrate affective distress, it is important to ask about exposure to traumatic events and to provide possible examples, such as, assault, rape, motor vehicle accidents, and childhood abuse (NICE, 2005). In the majority of individuals diagnosed with PTSD, there are comorbid conditions, such as depression, other anxiety disorders, or substance abuse (Kessler et al., 1995). Most individuals demonstrate PTSD symptoms within the 1st month of the traumatic event; however, some individuals (15%) may not demonstrate symptoms of PTSD for years after the event (McNally, 2003).

The mnemonic DREAMS (Detachment, Reexperiencing, Event had emotional effects, Avoidance, Month in duration, Sympathetic hyperactivity or hypervigilance) has been suggested as one way to help guide the screening of individuals who report an exposure to a traumatic incident (Lange, Lange, & Cabaltica, 2000).

The PTSD checklist (PCL; Blanchard, Jones-Alexander, Buckley, & Forneris, 1996) has been widely used to screen for PTSD; however, there are multiple forms of the PCL (i.e., civilian, military, specific trauma), and there is debate about the most appropriate cutoff score (e.g., Blanchard et al., 1996; Cook, Elhai, & Areán, 2005; Lang, Laffaye, Satz, Dresselhaus, & Stein, 2003; Yeager, Magruder, Knapp, Nicholas, & Frueh, 2007). NICE (2005) recommended the use of the Impact of Event Scale (IES; Horowitz, Wilner, & Alvarez, 1979); Startle, Physiological arousal, Anger, and Numbness (SPAN; Meltzer-Brody, Churchill, & Davidson, 1999); and the Trauma Screening Questionnaire (TSQ; Berwin et al., 2002). The IES, which was revised in 1997 (Weiss & Marmar, 1997) to be consistent with the *Diagnostic and Statistical Manual of Mental Disorders, Fourth Edition* (APA, 1994), is long at 22 items and can be challenging to score (e.g., one must add responses to items that are not next to each other on the measure); therefore, we do not recommend it as a primary screening measure. On the SPAN, a cutoff score of 5 provides a sensitivity of 84% and a specificity of 91% for PTSD (Yeager et al., 2007), whereas using a cutoff score of 6 on the TSQ yielded between 76% to 86% sensitivity and between 89% to 97% specificity (Brewin et al., 2002; Walters, Bisson, & Shepherd, 2007). In addition to these measures, the Primary Care PTSD Screen (PC-PTSD) may be a useful screening measure for PTSD, as it has been shown to have good test–retest reliability ($r = .84$) and optimal sensitivity and specificity (87%; Prins et al., 2003).The PC-PTSD is available in Figure 5.6, the TSQ can be obtained from the author and the original article (Brewin et al., 2002), and the SPAN can be obtained from Multi-Health Systems, Inc.

Advise.   In primary care settings, SSRIs will likely be a first line of treatment for the symptoms of PTSD, given the systematic review evidence supporting their use (Stein, Ipser, & Seedat, 2006). As

with depression, it is important to advise patients to use the medication as prescribed. In addition to medications, it is often necessary to recommend psychotherapy. A BHC can play a vital role in discussing what psychotherapy might involve and in advising the patient about the importance of pursuing treatment and the likelihood of improvement.

Agree.   The BHC can help the medical team by establishing a plan of treatment, even if it is a wait-and-see approach, as well as by maintaining appropriate medication use and/or pursuing psychotherapy. The BHC may also contribute by developing a treatment plan that the patient agrees to and by helping the patient to identify situations that may indicate that the treatment is not working. The BHC might say the following:

> So, you are going to continue with the medication and consider pursuing psychotherapy. If your symptoms worsen, such as if the nightmares

---

Primary Care Posttraumatic Stress Disorder Screen

A positive response to the screen does not necessarily indicate that a patient has posttraumatic stress disorder (PTSD). However, a positive response does indicate that a patient may have PTSD or trauma-related problems and further investigation of trauma symptoms by a mental health professional may be warranted.

Primary Care PTSD Screen (PC-PTSD)
In your life, have you ever had any experience that was so
frightening, horrible, or upsetting that, <u>in the past month,</u> you . . .

1. Have had nightmares about it or thought about it when you did not want to?

      YES   NO

2. Tried hard not to think about it or went out of your way to avoid situations that reminded you of it?

      YES   NO

3. Were constantly on guard, watchful, or easily startled?

      YES   NO

4. Felt numb or detached from others, activities, or your surroundings?

      YES   NO

Current research suggests that the results of the PC-PTSD should be considered "positive" if a patient answers, "Yes," to any three items.

FIGURE 5.6.   Primary Care Posttraumatic Stress Disorder screen (PC-PTSD). From "The Primary Care PTSD Screen (PC–PTSD): Development and Operating Characteristics," by A. Prins et al., 2003, *Primary Care Psychiatry, 9,* p. 10. Copyright 2004 by LibraPharm. Adapted with permission.

become more intense or more frequent, or if you notice your irritability negatively affecting your relationships at work or at home, we want you to come back to see what other services might be helpful. Does that seem reasonable to you?

Assist. Prolonged exposure techniques, as well as other treatments requiring extended and repeated appointments, are not appropriate for a primary care environment given the extended time necessary for such interventions. Data are insufficient to suggest that guided self-help or brief treatments for PTSD are effective (NICE, 2005). In addition to helping PCPs identify PTSD symptoms, there may be opportunities for BHCs to intervene with subclinical symptoms of PTSD and assist with monitoring symptoms that may indicate acute stress disorder. Once responses have been normalized for these individuals, the interventions, including relaxation exercises, cognitive disputation, and problem-solving (as discussed in chap. 3, this volume) may be particularly helpful for reducing symptoms associated with increased physiological arousal. In addition, writing down negative or worried thoughts, in a manner similar to strategies used with GAD, and using acceptance-based techniques may help in the management of the distressing symptoms.

Arrange. When making a referral to a specialty mental health provider for PTSD, it is important to ensure that he or she has experience treating PTSD. In addition to trauma-focused cognitive and behavioral treatments for PTSD, eye movement desensitization and reprogramming (EMDR; Shapiro, 1989) was also determined by NICE (2005) to be effective. However, empirical support for this treatment is not as strong as that for trauma-focused cognitive and behavioral treatments. There is significant controversy over whether the training and the eye movements required for EMDR add any effectiveness to the existing cognitive and behavioral treatments (e.g., Lohr, Tolin, & Lilienfeld, 1998); however, that discussion goes beyond the scope of this book. In short, a therapist practicing EMDR may be an appropriate provider for a patient with PTSD symptoms. In contrast, supportive and nondirective therapies, psychodynamic therapies, and hypnotherapies do not have sufficient evidence so that we may consider them as effective treatments for PTSD (NICE, 2005). Regardless of who is treating the patient, it is most important for PTSD symptoms to be treated as promptly as possible.

SLEEP

The prevalence of sleep complaints in primary care has been estimated to be as high as 69%, with 50% of patients reporting occasional insomnia and 19% reporting chronic insomnia (Schochat, Umphress, Israel, & Ancoli-Israel, 1999). Although the most commonly offered treatment for insomnia in primary care has been prescription medications (Chesson et al., 1999; Nowell et al., 1997), behavioral treatments (e.g., sleep hygiene, stimulus control, sleep restriction) have been shown to be just as effective and longer lasting (Morin et al., 1999). According to the *DSM–IV–TR* (APA, 2000), primary insomnia occurs when an individual has difficulty initiating or maintaining sleep or has nonrestorative sleep for at least 1 month with this sleep disturbance resulting in clinically significant impairment. The sleep disturbances cannot be due to other sleep or mental health disorders or to the physiological effects of an illicit drug, medication, or medical condition.

Specialty Mental Health

Evidence from meta-analyses generally concurs that cognitive behavior therapies for insomnia are effective (Irwin, Cole, & Nicassio, 2006) and superior to pharmacotherapy, including newer medications (Sivertsen et al., 2006), over the long-term (Morin, Colecchi, Stone, Sood, & Brink, 1999; Morin et al., 2006). Single 45-minute interventions have also been found to reduce insomnia (Germain et al., 2006). Cognitive and behavioral interventions usually involve a combination of sleep hygiene, stimulus control, sleep restriction, and relaxation. Sleep hygiene involves lifestyle (e.g., caffeine, nicotine, alcohol, diet, exercise) and environmental factors (e.g., noise, room temperature, body temperature, air quality, light, bed comfort) that patients can potentially control (Morin & Espie, 2003).

Increasing the degree to which the bed and bedroom are associated with sleep rather than other activities (e.g., watching television, eating, using the computer) is called *stimulus control* (Bootzin & Epstein, 2000). To maximize stimulus control, patients are encouraged to avoid all activities in the bedroom except sleep and sex, and they are encouraged to get out of bed in 15 minutes if they are not asleep. Sleep restriction requires that individuals reduce the amount of time that they are in bed to the amount of time that they are actually asleep. Therefore, if someone only sleeps 5.5 hours but typically stays in bed for 7 hours, the time between getting in and out of bed would be reduced so that the total time in bed would only be 5.5 hours. Developing a wind-down routine and engaging in relaxation training help reduce sympathetic arousal before bedtime, increasing the likelihood that the patient can fall asleep.

Behavioral Health in Primary Care

Evidence has shown that brief interventions, including self-help programs, can successfully reduce insomnia (Morin et al., 2006) and that these interventions can be successful in primary care environments (Edinger & Sampson, 2003; Goodie et al., in press; Isler, Hunter, Isler, & Peterson, 2003).

Primary Care Adaptation

Assess. Typically, in outpatient specialty mental health settings, sleep diaries are used as part of a sleep assessment; however, in primary care environments we rely more heavily on patient self-report. We suggest your primary assessment involves asking targeted questions to assess sleep behaviors, factors that may prompt and maintain insomnia (stimulus control), and sleep hygiene. Brief, standardized self-report measures exist that can be appropriate for the primary care environment. The Insomnia Severity Index (ISI; Bastien, Vallieres, & Morin, 2001) uses seven items to measure sleep impairment. Using a cutoff score of 14, the ISI distinguished between those with and without insomnia, with a sensitivity of 94% and specificity of 94% (Smith & Trinder, 2001), and is considered a valid

index of insomnia severity (Smith & Wegener, 2003). The ISI is presented in Figure 5.7.

The Epworth Sleepiness Scale (ESS; Johns, 1991) is a commonly used measure that has eight items measuring daytime sleepiness, regardless of the cause of that sleepiness (i.e., sleepiness may or many not be due to insomnia). The ESS has a 93.5% sensitivity and 100% specificity for detecting narcolepsy when using a cutoff score that is great than 10 (Johns, 2000); however, it is not considered to be a valuable tool for distinguishing between individuals who do and do not meet criteria for insomnia (Sanford et al., 2006).

A focused functional assessment of a sleep problem might focus on the following areas:

History.
- "When did you first start having difficulty with your sleep?"
- "Did anything happen that started your sleep problem?"
- "How many nights of the week do you have difficulty with your sleep?"

Sleep environment.
- "Is your bedroom generally quiet and comfortable?"
- "Is there anything that wakes you up throughout the night, such as noises, pets, children?"

Pre-sleep behaviors.
- "Do you take or use anything to help you fall asleep, including alcohol or sleeping medication?"
- "What time of day do you exercise?"
- "Do you use any tobacco? If so, what is the latest time you use tobacco before you go to bed?"
- "How much caffeine, including coffee, tea, soda, do you consume? What is the latest time you have any caffeinated beverages before getting into bed?"

In-bed behaviors.
- "What time do you go to bed? How long does it take you to fall asleep once you are in bed?"
- "How many times do you wake up throughout the night? How long are you awake? What do you do when you wake up? Do you worry about not sleeping?"
- "What time do you wake up? Is that before or after the time you set on your alarm?"
- "How many naps do you take during the day? For how long?"

The Insomnia Severity Index

Please rate the current (i.e., last 2 weeks) severity of your insomnia problem(s).

	None	Mild	Moderate	Severe	Very
a. Difficulty falling asleep:	0	1	2	3	4
b. Difficulty staying asleep:	0	1	2	3	4
c. Problem waking up too early:	0	1	2	3	4

How satisfied/dissatisfied are you with your current sleep pattern?

Very satisfied	**Satisfied**	**Neutral**	**Dissatisfied**	**Very dissatisfied**
0	1	2	3	4

To what extent do you consider your sleep problem to interfere with your daily functioning (e.g., daytime fatigue, ability to function at work/daily chores, concentration, memory, mood, etc.).

Not at all interfering	**A little**	**Somewhat**	**Much**	**Very much interfering**
0	1	2	3	4

How noticeable to others do you think your sleeping problem is in terms of impairing the quality of your life?

Not at all noticeable	**A little**	**Somewhat**	**Much**	**Very much noticeable**
0	1	2	3	4

How worried/distressed are you about your current sleep problem?

Not at all worried	**A little**	**Somewhat**	**Much**	**Very much worried**
0	1	2	3	4

Guidelines for Scoring/Interpretation
Add scores for all seven items (1a + 1b + 1c +2 + 3 + 4 + 5) =
Total score ranges from 0–28; if total score falls between:
    0–7 = No clinically significant insomnia
    8–14 = Subthreshold insomnia
    15–21 = Clinical insomnia (moderate severity)
    22–28 = Clinical insomnia (severe)

FIGURE 5.7.   The Insomnia Severity Index. From *Insomnia: A Clinical Guide to Assessment and Treatment* (p. 137), by C. M. Morin and C. A. Espie, 2003. New York: Kluwer Academic/Plenum Publishers. Copyright 2003 by Kluwer Academic/Plenum Publishers. Reprinted with permission.

- "When you are awake in bed, do you watch TV, read, or eat?"
- "How long do you stay in bed when you are awake?"
  Consequences.
- "Do you feel rested or tired when you wake up? Does that change during the day?"
- "Do you feel sleepy throughout the day?"
- "Have you fallen asleep in inappropriate places? Do you have difficulty concentrating?"
- "What are some ways that your sleep affects your functioning?"
- "Do you nap? If so, how long are your naps?"
  Exclusions.
- Sleep apnea: "Do you snore at night? Do you wake up with a headache? Has anyone told you that you gasp for air when you are sleeping?"
- Periodic limb movements: "Has a bed partner ever told you that you kick them at night? Do your legs suddenly move and wake you up?"

■ Restless leg syndrome: "Do you experience uncomfortable feelings in your legs, such as burning, itching, or crawling sensations that might go away for a little bit when you move your legs but make it difficult to fall asleep?"

Advise.   Similar to dealing with individuals with depressive and anxiety symptoms, BHCs need to be prepared to discuss the role of medication in managing sleep. In primary care settings, we see a wide range of individuals with sleeping problems, from those who have recently developed insomnia to those who have had insomnia for decades. We discuss the value of trying to minimize the use of medications to manage sleep over the long-term although acknowledging the possible short-term benefits of medications. We encourage patients to consider behavioral changes as alternatives to medications and explain that these behavioral changes have been shown to work for 70% to 80% of patients struggling with insomnia. In a discussion about sleep medication, the BHC might say the following:

> In the short-term, sleep medications can be very useful for helping people to get sleep when they really need to sleep. However, we know that for the majority of people with sleep problems, there are things that they can do differently that can significantly improve their sleep if they stick with those changes for about a month. By making these changes, most individuals don't need sleep medications.

We believe it is important to make clear the types of behaviors the individual can change and why those changes are important to improve sleep. We might say the following:

> There are several things you might consider doing to improve your sleep. I'd like to tell you what those are and how they might work, and then you can tell me whether you think you want to do them.
> Going to bed when you are not sleepy and lying in bed awake is a sure

way to make your sleep problem worse. The longer you stay in bed awake, the more you associate your bed with a place to be awake; the bed becomes a signal to be awake instead of asleep. I'd suggest you stop watching TV in bed as well. Watching TV is not compatible with sleep, so your bed becomes your couch or easy chair and is a reminder to watch TV, not sleep. I would also recommend stopping your 2-hour nap in the afternoon. That nap interrupts your sleep-wake cycle so you are not sleepy at night or, if you do fall asleep, your sleep is light and you wake frequently.

> Increased stress and worry is also a target for change. Stress and worry are not compatible with sleep, and, in fact, you have experienced this so much, that often when you are sleepy and get into bed, you immediately wake up and start worrying about the next day. Your bed has become your worry place. Learning relaxation strategies and getting out of bed when worry starts can help improve sleep and allow the bed to become a place to sleep and not be awake.

Agree.   Typically, patients will agree to start the recommended changes; then you can begin to help them learn what they need to do, set a specific plan, and teach them the skills required. Behavioral interventions for sleep require commitment, and sometimes the prospect of getting out of bed if the patient does not fall asleep or fall back to sleep after waking can be concerning. It is important to answer all questions and discuss the reasons why it is important to change. If the patient continues to hesitate over the recommended change(s), you can ask, "Is what you are currently doing to manage your sleep working?" When they say, "No," then say the following:

> The one thing we know for sure is that if you keep doing what you are doing it will continue to not work. In fact,

you've really proven this by doing it for the last 6 months. To get a different outcome, you are going to have to do something different. Are you willing to try these recommendations for the next 3 weeks to see what happens?

Assist.   We suggest using the handout in Figure 5.8, "Improving Sleep Through Behavior Change," to help patients learn about sleep and interventions for improving sleep. When reviewing the handout, target those areas that appear to be of particular concern on the basis of the functional assessment.

Sleep Hygiene.   Focus on prebedtime rituals that may be influencing sleep as well as possible influences of the substances that the patient is using. For example, if we were discussing alcohol, we might say the following:

> Although alcohol can help you fall asleep, it can disrupt the quality of your sleep and contributes to less restful sleep. Having one to two drinks with dinner is probably OK, as long as you're not getting into bed for 4 hours. Is it reasonable for you to avoid alcohol before bedtime?

We suggest going through each lifestyle and environmental factor that may be contributing to the sleep problem and briefly discussing what and how these factors can be changed.

Stimulus control.   When discussing stimulus control, we emphasize using the bed only for sleep and sex and avoiding all other activities in bed. We focus on the activities that patients indicated that they do in bed and discuss alternatives for those activities. For example, we might say the following:

> You mentioned that you sometimes watch TV in bed before trying to fall asleep. Sleep is an automatic process, and our bodies can learn to stay awake in bed, rather than associate the bed with sleep. It is important to reteach your body that the bed is a place where

you sleep. Would you be willing watch TV in another room before getting into bed?

If patients tend to stay in bed when they are not asleep we discuss possible alternatives, as follows:

> You mentioned that when you cannot fall asleep, you tend to lie awake in bed. Because we want you to associate your bed with sleep and sex, and nothing else, it is important to get out of bed and do something boring when you cannot sleep. We recommend that if you've been awake for longer than 15 minutes, that you get out of bed and go into another room where you can sit quietly until you feel sleepy, that is, when you eyes feel heavy and you think that you'll fall asleep.

Sleep Restriction.   Most often we do not have a sleep diary to estimate total sleep time. On the basis of self-reports of how long it takes to fall asleep, whether the patient is waking before his or her alarm clock, and his or her estimated total sleep time, we develop a plan for when the patient should get into bed and plan to wake. Figure 5.9, "Sleep Restriction," is an interactive handout. We suggest having the patient read it and to then explain it to him or her verbally, as follows:

> The idea of sleep restriction is to take the amount of time you are asleep in bed—for you it is 5 hours—and limit the time you can be in bed to that— 5 hours. Because you get up at 8:00 a.m. every morning, the earliest you would be able to get into bed would be 3:00 a.m. By staying up so late you will get very sleepy and are more likely to fall asleep quickly and limit the time you are awake in bed, both of which will help improve your sleep. Once you are falling asleep within 15 minutes, we can move back your bedtime by about 20 minutes and continue to do that until we get the best time range determined.

Improving Sleep Through Behavior Change

Stimulus Control Procedures

Go to Bed Only When You Are Sleepy
The longer you are in bed, the more the bed is associated with a place to be awake instead of asleep. Delay bedtime until sleepy.

Get Out of Bed When You Can't Fall Asleep or Go Back to Sleep in About 15 Minutes
Get out of bed if you don't fall asleep fairly soon. Return to bed only when you are sleepy. When you feel sleepy, return to bed. The goal is to reconnect your bed with being asleep.

Use the Bed for Sleep and Sex Only
Do not watch TV, listen to the radio, eat, or read in your bed or bedroom.

Sleep Hygiene Guidelines

Caffeine
Avoid caffeine 6 to 8 hours before bedtime. Caffeine disturbs sleep. Thus, drinking caffeinated beverages should be avoided near bedtime.

Nicotine
Avoid nicotine before bedtime. Nicotine can keep you awake. Avoid tobacco near bedtime and during the night.

Alcohol
Avoid alcohol after dinner. Alcohol often promotes the onset of sleep, but interrupts your natural sleep pattern. Do not consume it any closer than 4 hours before going to bed.

Sleeping Pills
Sleep medications are effective only temporarily. Sleep medications lose their effectiveness in about 2 to 4 weeks when taken regularly. Over time, sleeping pills actually can make sleep problems worse; withdrawal from the medication can lead to an insomnia rebound. Keep use of sleeping pills infrequent, but don't worry if you need to use one on an occasional basis.

Regular Exercise
Do not exercise within 2 hours of bedtime as it may elevate nervous system activity and interfere with your ability to fall asleep

Bedroom Environment
Your bedroom should have a moderate temperature and be quiet and dark. Noises can be masked with background white noise (e.g., the noise of a fan) or with earplugs. Bedrooms may be darkened with black-out shades, or sleep masks can be worn.

Eating
A light bedtime snack, such a glass of warm milk, cheese, or a bowl of cereal can promote sleep. Avoid snacks in the middle of the night because awakening may become associated with hunger.

Avoid Naps
The sleep you obtain during the day takes away from the amount of sleep you need that night. If you must nap, schedule it before 3:00 p.m. Don't sleep more than 15 to 30 minutes.

Allow Yourself at Least an Hour Before Bedtime to Unwind
Find what works for you to wind down, and perhaps give yourself an hour to do so.

Regular Sleep Schedule
Keep a regular time each day, 7 days a week, to get out of bed. Keeping a regular waking time helps set your circadian rhythm so that your body learns to sleep at the desired time.

Set a Reasonable Bedtime and Arising Time and Stick to Them
Set the alarm clock and get out of bed at the same time each morning, weekdays and weekends, regardless of your bedtime or the amount of sleep you obtained on the previous night. This guideline is designed to regulate your internal biological clock and reset your sleep–wake rhythm.

FIGURE 5.8. Improving sleep through behavior change handout.

Sleep Restriction: One of the Keys to Changing Your Sleep Behavior

---

What Is It?

Sleep restriction involves restricting the amount of time you spend in bed to the amount of time that you currently spend asleep.

Why Would This Be Helpful?

Research has shown sleep restriction to be an effective technique for improving sleep. In general, most people notice their sleep improves within just a few weeks. Sleep restriction initially produces a mild state of sleep deprivation, which helps people fall asleep faster, stay asleep longer, and improves their overall quality of sleep.

How Do I Do It?

Consider the following example: Your usual bedtime is 10:00 p.m. and you get out of bed in the morning at 6:00 a.m. (8 hours in bed). However, it takes you 1 hour to fall asleep, and you wake up for 30 minutes in the middle of the night, and 30 minutes before you get out of bed. Therefore, you spend 6 hours sleeping and 2 hours awake. Your sleep efficiency (the percentage of time you are actually asleep during the time period you are trying to sleep) is 75%. Sleep restriction in this case would mean decreasing time in bed (8 hours) to the estimated time actually spent sleeping (6 hours).

   In this example, you would adjust either your bedtime or the time you get up in the morning, so that the maximum amount of time you spend in bed is 6 hours. You could go to bed at 12:00 midnight and get up at 6:00 a.m., or continue to go to bed at 10:00 p.m. and get up at 4:00 a.m. After sleep efficiency reaches 85% or greater, time in bed can be increased in 15 to 20 minute blocks. Time in bed each week is increased if 85% sleep efficiency or greater is achieved. This pattern continues until sleep efficiency starts to fall below 80%, at which point time in bed is decreased by 15 to 20 minute blocks. This process of increasing or decreasing time in bed is continued until sleep efficiency falls between 80% and 85% on a regular basis.

FIGURE 5.9. Sleep restriction handout.

Relaxation.   If patients report sympathetic arousal before bedtime, we may teach them the brief relaxation techniques presented in chapter 3; however, this often requires a separate follow-up appointment. Similarly, if patients report that they worry in bed, we may discuss using a worry log in which to write their worries before getting into bed. You should inform patients that it may take 2 to 4 weeks for their sleep to improve and that their sleep may get worse before it improves. Identify with patients' barriers to implementing the recommendations and set appropriate follow-up appointments to assess change and solve difficulties. A typical follow-up might occur about 2 weeks after the previous appointment.

Arrange.   Most cases of insomnia likely can be treated in primary care. One or two return appointments after the interventions for sleep have been taught can help the PCP assess whether the interventions are working for the patient. If interventions in primary care are not effective and the patient is being referred to a specialty mental health care setting, consider making the referral to a provider who has experience treating sleep disorders, such as a clinical health psychologist.

SUMMARY

Subclinical and clinical depression, anxiety, and sleep problems will be the mainstays for most BHCs in primary care settings. There is evidence that brief interventions can help many of these symptoms. Currently we do not have good data about what can be done for PTSD in primary care. The recommendations and handouts in this chapter provide a place to start; building on these ideas to develop time-limited effective interventions for these problems will be essential for any BHC.

CHAPTER 6

HEALTH BEHAVIORS: TOBACCO USE, OVEREATING, AND PHYSICAL INACTIVITY

Together, tobacco use, poor dietary habits, and physical inactivity are responsible for 34.7% of morbidity (Mokdad, Marks, Stroup, & Gerberding, 2004) in the United States. These numbers will likely rise considering that 87.5% of the U.S. population either smoke, are overweight, or are physically inactive, with an estimated 9.8 million Americans having all three risk factors (Fine, Philogene, Gramling, Coups, & Sinha, 2004). It is surprising that many individuals who demonstrate these health risks are not targeted by health care professionals. Among those who had a general physical exam or routine medical checkup, only half were asked about their health risk behaviors (Coups, Gaba, & Orleans, 2004). Only 40% of women and 25% of men who were overweight or obese reported ever having been counseled about the adverse consequences of increased weight (Galuska, Will, Serdula, & Ford, 1999). Similarly, only 31.3% of those who were physically inactive were encouraged to increase their physical inactivity (Kreuter, Scharff, Brennan, & Lukwago, 1997), and only 55% of smokers were encouraged to quit at their medical office visits (Lucan & Katz, 2006).

Physicians report multiple barriers to assessing and intervening in these health behaviors, including lack of time, perceived ineffectiveness of behavior change strategies, and low confidence in their abilities and knowledge to affect behavior change (Rosal et al., 2004; Tully, Cupples, & Young, 2004; Vogt, Hall, & Marteau, 2005). Despite these barriers, the primary care setting is an important place, if not the most important place, to target health behavior change, given the full range of care that occurs in this environment. In this chapter, we provide systematic methods for addressing these health behavior problems in a busy primary care setting.

TOBACCO USE

Tobacco use is the single largest cause of morbidity and mortality and accounts for more than 400,000 deaths every year (Mokdad et al., 2004). Despite increased awareness of the dangers of tobacco use, 20.9% of Americans continue to use smoke cigarettes, 2.2% smoke cigars, and 2.3% use smokeless tobacco (Centers for Disease Control and Prevention [CDC], 2006). According to the CDC, of the 45.1 million adult cigarette smokers, 42.5% stopped smoking at least 1 day within the previous 12 months in an attempt to quit tobacco use, suggesting that many smokers want to quit but have difficulty doing so. To help individuals stop using tobacco, a variety of behavioral and pharmacological treatments have been developed and used in tertiary and primary care settings.

Specialty Mental Health
In specialty mental health settings a variety of interventions and delivery formats are used. Interventions are typically behavior-change focused, use pharmacological agents or some combination of these interventions.

Behavior change interventions. Tobacco cessation counseling has been found to be helpful for increasing quit rates compared with no counseling (Lancaster & Stead, 2005) and medication alone (Ranney, Melvin, Lux, McClain, & Lohr, 2006). Participants in group therapy are approximately 2 times more likely to quit tobacco use than those using no intervention or a self-help program; however, it is unclear whether there is a difference between individual counseling and group counseling (Stead & Lancaster, 2005). Overall, having at least four or more individual appointments, even if those appointments are brief, substantially improves abstinence rates (Fiore et al., 2000). Therefore, brief and frequent contacts (e.g., multiple 10–15-minute appointments) with individuals who are quitting tobacco may provide the best results for successful cessation attempts. Although more research is needed, the available evidence does not support the use of acupuncture, acupressure, laser therapy, or electrostimulation as effective smoking cessation treatments (White, Rampes, & Campbell, 2006).

Pharmacological agents.   Pharmacological agents, including nicotine replacement therapy (NRT) and non-nicotine medication, are efficacious for tobacco cessation (Ranney et al., 2006). Current NRT agents, including chewing gum, transdermal patches, nasal spray, inhalers, and tablets, provide a 1.5- to 2-fold increase in cessation rates compared with placebo and non-NRT groups (Silagy, Lancaster, Stead, Mant, & Fowler, 2004). Non-nicotine medications that have been found to assist with tobacco cession include bupropion SR (i.e., Zyban, Wellbutrin), nortriptyline (e.g., Elavil), and varenicline tartrate (e.g., Chantix; Keating & Siddiqui, 2006). These medications double the chances of quitting successfully (Hughes, Stead, & Lancaster, 2007; Ranney et al., 2006). Compared with placebo, individuals taking varenicline were 3.2 times more likely to remain tobacco-free (Cahill, Stead, & Lancaster, 2007). Therefore, it is important for behavioral health professionals to be familiar with these options and their contraindications, as pharmacological therapies are an important addition to behavior change strategies for tobacco cessation.

Behavioral Health in Primary Care

Messages to quit tobacco use delivered in the primary care setting combined with self-help or pharmacologic agents can lead to 10% of patients successfully quitting tobacco use, which is significantly higher than the 3% to 5% of smokers who quit on their own. Even brief advice to quit smoking (e.g., simply being told to quit) produces abstinence rates of 5% to 10% (CDC, 2000). However, spending just 31 to 90 minutes with patients intervening with tobacco cessation could increase the abstinence rate from 21.5% to 31.4% (Fiore et al., 2000). Overall, counseling and medication intervention is most effective for tobacco cessation (Fiore et al., 2008). Other than this chapter, there are multiple resources, including practical handbooks, that one can use to develop effective assessment and treatment plans in a primary care setting (e.g., Shadel & Niaura, 2003).

Primary Care Adaptation

Assess.   Existing guidelines recommend that all patients entering a clinic should be screened for tobacco use (Fiore et al., 2008). Incorporating screening questions into intake forms is one method of instituting a clinic-wide change. Asking tobacco users at every appointment about whether they are considering quitting is also important for a population health approach to decreasing tobacco use. Patients who have denied being ready for change at previous appointments may be ready to quit at the moment that they are sitting with a provider. It is important to understand the situations that are conducive to tobacco use and why the person chooses to use tobacco. Successful tobacco cessation will often involve finding healthier alternatives that serve similar functions as tobacco.

Establish a pattern of use. For tobacco cessation, it is important to establish the pattern of tobacco use. The behavioral health consultant (BHC) will need to determine what happens when patients use tobacco, what situations are associated with tobacco use, and the perceived benefits of tobacco use. Examples of questions to ask include the following, What kind of tobacco do you use? How much tobacco do you use? How often do you use tobacco? Everyday or on the weekends only? The BHC should also attempt to find out what factors predispose the individual to use tobacco (i.e., what the antecedents are). Examples of questions to ask include:

- Are there situations, such as in the car, at home, or when you are with others when you are more likely to use tobacco?
- How often do you smoke at work? What determines when you take a break to smoke?
- Are there certain emotions or thoughts that seem to be related to when you use tobacco? Stress? Sadness? Worry? Feeling overwhelmed?
- Physically, do you notice changes, such as your heart racing, muscle tension, sweatiness before you use tobacco?
- Are there other household members who smoke? Do your friends use tobacco? Do you have any friends who do not use tobacco?
- How does using tobacco help you?
- How do you feel when or just after you've used tobacco? Relaxed? Calmer? More stressed? What do you like about using tobacco? What do you dislike?

Establish a history of cessation attempts. Understanding whether someone has quit and what has and has not worked in the past can be valuable for developing a treatment plan. These questions are examples of what you might ask to establish a patient's history of quit attempts:

- How many times have you quit before? When was the last time you quit? What is the longest amount of time you have remained tobacco-free? How did you stay tobacco-free for that long?
- What contributed to you going back to tobacco use?
- Did you use the patch, gum, or any other nicotine replacement? Did you use any medication, such as Zyban, or any herbal supplements to help you quit?

Ultimately, your assessment should provide a brief understanding of why the individual chooses to use tobacco, what makes it difficult to quit, and what has and has not worked in the past. The most

common reason a former smoker goes back to tobacco use is perceived stress (Baer & Lichtenstein, 1988). Therefore, specifically determining potential alternatives for managing stress will be an essential component to a successful tobacco cessation plan. So you may ask the following:

- What do you do for enjoyment?
- When you are stressed, is there anything else that you do to manage the stress other than tobacco use?
- What do you do to relax? Have you ever learned ways to help you relax?

Advise. Consistent with recent guidelines (Fiore et al., 2008), regardless of how much someone is using tobacco, we inform patients that quitting tobacco is the most important change they can make for their long-term health. Even if the individual was not specifically referred for tobacco use, we advise them to consider quitting. For those individuals who demonstrate no interest in quitting, we say the following:

> It doesn't sound like you are interested in quitting right now, but if you ever change your mind and want to consider quitting, Dr. Smith [the patient's primary care provider (PCP)] and I would be happy to help you quit. We can help you right here in the clinic or we can refer you to a more intense treatment program. We both consider quitting tobacco to be the most important change you can make for your health.

With patients who appear to be more ambivalent or who are interested in change, we move to the agree phase, in which we discuss their motivation for change.

Agree. Tobacco use, like any behavior change, requires a willingness to change. When attempting to initiate a health behavior change with a patient, it is necessary to determine the patient's motivation for change. Despite having multiple medical problems that are affected by health behaviors, individuals may still not be motivated to change those behaviors. The stages of change model

(Prochaska & DiClemente, 1983; Prochaska & Velicer, 1997) is perhaps the most ubiquitous model for examining readiness to change. A central tenet of stages of change is that individuals are unlikely to change their behaviors unless they decide to make a change. Motivational interviewing (MI) strategies (Miller & Rollnick, 2002; Rollnick, Mason, & Butler, 1999), which we discussed in chapter 3, have been shown to increase the likelihood of behavior change across a range of behaviors, including tobacco use, diet, and exercise (Burke, Arkowitz, & Menchola, 2003).

In addition to assessing an individual's motivation to quit, it is important to establish whether the primary care setting is appropriate for his or her cessation attempt. For individuals who report that they participated in a tobacco group or more intensive treatments in the past and were successful, we discuss the possibility of using those treatment modalities again or using the program that we can offer in primary care.

Assist. Helping a patient quit tobacco use should involve establishing a plan that identifies when the patient is going to quit, working to prepare for that quit date, and developing skills to manage challenges the patient will face after he or she has quit. In Figure 6.1 we provide an example of a handout that we use to guide our tobacco intervention.

Preparing to quit. Consistent with the U.S. Surgeon General's recommendations (Fiore et al., 2000) for behavioral and cognitive interventions, a specific quit plan should be developed. To establish such a plan, tobacco users should be asked the following: "It is important to have a specific date and time when you will quit tobacco use. Considering your schedule, when would be the best time for you to use tobacco for the last time? [Elicit a specific date and time from the patient]."

Once a date and time is established, discuss how the individual is going to facilitate the quit attempt by preparing his or her environment during the time before the quit date. We use the handout in Figure 6.1 to record the patient's quit date and to review strategies for quitting. Strategies include not buying tobacco in bulk; cleaning the areas where they are most likely to use tobacco, such as their

house, garage, and/or car; and eliminating materials such as lighters and ashtrays. Patients may be reluctant to throw away ashtrays. If this is the case, you could ask them the following:

> What can you do to make it harder for yourself to use tobacco if you suddenly got an urge to do so? If you are not willing to throw away your ashtrays, is there a place you can store them where they would be difficult to get to, such as at a neighbor's house?

Tobacco users should consider how they will live their life differently after they quit and become nontobacco users. You could ask the following questions: "Will you stop carrying lighters in your pockets?" "Will you be able to drink alcohol without using tobacco?" "Will you still take breaks at work without using tobacco?"

Patients should decide whether they are going to enlist the support of people around them. Identifying individuals to serve as social supports can help facilitate the cessation attempt (Fiore et al., 2000). BHCs can encourage patients to enlist the support of others by saying the following:

> It is often helpful to get the support of others when you art trying to quit. How would you feel about asking your significant other/spouse and coworkers to help you quit? Could you let your friends and coworkers know that you are quitting?

Tobacco users should also examine whether there are certain individuals they should avoid, particularly other tobacco users. If others in the household smoke, they could be encouraged to smoke away from the patient or even to quit tobacco use at the same time as the patient. To accomplish this, patients might be asked, "Could you ask your (significant other/spouse/housemate) to avoid you when he or she smokes? Could you ask coworkers not to invite you out to the smoking area?"

Before the quit attempt is made, if bupropion or varenicline is going to be used, patients should begin to take that medication approximately 1 week before their quit date according to the prescription of their PCP.

Tobacco Cessation

How to Change?

To effectively change your tobacco use, consider all of the factors that contribute to using tobacco. It can be helpful to group these factors into three main categories: physical factors, habits, and psychological factors (i.e., your thoughts and emotions).

Physically, nicotine is the most addictive substance on the planet. Your medical provider will tell you whether it is appropriate for you to use a nicotine replacement product, such as the patch or gum. Some medications, like Zyban, don't seem to help some people with their nicotine cravings.

Behaviorally, you will need to change your habits and the situations that you typically associate with tobacco. Undoubtedly, you will experience situations that cause you to crave tobacco, but you can learn skills that will help you choose alternatives other than using tobacco.

Thoughts and emotions are some of the hardest aspects of tobacco use to change. Often, individuals think that they need tobacco to get through a difficult situation. Changing these thoughts to cope with stress and negative emotions is an essential aspect of successful tobacco cessation.

Preparing to Quit

Your Quit Date

When is the last day and time that you are going to use tobacco?

Month_____ Day_____ Year_____ Time_____

Preparing Your Surroundings

What are the things that remind you to use tobacco? It is important to change your surroundings so that you won't be reminded about tobacco use as frequently. Before your quit date consider the following:

- Don't buy tobacco in bulk (e.g., don't buy cartons).
- Find all of your hidden stashes of tobacco. Check in the couch, the glove compartment, in your drawers at home and at work. It is unwise to keep an emergency stash once you quit.
- Get rid of tobacco-related materials—things like ashtrays and lighters. You may need lighters for candles or fireplaces, but you likely don't need to carry lighters wherever you go.
- Prepare family and friends. Let them know that you are planning to quit and ask for their help. If you have friends and family who do use tobacco, ask them to avoid using tobacco around you.
- Choose a method to quit. There are several ways to consider quitting, but one of the most important considerations is to avoid romanticizing your last tobacco use. If you remember your tobacco fondly, then you may be more likely to go back to tobacco use when you perceive that you need it. The following are some ways to avoid romanticizing your last use of tobacco.

Nicotine fading. Gradually decrease the amount of tobacco you are using. You can do this by decreasing how often you use your current tobacco, or you can switch to another brand of tobacco that has less nicotine.

Brand switching. On the day that you are planning to quit, use a different brand of tobacco, preferably a brand that tastes stronger or significantly different from the brand that you use today. Rather than the pleasant sensation you associate with you current brand, you'll remember the more unpleasant taste of the new brand.

Aversive tobacco use. The last time that you use tobacco, use a lot of it or use it quickly. Again, the idea is to have your last memory of tobacco be an unpleasant memory. So you might decide to smoke your last cigarette very rapidly, or use two or three times as much chewing tobacco than you normally would.

Using the Four As to Outsmart Tobacco Urges

Avoid. What are the situations or places that you need to avoid over the next month?

1. _____

2. _____

3. _____

FIGURE 6.1. Tobacco cessation handout. (*Continued*)

Alter. What situations will you need to change to help you be more successful?

1. _____

2. _____

3. _____

Alternatives. What can you put in your mouth or hands instead of using tobacco?

1. _____

2. _____

3. _____

Action. When you get an urge to use tobacco, what can you do to be active or busy?

1. _____

2. _____

3. _____

FIGURE 6.1.　*(Continued)* Tobacco cessation handout.

Quitting. As they approach the quit date, there are multiple behavioral techniques for patients to consider to help them quit. These methods include nicotine fading, aversive smoking, and brand switching. Nicotine fading involves gradually decreasing the amount of nicotine that is being consumed. Fading can be done by tapering the frequency of tobacco use over time or by switching to a different brand of tobacco that contains less nicotine. Aversive tobacco use and brand switching are intended to make the last experiences with tobacco unpleasant to decrease the likelihood that the patient will return to tobacco use. Aversive smoking (or aversive chewing) involves the rapid consumption of tobacco (e.g., rapidly smoking the last cigarette). Brand switching requires that the patient select a different brand of tobacco to consume on the last day of tobacco use. Any of these techniques can be quickly described to the patient, who could then choose the preferred method of quitting. Ultimately, the BHC should decrease the likelihood that the patient will romanticize his or her last use of tobacco. Individuals who view quitting as "losing a good friend" and who remember that friend fondly may be more likely to return to the friend during a crisis period.

When patients reach their quit date, they should start using their nicotine replacements (i.e., patch,

gum, and/or spray). The quit date, or shortly after, is a good time to meet with the patient to discuss any concerns he or she might have as they begin to quit.

Maintaining cessation. Once the patient has quit tobacco, the goal is to "not have a single puff or chew." Withdrawal symptoms, negative affect, and cravings are three of the most important reasons individuals return to tobacco use (Piasecki, 2006). Once individuals quit tobacco use, they will need to consider what they will do when they feel a strong urge to use tobacco again. NRT can help significantly with moderating withdrawal symptoms. Patients can use the mnemonic of the four A's (not to be confused with the 5A's) to help them to overcome tobacco urges. The four As guide the individual to consider ways to avoid, alter, use alternatives, or stay active to cope with urges to use tobacco. Patients should be encouraged to plan ahead for situations that are closely paired with tobacco use. Using the handout in Figure 6.1, you can guide the patient by asking the following:

> What situations (e.g., bars, sporting events, smoking areas) do you need to avoid during the next month to limit your urges to use tobacco? How can

you change situations that you can't avoid so that you'll be more successful with your quit attempt? When you feel an urge to put tobacco in your mouth, what could you use instead (e.g., gum, hard candies or mints, toothpicks, cinnamon sticks)? Are there activities (e.g., going for a walk, doing push-ups, running) you can do or ways you can keep busy if you feel an urge to use tobacco?

Cognitively, patients can be encouraged to consider themselves a tobacco user, and when they encounter situations that result in increased urges to use tobacco, to ask themselves, "What would a nontobacco user do?" It will be important to ask patients what they will do when they believe that they must or have to use tobacco. Briefly discuss methods to challenge these beliefs, such as telling themselves, "I'd like to have a cigarette, but I don't need to have one." Discuss how they can "ride the emotional wave" of the urge to use tobacco by deep breathing and by recognizing that such urges will subside over time.

The most common reason individuals return to tobacco use is negative affect (e.g., stress). Therefore, it can be valuable to talk specifically about what they can do in response to stressful situations. Ask what they currently do, besides using tobacco, to manage stress and whether they can use those techniques when they feel stressed. In addition, it may be useful to consider teaching brief relaxation methods and cognitive strategies (see chap. 3, this volume) as well as increasing physical activity to manage stressors without tobacco.

Although the goal is for the patient to not use any tobacco, the likelihood that the individual will slip is very high; most lapses occur within the first 5 to 10 days after quitting, and 90% of lapses lead to a relapse (e.g., Piasecki, 2006; Westman, Behm, Simel, & Rose, 1997). Therefore, it is important to consider a relapse prevention plan. Remind the patient as follows:

> The goal is not to use any tobacco, not a single puff/dip/chew, but if you do slip, what can you do to keep the slip from becoming a total collapse? A slip doesn't mean that you've failed. How can you recommit yourself to not using tobacco?

Despite the best relapse prevention plans, tobacco cessation attempts often are accompanied by relapses and return to previous tobacco use levels (Piasecki, 2006); it often takes multiple attempts for someone to successfully quit. Therefore, it is imperative that providers and patients do not become hopeless after a failed cessation attempt. Even in specialty mental health settings, the best relapse prevention plans do not appear to result in a significant reduction in relapse (Hajek, Stead, West, Jarvis, & Lancaster, 2006). Therefore, continuing to target tobacco use at all appointments is the best way to help patients return to their commitment to quit tobacco use and become nontobacco users. Even providing self-help print or Web-based material that is tailored to the patient can be effective for helping patients to quit tobacco (Fiore et al., 2008).

Arrange. At a minimum, you will want to meet with patients for 15 to 30 minutes at least four times during their quit attempt. Your schedule might be arranged as follows:

- Appointment 1. Preparing for the quit attempt
- Appointment 2. On or around the quit date
- Appointment 3. Approximately 1 week after the quit date
- Appointment 4. Approximately 1 month after the quit date

You may want to consider more frequent appointments because the number of contacts with the patient is positively associated with quitting (Fiore, 2000). However, the appointments do not have to be with you. Instead, consider ways to incorporate the entire primary care team to facilitate tobacco cessation. Most patients can be appropriately targeted for cessation of tobacco use in primary care settings. However, individuals who have significant medical conditions or upcoming surgeries necessitating close monitoring of the patient during the quit attempt may be better served in the tertiary care setting. Individuals who have attempted to quit tobacco use through primary care in the past and have failed to remain tobacco-free may also benefit from tertiary care treatments.

OVEREATING

Over 66% of the U.S. population is considered either overweight or obese (Ogden et al., 2006). The primary causes for the recent increase in obesity are believed to be decreased energy expenditure and increased food intake, in part because of technological advancements in Western cultures (Finkelstein, Ruhm, & Kosa, 2005). Obesity-related costs exceed $139 billion per year (Finkelstein et al., 2005). Most patients who are overweight and obese want to lose weight and believe that their PCP could be of more help in this area (Potter, Vu, & Croughan-Minihane, 2001). As with tobacco use, the primary care environment is an ideal place to start to target weight loss.

Specialty Mental Health

Studies over the last 30 years in specialty weight loss clinics and university settings have shown a variety of weight loss programs and strategies to be effective (e.g., Ayyad & Andersen, 2000; Wing, 1997). The best current evidence-based recommendations for weight loss include setting realistic goals (e.g., 1–2 pounds per week), self-monitoring of calories, stimulus control to change the environmental cues for eating, and introducing physical activity to maintain weight loss achievements (Faith, Fontaine, Cheskin, & Allison, 2000; National Institutes of Health/National Heart, Lung, and Blood Institute, 1998; Wing & Polley, 2001).

Behavioral Health in Primary Care

Only 5.6% of primary care visits involve weight-related counseling (McAlpine & Wilson, 2007). PCPs report multiple reasons for not discussing weight loss, including trying to manage time, inadequate access to resources that would support weight interventions (e.g., psychologists, health educators, dietitians), patient motivation, and perceived lack of treatment effectiveness for weight loss (Leverence, Williams, Sussman, Crabtree, &

RIOS Net Clinicians, 2007). Little is known about the most effective ways to target weight loss in primary care settings. Research has shown a minimal effect on weight loss with medications and brief counseling (Poston et al., 2006). Integrating behavioral health providers into primary care would undoubtedly help physicians overcome some of the barriers to targeting weight loss and would expand the opportunities for targeting weight loss in primary care.

Primary Care Adaptation

The following recommendations focus on behavioral and cognitive assessments and treatments for weight loss, which will serve as the first step in a stepped-care approach, as encouraged by Wadden, Brownell, and Foster (2002). These approaches could be followed by more intensive treatments offered in specialty mental health settings, if necessary. The approaches may also be paired with medication management.

Assess. Body mass index (BMI; BMI = $(703 \times$ weight (pound)) / (height (inch))^2) offers a fast, simple way to identify those who might benefit from weight loss interventions. A free chart for quickly determining BMI can be downloaded at http://www.nhlbi.nih.gov/guidelines/obesity/bmi_tbl.pdf. Posting a BMI chart in the area where patients are weighed encourages the medical personnel who weigh the patient to quickly identify patients who fall in the overweight ($25 \leq$ BMI < 30) or obese (BMI ≥ 30) category and then report that information to the patient's provider.

Once overweight or obesity is identified as a health concern for the patient, it is important to ask whether the patient is willing to discuss their weight and weight history. If so, it is useful to determine the patient's pattern of weight gain and weight loss to establish the learning history related to weight changes. If the individual has successfully lost weight in the past, there may be skills that can be built on when developing current recommendations. For instance, you might ask the following:

> As an adult, what is the most you have weighed? What was the least? Have you

lost weight in the past? Did you use a special program? What was it? Have you tried monitoring calories or increasing exercise? What has been your weight pattern over the last year? Have you been gaining, losing, or maintaining a steady weight?

Assessing thoughts associated with weight loss can be helpful for determining the individual's self-efficacy regarding controlling his or her weight and motivation for weight change. Questions might include, "Do you feel like you have control over your weight? Do you worry about gaining weight? What health effect has weight had on you? Are you concerned about the effect of weight on your appearance?"

We recommend assessing current eating habits to include establishing where patients eat, whether they are distracted while they are eating, what situations tend to be associated with eating more, how much time elapses between meals or eating times, and what the individual typically eats and drinks. You might ask the patient the following:

> Do you eat while you are watching TV or doing other things? How often do you eat out? Do you eat breakfast, lunch, and dinner? Do you snack during the day? Do you find that you are more likely to eat when you're upset or stressed?

Given that 10% to 30% of obese individuals seeking treatment engage in binge eating (Spitzer et al., 1993), it is important to rule out eating patterns that may be associated with an eating disorder (e.g., binging, purging) and symptoms related to negative moods (e.g., depression, anxiety). Ask short, clear questions to determine whether patients binge and engage in compensatory behaviors following a binge, such as the following: "Do you ever binge eat? That is, do you eat a lot at one sitting with a feeling that you have lost control over your eating?" If they say that they do, you might ask the following:

> How often do you binge? Once a month, once a week, every day? Do you ever make yourself vomit after you binge or do things soon afterwards to try to eliminate the food you took in, such as exercise a lot or take laxatives? Do you feel guilty or disgusted after you binge? Are you secretive about your binges? Are you sad more days than not? Do you tend to eat more when you are sad? How often do you feel nervous or upset? Do you eat more when you are stressed?

Individuals engaging in binging and purging behaviors will need to be monitored closely for physical complications, such as damage to the teeth and throat as well as electrolyte imbalances and may be better served in an specialty mental health clinic. However, if the patient is motivated to target these behaviors and the PCP is interested in managing the care in the primary care clinic, binging and, possibly, purging behaviors could be targeted in primary care (Williams, Goodie, & Motisinger, 2008).

Advise. When advising patients about losing weight, we emphasize that a relatively small amount of weight loss, such as losing 5% to 10% of their current weight, can have significant benefits for their health. We also discuss the recommendations that safe and effective weight loss strategies involve losing about 1 to 2 pounds per week. For some patients, this information can be disheartening, as they have been exposed to advertisements and television shows claiming rapid and large weight loss over the course of several weeks. We emphasize that to be able to sustain their weight loss they should lose the weight slowly. Thus, we would say the following:

> To lose weight, and be able to keep the weight off, we recommend a plan in which you will lose weight at the rate of about 1 to 2 pounds per week. For some people this might not seem like it is fast enough, but we want you to be able to keep the weight off once you lose it, and we believe that this is

the best way to do that. Over the course of about 6 months, we would expect that you would lose about 5% to 10% of your weight, which would significantly decrease the risk that your weight poses to your health.

Similar to other chronic conditions, overweight and obesity require regular follow-ups to ensure that they are being managed effectively. Therefore, we also let the patient know that, to maximize success, it will likely be important for them to follow up regularly (e.g., once per month) with us throughout their weight loss efforts.

It is not uncommon for patients to be using a self-help program (e.g., Atkins, The Zone, South Beach) or a more formalized commercial program (e.g., Weight Watchers). The available research suggests that these programs can help patients lose weight (Dansinger, Gleason, Griffith, Selker, & Schaefer, 2005; Gardner et al., 2007), at least in the short-term (e.g., 6–12 months). We know less about the effectiveness of these programs over the long-term. We support patients using these programs if they are finding the program helpful. Unless it appears that they would benefit from additional help (e.g., they express difficulty implementing the program) or there are medical contraindications to their diet plan, we encourage patients to make a follow-up appointment within 3 to 6 months to evaluate whether they are continuing to be successful in their weight loss attempt.

The patient's PCP may also consider medications to help with weight loss. A systematic review has shown sibutramine (e.g., Meridia) and orlistat (i.e., Xenical, Alli) to be effective medications for assisting with weight loss (Padwal, Li, & Lau, 2003); however, these medications are associated with side effects that can contribute to discontinuation of the medication before achieving the desired weight loss.

Agree. Once you have completed your assessment and advised patients about the benefits of losing weight, it is helpful to summarize for patients your understanding of their difficulties and concerns as well as their hopes and expectations for weight loss. Asking whether they are interested in developing a plan to start targeting weight loss can help to bridge

the gap between the assess and assist phases. For example, you might say the following:

> It sounds like you've struggled with weight loss for a long time. You've tried a variety of programs that have helped you lose weight initially, but you have put the weight back on, which has been frustrating. Now that your doctor has suggested your weight might affect your health, you're concerned about your weight and want to do something about it. Are you interested in working with me to develop a plan that would help you lose weight and keep it off?

Again, the motivational enhancement questions that we discussed in chapter 3 and in the tobacco cessation section of this chapter are important to ask when starting a weight loss program. DiLillo, Siegfried, and West (2003) presented specific examples of how motivational enhancement questions could be used to facilitate a weight loss treatment. Such techniques have been shown to enhance adherence to weight control programs (Smith, Heckemeyer, Kratt, & Mason, 1997). For example, it is particularly important to elicit self-motivational statements associated with the patient's decision to lose weight. So you could ask, "What would make this weight loss attempt different from previous attempts? How would your life be different if you lost weight?" With this information, you can then tailor the recommendations in the assist phase to enhance the motivators and decrease the barriers to maintaining weight loss behaviors.

Assist. Evidence-based interventions for losing weight and keeping weight off can be tricky in the primary care setting. Often, the patient has tried many methods and may have had some short-term success, but like most who struggle with weight problems, keeping the weight off in the long-term is a challenge. Most individuals know the mantra of weight loss programs, "Eat less, exercise more." In the primary care setting, interventions are focused on putting this mantra into practice in a manageable way, by providing specific, concrete recommendations that help patients adapt their behaviors to the specific situations they encounter. The primary focus of these interventions is to reduce the number of calories consumed and incorporate lifestyle changes, such as being mindful of portion sizes, which will help control the number of calories consumed. Because exercise can be a helpful addition to a weight loss regimen and is important in weight maintenance, we also encourage a gradual increase in physical activity. The details of these recommendations are addressed in the next section. In addition, we recommend that being overweight and obese be conceptualized as chronic medical conditions. Therefore, like those for other chronic medical problems, such as hypertension and diabetes, intervention plans for weight loss are made both for the short term and long term. The best outcomes are typically consistent, with long-term follow-up care over years, not just months (Wadden et al., 2002). Unlike specialty care, in which an individual might be seen in a group setting for 16 consecutive weeks and then discontinue treatment, the goal in primary care is to establish a program that the individual understands and can self-manage with assistance from the primary care team. Although the visits may be less frequent, they often occur over a longer span of time.

Goal setting. Once patients are motivated to change behaviors, the first step for effective weight loss is to set realistic, doable goals. We set goals with patients that are consistent with the data from the National Heart, Lung, and Blood Institute (1998), which suggest that the best way for them to lose weight and maintain the loss is to lose 1 to 2 pounds per week, with the goal of losing no more than 10% of their current weight in a 6-month period. After those 6 months, they should focus on maintaining their weight loss for another 6 months. Although this may not be as appealing as the rapid weight loss promised in infomercials, patients are often reassured to know that this strategy can result in sustainable weight loss, whereas other plans likely will not. Questions to help patients set realistic goals might include the following: "If you were to lose 10% of your current weight, how many pounds would that be? Would it be realistic to lose 10% of your weight over the next 6 months?"

Calorie education. The second step is to educate patients about the number of calories they need to consume to lose weight effectively. One simple method of estimating calorie needs is to multiply the weight of the individual by a factor of 10 for sedentary individuals, 12 for moderately active individuals, and 14 for very active individuals to determine the number of calories needed to maintain their current weight. For example, a sedentary person weighing 200 pounds would need to consume 2,000 kilocalories a day to maintain their current weight. Although this is just a rough estimate, it provides a good starting place for setting calorie goals. To lose weight at the recommended rate of approximately 1 to 2 pounds per week, the individual would need to consume 500 kilocalories less per day (i.e., 7 days per week × 500 kilocalories = 3,500 kilocalories, which is equivalent to 1 pound). For health and safety reasons, we rarely recommend a goal of less than 1,200 kilocalories a day unless specifically prescribed and monitored by a physician. Finally, we have found that educational materials, such as those in Figure 6.2, can be used to clarify the goal with the patient.

Behavior change planning. Once the number of calories patients should consume is established, the next step is to help identify methods for meeting that calorie goal. One effective method is to encourage daily calorie monitoring using a food diary (Wadden et al., 2002). Using a simple food diary or calorie log and encouraging the purchase of a calorie guide can help patients start to monitor their calorie intake. We suggest patients complete a food diary for 1 week (see Figure 6.3) and then return to discuss the contents to identify eating habits that could be changed.

Patients may find counting calories to be overwhelming or too time consuming. If they demonstrate a reluctance to monitor their calorie intake, reassure them that they can still lose weight by focusing on making behavior changes that will reduce their calorie intake. Reducing their intake of calorie dense foods (e.g., meats) and increasing their intake of fruits, vegetables, and whole grains while reducing portion sizes will reduce their calorie intake. If the patient keeps a food diary, it can help the BHC to make recommendations for changes that are more specific.

Goal Setting for Weight Loss

Recommended weight loss is 10% of one's weight over 6 months.

1. Your current weight is _____ pounds.

2. Your current activity level is: Sedentary (10) Moderately Active (12) Very Active (14)

3. _____ × _____ = _____

    Current weight   Current activity   Total calories needed to
                                                          maintain weight

4. _____ − 500 = _____

    Total calories needed to   (3,500 kilocalories per   Total calories to consume
    maintain weight   pound / 7 days per week)   each day

    If you consume _____ calories every day, you should lose approximately 1 pound per week, which
    is a healthy weight-loss rate.

Total calories to consume each day should not be below 1,200 calories.

FIGURE 6.2. Goal setting for weight loss handout.

Date:_____   **Personal Food Diary**

Time of day	Food or beverage item	Serving size	Estimated calories	Comments (e.g., stressors, eating because of boredom or emotions, high risk eating situations)

Exercise and Activity Log

Type of exercise or activity	Total duration in minutes	Intensity (low, medium, high)	Estimated calories burned	Comments

FIGURE 6.3. Personal food diary handout.

The focus should be on simple changes related to what the patients ate. Suggesting dramatic changes or placing certain foods off-limits may decrease motivation for treatment and the likelihood that the patients will follow through with the changes. Focusing on small, concrete changes may contribute to the belief that a sustained weight loss is possible. Using the information obtained during the assessment can be helpful to point out specific foods that patients could reduce, modify, or eliminate to reduce their calorie intake by 500 calories. For example, by eliminating two non-diet sodas or two beers a day, patients could reduce their caloric intake by approximately 250 to 350 kilocalories. One way to target these changes is to discuss what foods to *cut, add, move, eliminate, or substitute* (i.e., the C.A.M.E.S. approach; McKnight, 2006). A handout to guide this discussion is presented in Figure 6.4. Some questions you can ask include the following: "What foods could you eat less of or modify to help you meet your goal? Are there other foods that you could eat? Is there a sugar-free version of some of the foods that you enjoy? Are there foods you would like to eat more of?"

In addition to recommending changes about what patients eat, it can be helpful to recommend changes to how they eat. Using a handout, such as the one in Figure 6.5, can help to highlight doable behavioral changes. Ultimately, patients should be encouraged to avoid distractions while eating (e.g., eat at a dining room table, avoid watching TV while eating). Distractions during eating may interfere with patients' awareness of how much is eaten and feelings of being full. Reeducating patients about standard serving sizes (e.g., a supersized drink is not a standard serving size) and suggesting the use of their fist or palm as a guide for the serving size of most foods provides a "portable" means for measuring how much they should eat, no matter where they are eating. Slowing eating rates (e.g., placing utensils down between bites) and making food less accessible (e.g., keeping serving dishes off the dining table) give patients more time to

---

The CAMES™ Principle for Improvement (Cut, Add, Move, Eliminate, Substitute)

Evaluate the foods in your diet. Make decisions about what you would like to do with those foods to meet your calorie goals.

TOP 10 FOODS / MENUS IN MY DIET

List of Foods	C.A.M.E.S.
Example: 1. Donuts	1. C & S
2. Vegetables	2. A
1.	1.
2.	2.
3.	3.
4.	4.
5.	5.
6.	6.
7.	7.
8.	8.
9.	9.
10.	10.

FIGURE 6.4. The CAMES™ Principle for Improvement handout. From *Obesity Management in Family Practice* (p. 33), by T. L. McKnight, 2006. Copyright 2006 by Springer Publishing Company. Reprinted with permission.

Modifying Eating Habits

1. Do nothing else while eating.
2. Eat in the same place each time.
3. Do not clean your plate.
4. Eat on a schedule.
5. Slow your eating rate. Put your fork down between bites. Pause during the meal.
6. When shopping for food, shop on a full stomach, shop from a list, and get foods that require preparation.
7. When storing foods, store high-calorie foods out of sight ("Out of sight, out of mouth") and keep healthy snacks available.
8. When serving and dispensing food,
   - Remove serving dishes from the table
   - Leave the table after eating
   - Serve and eat one portion at a time
   - Wait 5 minutes before getting second servings
   - Avoid dispensing (serving) food
9. When eating away from home,
   - Order a la carte meals
   - Watch the salad dressing
   - Beware of the breadbasket
   - Be wise with dessert
   - Share your meal with your friend/spouse/partner
   - Take a portion of the meal home to eat at another time

FIGURE 6.5. Modifying eating habits handout.

become aware of being full, meaning they will likely eat less.

Situations typically associated with unhealthy eating (e.g., buffets, parties) cannot be avoided completely, so identifying simple, concrete methods for modifying the situation may help to reduce unplanned eating. For example, eating at restaurants may be particularly difficult for some patients. Encouraging them to split their meals with someone, to place half of their meal in a take-out container, and avoid having bread on the table could reduce unwanted eating. Similarly, some may find that they eat more when they are stressed or when they experience heightened emotions, such as anxiety or depression. Discussing methods for delaying eating and engaging in alternative behaviors (e.g., relaxation techniques) may be helpful for decreasing the likelihood that they will eat as a way to distract themselves from unwanted emotions.

Physical activity, which is discussed more extensively in the next section, is another important component of an effective weight loss/maintenance program. Research suggests that although physical activity may be helpful, but not necessary, for initial weight loss, it plays an important role in the maintenance of weight loss (King, Haskell, Young, Oka, & Stefanick, 1995; Perri, Martin, Leermakers, Sears, & Notelovitz, 1997; Pronk & Wing, 1994). In our experience, it has been helpful to encourage patients to modify their activity level throughout the day as an initial first step as opposed to developing a specialized exercise program.

Arrange.   After you have met with patients one or two times to assess the problem and start a behavior change plan, determine how and when the patient will follow up. The purpose of these follow-up appointments is to assess progress, resolve difficult situations or lapses, and possibly introduce a new skill (e.g., communication). Initially (i.e., for the first 2–4 weeks), it may be helpful to meet with the patient on a weekly basis to assess progress and eliminate barriers to sticking to the established plan. At each appointment, the patient's weight should be recorded and compared with the previous weight. Throughout the remainder of the 6 months, monthly appointments may be possible for maintaining weight loss progress. However, given the patient loads in primary care settings, it is impractical in terms of time and cost to maintain the

frequency of such visits with the PCP or yourself; therefore, consider health care extenders (e.g., nurses, medical technicians) and alternative methods (e.g., telephone contact) to help meet the needs of patients as they progress with their weight loss plan.

Once individuals have lost 10% of their initial weight, the focus of the plan should turn to maintaining their weight loss by continuing to implement the behavior changes they have found to be successful. Again, the primary care environment provides an ideal setting in which individuals can continue to monitor and maintain their weight loss. If weight is managed similar to other chronic illnesses, such as hypertension and diabetes, regular check-in appointments can be scheduled to help ensure that individuals are maintaining their weight loss and help them deal with lapses. Each individual will have different requirements regarding the frequency of their follow-up appointments (e.g., monthly, quarterly, semi-annually). To help patients recognize when they are having difficulty managing their weight, it may be useful to use a handout, such as the one in Figure 6.6, which establishes zones of care. If an individual is in the green zone, that is, they are at or below target weight, they should continue with their lifestyle. If they find that they are entering the yellow zone or the red zone (i.e., they are above their target weight), they may need to change their lifestyle or schedule an appointment with their PCP.

Individuals should be considered for management in specialty mental health care if binging and/or purging behaviors do not resolve or their BMI exceeds 40 (or 35 if they are managing multiple, serious weight-related medical problems). Individuals in this weight range may be appropriate for surgical interventions (National Institutes of Health, 1991; Saltzman et al., 2005) or may need the closer contact that a specialty mental health care setting can provide. Individuals who do not lose weight after a primary care intervention should also be considered for specialty mental health referral.

PHYSICAL INACTIVITY

Physical inactivity is not only a significant contributing factor to some of the most prevalent diseases (e.g., Mokdad et al., 2004; Paffenbarger, Hyde,

---

Weight Maintenance

Zones for timely intervention before weight is regained.

Green Zone

Minimal monitoring (within 4 pounds of your target weight).

  If your weight is in the green zone, then simply monitor your weight periodically (e.g., once a week). Maintain your current eating and physical activity habits.

Yellow Zone

Adjust either eating behavior or physical activity (within 7 pounds of your target weight).

  If your weight enters the yellow zone, then it is time to consider modifying your calorie intake or your physical activity levels, to use more energy.

Red Zone

Adjust both eating behavior and physical activity; consider follow-up appointment with provider (more than 7 pounds above your target weight).

  If your weight enters the red zone, consider modifying your calorie intake and your physical activity level. You may want to consider coming back to the clinic to get assistance if you have difficulty making these changes.

My Zones

Green: _____ to _____ (Maintain current eating and physical activity habits)

Yellow: _____ to _____ (Decrease calorie intake **or** increase physical activity)

Red: _____ or higher   (Decrease calorie intake **and** increase physical activity)

FIGURE 6.6. **Weight maintenance handout. Adapted from** *Obesity Management in Family Practice* (p. 132), **by T. L. McKnight, 2005, New York. Springer Publishing. Copyright 2005 by T. L. McKnight. Adapted with permission.**

Wing, & Hsieh, 1986), including cardiovascular disease, hypertension, obesity, and colon cancer but there is also growing evidence that increasing physical activity improves mental health disorders such as depression (Blumenthal et al., 2007; Palmer, 2005). To improve the health of the nation, multiple health organizations, including the U.S. Surgeon General, CDC, and the American College of Sports Medicine (Pate et al., 1995; U.S. Department of Health and Human Services, 1996) have recommended that individuals engage in at least 30 minutes of moderate physical activity most days; however, only 25% of Americans achieve that level of activity (CDC, 2001). In 2007, the American College of Sports Medicine and the American Heart Association updated recommendations for physical activity for adults (Haskell et al., 2007) and older adults (Nelson et al., 2007). These organizations continued to promote 30 minutes of moderate physical exercise at least 5 days a week or vigorous exercise 20 minutes a day 3 days a week; however, they also introduced a new recommendation that adults engage in activities that maintain or increase muscular strength or endurance at least 2 days a week (Haskell et al., 2007). To enhance weight control, even higher levels of physical activity (i.e., 60–90 minutes per day of moderate to vigorous activity) are needed (Jakicic et al., 2001; U.S. Department of Health and Human Services & U.S. Department of Agriculture, 2005).

Specialty Mental Health

Research on ways to increase physical activity has not been a focus in specialty mental health. Instead, more research has been done on community interventions. Kahn et al. (2002) conducted a systematic review of interventions designed to increase physical activity, such as point of decision prompts (e.g., signs by elevators to encourage using the stairs), communitywide campaigns, mass media campaigns, classroom-based interventions, increasing social support, individually adapted behavior change programs, and environmental and policy changes. Among the interventions that the authors determined had strong evidence supporting use was individually adapted behavior change programs, suggesting that working individually with patients is one important way to target physical activity levels in the population.

Behavioral Health in Primary Care

Findings have been mixed regarding the effectiveness of behavioral counseling in primary care to promote physical activity. Physician counseling increased physical activity in several studies (e.g., Calfas et al., 1996; Elley, Kerse, Arroll, & Robinson, 2003) but produced no such effect in others (e.g., Norris, Grothaus, Buchner, & Pratt, 2000). These mixed findings contributed to the conclusion that there is insufficient evidence to recommend or not recommend behavioral counseling in primary care settings to promote physical activity (United States Preventive Services Task Force, 2002a). Therefore, unlike tobacco use, it is unclear which interventions to use in primary care and whether physical activity can be effectively targeted in this setting. A review of cognitive and behavioral interventions used in primary care settings found that education and feedback about physical activity guidelines, advice, and self-monitoring can increase physical activity among adults (Smitherman, Kendzor, Grothe, & Dubbert, 2007).

Primary Care Adaptation

On the basis of the evidence that individual counseling using cognitive and behavioral strategies can help increase physical activity, we discuss ways that we have incorporated these skills into primary care settings. Before encouraging increases in physical activity, ensure that the patient's PCP has medically cleared the patient for increased activity levels. In addition to these recommendations, the American Academy of Family Physicians has developed the American in Motion (AIM) program (http://www.aafp.org/online/en/home/clinical/publichealth/aim/foryouroffice.html) which has many resources for the primary care environment.

Assess. Individuals often equate physical activity and exercise. The term *exercise* may conjure up images of sweaty, burly men groaning as they lift hundreds of pounds in a smelly gym. This may not be an appealing image to many patients; therefore, we use the term *physical activity* when discussing ways to increase activity levels.

Unlike tobacco use and weight, which are parts of standard assessments in primary care, physical inactivity is not assessed as a routine measure of physical functioning. In addition, there are no medications or medical interventions that can increase an individual's physical activity. Most likely, a patient will be identified as sedentary during the assessment of other chronic conditions, such as diabetes or hypertension, rather than receiving a specific referral to help the patient increase his or her physical activity. To begin assessing physical activity you could ask, "What do you do for physical activity? Do you participate in any individual or team physical activities, such as basketball, running, tennis, or swimming? Do you go to the gym?"

It can also be informative to assess whether the patient has ever engaged in physical activities. When we are developing the most effective ways to assist patients with increasing physical activity, it can be helpful to build on what they have already done. So you could ask, "Was there ever a time when you engaged in more physical activities? What activities did you participate in? Did you enjoy those activities?"

Often patients will point to housecleaning or walking around at their job as evidence that they are engaging in sufficient physical activity. It is important to determine whether these activities would actually be classified as a moderate (i.e., the equivalent walking at 3.0 miles per hour) or vigorous (e.g., walking at a brisk pace of 4.5 miles per hour or faster; look to the Centers for Disease Control and Prevention at http://www.cdc.gov/nccdphp/dnpa/physical/pdf/PA_Intensity_table_2_1.pdf for examples of moderate and vigorous activities). You could ask, "What activities do you do that you would consider moderate or vigorous? Do you notice your heart rate increasing when you are doing those activities?"

Once you know what activities individuals are engaging in, it is helpful to assess the duration and frequency of those activities. Patients may over-estimate the amount of time that they engage in these activities or the distance involved, so it may be informative to ask how they know how much time they are engaged in the activity or how far they go. For example, you could ask the following:

> How much time do you spend walking outside? When do you engage in moder-ate or vigorous activity? How long do you engage in that activity? Is there any-thing that you do to make sure that you engage in that activity (e.g., walk with a friend or family member, walk a pet)? Have you measured the distance? Do you keep track of the time on your watch?

There are brief assessment measures that are available to help obtain a standard assessment of physical activity, such as the Rapid Assessment of Physical Activity (RAPA; University of Washington Health Promotion Research Center, n.d.) and the International Physical Activity Questionnaire (Booth, 2000). The RAPA has been recommended for use in primary care to screen for physical activity levels (Topolski et al., 2006). The RAPA has good sensitiv-ity (81%) but lower specificity (69%) in a sample of older adults for distinguishing exercisers from non-exercisers. The RAPA and scoring instructions can be downloaded for clinical use from (http://depts. washington.edu/hprc/docs/rapa_03_06.pdf). The International Physical Activity Questionnaire has been used throughout the world to assess physical activity across cultures and nations.

Advise. Usually, we advise individuals to increase their physical activity as a way of helping them to manage other conditions, such as depres-sion, hypertension, insomnia, overweight, obesity, or stress management. For individuals who are overweight or obese, increased physical fitness may help protect against all-cause and cardio-vascular disease mortality (Lee, Blair, & Jackson, 1999), even if they are not able to engage in a level of physical activity that would help them lose weight. Our focus during the advise period is to inform patients about recommended goals for physical activity and let them know that we are

looking for ways that they may be able to build on what they already do. Therefore, we could say the following:

> To help you improve your health and to help you avoid developing significant health problems, we know that it is important for you to engage in a moder-ate activity for 30 minutes at least 5 times per week or a vigorous activity for 20 minutes at least 3 times per week. In addition, for optimal health, it is important to discuss ways to engage in muscle strengthening exercises 2 times per week. We don't have to start at these levels, but we can work together to figure out a plan of how to get there. We want to build on what you are already doing and figure ways to incorporate physical activity into your daily life.

It is also important to set realistic expectations. Physical activity, by itself, may not lower blood pressure, decrease weight, or improve glucose con-trol, but it is an important aspect of managing health, so you might say the following:

> We know that physical activity is one of the most important behaviors for overall health. Physical activity can help manage your (hypertension/ diabetes/weight/etc.). It will be important to take an activity that you enjoy and gradually try to increase the amount of time that you engage in that activity. We may not see immediate changes in your (hypertension/diabetes/ weight/etc.), but in the long run you will be healthier and you may help prevent this condition from getting worse.

Agree. In the agree phase, we evaluate whether patients accept that increasing physical activity would be important for them. As with tobacco use and weight, assessing importance, confidence, and patients' readiness to change are important aspects of determining whether patients are interested in changing their physical activity. Ultimately, you want to know whether patients want to discuss a plan for targeting their physical activity. Thus, you could ask the following:

> I've talked about how increasing physical activity could help you manage your blood pressure and weight. Do you think it would be valuable for us to take some time to discuss how you might be able to increase your physical activity?

Assist.   Figure 6.7 can be used as handout that might be useful when setting the patient's activity plan.

Identify the activity.   The first step in the assist phase is to identify how the individual is going to increase his or her physical activity. We then discuss different options that we could consider for increas-

ing physical activity. The individual may be engaging in an activity but not at the frequency or duration that is recommended, so we can easily discuss ways to increase the frequency or duration of those activities. If individuals have previously engaged in an activity or sport or if they previously used a gym, then we might discuss how they could reinitiate that activity. Figure 6.7 is provided as an educational handout that can be used while developing the activity plan. We find it easiest to build on what someone is doing or what they have done in the recent past. Therefore, we might say, "You indicated that you used to play tennis with your neighborhood friend. Is that something you think you might be interested in starting again?" If the person has not regularly engaged in physical activity, we might say the following:

> It doesn't sound like you regularly engaged in a physical activity in the past. One of the easiest activities to start is walking. Is that something you might be interested in starting? If not, are there other physical activities you would consider increasing? We can talk about ways to integrate walking into your daily activities.

Some individuals may have difficulty leaving the home to engage in physical activities (e.g., a parent with a small child). In those situations, it is necessary to identify activities in the home, such as DVD-guided activities (e.g., home aerobics) that can be used to facilitate physical activity.

Set specific goals.   Once you've identified the activity or multiple activities in which the patient is going to engage, it is necessary to set specific goals about when and how long the patient will engage in the activities. We find it useful to establish the days when they will engage in the activity and then gradually increase the duration of the activity. We ask the following:

> To ensure that you get in 5 days of walking, which days of the week are generally going to be the best days for you to walk? What time during the day

---

Increasing Physical Activity

Do you need to change?

Individuals who engage in at least 30 minutes of moderate physical activity at least 5 days a week are healthier overall compared with those who do less physical activity. If keeping extra weight off is important to you, then 60 to 90 minutes of moderate activity might be an important goal. Examples of moderate physical activities include brisk walking, riding a bicycle, and raking leaves. You might think it would be difficult to find 30 minutes, much less 90 minutes, to engage in physical activity or exercise.

How do you change?

Check with your physician. Make sure you physician has given you the OK.

Have fun. Choose an activity that you enjoy.

Set goals—short term and long term. Specify days, times activities, and duration.

Start slowly and gradually increase. Generally you don't want to increase by more than 10% each week.

Track your progress. This will help you to know whether you are staying on your plan.

Have a plan B. If you are planning to do you physical activity outside, what are you going to do if the weather is bad outside? What about on vacation? How about during the holidays? Think ahead about the week and consider what you can do to meet your goals if something (e.g., bad weather) gets in the way.

Reward yourself. When you meet your goals, reward yourself.

FIGURE 6.7.   **Increasing physical activity handout.**

are you going to walk? How long are
you going to walk?

Once we establish a plan for starting the activity, we discuss how the patient will gradually increase their activity level as follows:

> We've agreed that you will walk each
> weekday for 10 minutes at 7:00 a.m. It
> will be important to gradually increase
> the amount of time you are walking.
> Would it be reasonable to increase your
> walking by 2 minutes each week?

The rate of increase should be gradual and at a rate that the patient can sustain.

Measure progress. The simplest way to have patients measure their progress is to write down the days and the duration of their planned physical activity on a tracking form. Increasingly, pedometers are also being used to help monitor and promote physical activity. Pedometers can provide immediate and objective feedback regarding the number of steps taken by an individual. One method of attaining the recommended 30 minutes of physical activity is to accumulate 10,000 steps per day (Hatano, 1993; Wilde, Sidman, & Corbin, 2001). Relying on a step count with the feedback of a pedometer may be a more reliable method of increasing physical activity than suggesting individuals walk for 30 minutes. Hultquist, Albright, and Thompson (2005) found that inactive women who were told to walk 10,000 steps and who were provided with a pedometer walked more compared with those who were told to take a brisk 30-minute walk and were not provided with feedback about how far they had walked. Inexpensive, valid pedometers can be found for less than $20 (Schneider, Crouter, & Bassett, 2004).

Prevent relapse. As with other behaviors, individuals are likely to lapse and not engage in their physical activity as they planned. We discuss with the patient foreseeable barriers to engaging in the physical activity and what the patient will do if they miss a day of the physical activity. In this case, we would say the following:

> Is there anything coming up that might
> get in the way of you walking when you

are planning to walk? What will you do if you miss a day of walking? Sometimes it is useful to establish a make-up day; that is, a day when you would walk if you couldn't walk one day. So, for you, would it make sense to set Saturday as your make up day? What time would be the best time for you to walk on Saturday if you missed a day during the week?

Alternatively, you could establish another time during the day to walk, so if the patient did not walk at 7:00 a.m., he or she would plan to walk after work at 5:00 p.m. It is most important to take time to discuss a plan to help prevent a lapse from become a total collapse of the physical activity plan.

Arrange. As with other health behavior changes, following up with patients to assess progress is critical. We find it helpful to briefly meet with patients soon after starting an increase in physical activity (e.g., 1–2 weeks). If there are problems starting the program, we spend time discussing how to overcome those barriers. For individuals who appear to be doing well, we recommend following up in about a month with the primary care team to ensure that progress is continuing. We encourage the PCP to ask the patient about his or her physical activity levels at each follow-up appointment.

It is unlikely that most individuals will need specialty care to target physical activity. Of course, as we mentioned, other, more serious chronic medical conditions might necessitate referral to a specialty care setting. Patients who are interested in starting an exercise program would likely benefit from meeting with an exercise specialist who could help develop a specialized program.

SUMMARY

In the end, the time spent on targeting health behavior changes will likely save time in the future as chronic medical conditions may be avoided or more easily managed. Similar approaches to health behavior change can be used regardless of the health behavior. Informing patients of the need to change, assessing and enhancing patients' motivation to change, developing a change and relapse prevention plan, tracking changes, and establishing follow-up appointments in the clinic to help monitor progress will likely help patients change a behavior, whether it is tobacco use, overeating, or physical inactivity.

Lack of training and lack of time hinders a PCP's ability to begin these changes with patients. Behavioral health professionals integrated into primary care can enhance the effectiveness of the primary care team in targeting the health behaviors that are the most significant contributors to morbidity and mortality.

CHAPTER 7

DIABETES

In the United States, 9.6% of the entire population and 20.9% of adults 60 years of age or older have diabetes (National Institute of Diabetes and Digestive and Kidney Diseases [NIDDK], 2005). The prevalence of diabetes is considerably higher among non-Hispanic Blacks (1.8 times), Hispanic/Latino Americans (1.7 times), and American Indians and Alaska Natives (2.2 times), compared with non-Hispanic White counterparts (NIDDK, 2005). Diabetes was the sixth leading cause of death in the United States in 2004 and is associated with multiple complications, including heart disease, strokes, high blood pressure, blindness, kidney disease, nervous system disease, amputations, dental disease, and complicated pregnancies (Centers for Disease Control and Prevention [CDC], 2005). In the United States, the estimated 1-year cost of diabetes is $174 billion, without considering the costs associated with pain and suffering, nonpaid caregivers, and undiagnosed diabetes (CDC, 2005).

Diabetes is frequently diagnosed by measuring fasting blood glucose levels. Glucose is a sugar that cells need for energy. After one eats, pancreatic β-cells stimulate the secretion of insulin, which facilitates the transport of glucose into cells. The amount of glucose that stays in the blood is determined by how much insulin is available to transport glucose to the cells and whether there is a sufficient number of receptors on the cells to allow the glucose to enter. An insufficient number of cell receptors results in *insulin resistance* and increases blood glucose levels. If a person's fasting blood glucose level is higher than 126 mg/dl, the person is diagnosed with diabetes; a fasting blood glucose

level between 100 mg/dl and 125 mg/dl indicates prediabetes.

Diabetes is classified into four major groups: Type 1, Type 2, gestational, and other causes. Type 1 diabetes, previously known as insulin-dependent diabetes mellitus or juvenile-onset diabetes, accounts for approximately 5% to 10% of diabetes cases (American Diabetes Association [ADA], 2007a). Type 1 diabetes is caused by the autoimmune destruction of β-cells in the pancreas. The destruction of β-cells can happen rapidly or quite slowly; therefore, although Type 1 diabetes is typically diagnosed in childhood or adolescence, it may not be diagnosed until much later in life (ADA, 2007a). Individuals with Type 1 diabetes typically require exogenous insulin for survival.

Individuals with Type 2 diabetes, previously referred to as noninsulin dependent diabetes or adult-onset diabetes, demonstrate some insulin resistance but typically do not initially demonstrate absolute insulin deficiency. These individuals represent 90% to 95% of all diagnosed diabetes cases (ADA, 2007a). People with Type 2 diabetes do not always need to take injectable insulin and can often manage their diabetes through healthy eating, weight loss, increasing physical activity, and oral medications.

Gestational diabetes is diagnosed in women who demonstrate glucose intolerance after becoming pregnant (Expert Committee on the Diagnosis and Classification of Diabetes Mellitus, 1997). On average, 7% of all pregnancies are associated with gestational diabetes (ADA, 2008). There is evidence that maternal, fetal, and neonatal risks increase as maternal glycemia increases at 24 to 28 weeks of pregnancy

(ADA, 2008). For the fetus, the major risk is that it will grow to a larger than normal size and may experience hypoglycemia after it is born. Women with a history of gestational diabetes are at a greater risk of developing Type 2 diabetes later in life.

Other types of diabetes can result from genetic conditions, malnutrition, surgery, medication, and other illnesses. The remainder of this chapter focuses primarily on Type 2 diabetes, because this type of diabetes is most often managed in the primary care setting.

KEY BIOPSYCHOSOCIAL FACTORS IN TYPE 2 DIABETES

A behavioral health consultant (BHC) should be familiar with Type 2 diabetes because of how common it is in primary care. Considering the biopsychosocial factors that affect and that are affected by diabetes can help BHCs more effectively use the 5A's.

Physical Factors

Patients with diabetes must manage their blood glucose levels to avoid becoming hypo- or hyperglycemic. Hypoglycemia (i.e., blood glucose <60 mg/dl) may result in increased heart rate, headaches, hunger, shakiness, sweating, decreased concentration, mood changes, and confusion. If untreated, it may lead to coma and death. Conversely, hyperglycemia (i.e., blood glucose >140 mg/dl) results in increased thirst, increased urination frequency, and glucose in the urine. People with diabetes typically notice the symptoms of hypoglycemia and take corrective action to raise blood sugars to normal levels. However, symptoms of hyperglycemia may not be noticed. Unless the patient identifies hyperglycemia through monitoring of blood sugar, the levels may remain high for extended periods, leading to the development of future complications.

Over the long term, the hyperglycemia associated with undiagnosed or inadequately managed diabetes can result in macrovascular and microvascular diseases. Macrovascular problems result in increased risk of heart disease, stroke, and high blood pressure. The microvascular problems contribute to the development of blindness, kidney failure, and neuropathy, which in turn contribute to pain, loss of feeling, and

possibly paralysis. To measure how well patients manage their blood sugars, physicians examine a patient's glycated hemoglobin, technically their HbA1c, but usually referred to as their *A1c* level. This test, rather than measuring current blood sugar level, yields information regarding average blood sugar control in the preceding 2 to 3 months and thus is a good measure of how well the patient has been managing his or her diabetes. Although the ADA recommends that patients maintain A1c levels below 7, this may be challenging for some patients with diabetes (Qaseem et al., 2007).

The risk of diabetes is increased in overweight and obese individuals who are insulin-resistant; however, weight loss is associated with decreased risk (ADA, 2007a). Compared with normal weight individuals, those who were overweight were 1.59 times more likely to have diabetes, whereas those with a body mass index above 40 were 7.37 times more likely to have diabetes (Mokdad et al., 2003).

Currently there are five types of medications used to treat diabetes, including sulfonylureas (e.g., Glucotrol, Micronase), metformin (e.g., Glucophage), troglitazone (e.g., Rezulin), alpha-glucosidase inhibitors (e.g., Precose, Glyset), and repaglinide (e.g., Prandin; Florence & Yeager, 1999). These medications may affect insulin production, the body's sensitivity to insulin, or change blood sugar absorption.

Emotional and Cognitive Factors

Individuals with diabetes may be at greater risk of depressive symptoms (Anderson, Freeland, Clouse, & Lustman, 2001; Eaton, 2002; Golden et al., 2007; Nichols & Brown, 2003). Depressive symptoms interfere with self-management, decrease the likelihood of maintaining physical activity, and increase social isolation (Ciechanowski, Katon, Russo, & Hirsch, 2003). In addition, depression may be an independent risk factor for the development of diabetes (Golden et al., 2008; Lustman, Penckofer, & Clouse, 2007). The evidence for a relation between anxiety and diabetes is less strong. One systematic review suggested that 14% of patients with diabetes will experience generalized anxiety disorder and 40% will experience elevated anxiety symptoms (Grigsby, Anderson, Freedland, Clouse, & Lustman, 2002). Stress has also been linked to diabetes. The data regarding the relationship of stress and the onset of diabetes have been mixed and inconclusive; however, stress appears to negatively affect the control of diabetes (Lloyd, Smith, & Weinger, 2005). In patients with Type 2 diabetes, stress increases blood glucose levels (Surwit & Schneider, 1993) and is related to decreased self-management behaviors (e.g., poorer diet, physical inactivity; Albright, Parchman, Burge, & the RRNeSt Investigators, 2001). Stress management techniques have been shown to improve glycemic control in patients with diabetes (Surwit et al., 2002).

Behavioral Factors

The development and course of diabetes, particularly Type 2 diabetes, is strongly related to multiple behavioral factors including blood glucose monitoring, dietary habits, physical activity, and medication adherence. Regular blood glucose monitoring is necessary to maintain a healthy blood glucose range. Older, less accurate, methods of monitoring blood glucose levels involved the use of urine dipsticks. Today, most use small devices that analyze the glucose content in small amounts of blood, typically one drop obtained through pricking a finger. Patients may need to test their blood sugar from one to seven or more times per day. According to the ADA (2007b), managing nutritional intake is important for preventing and managing diabetes. Monitoring and limiting carbohydrate intake is a vital diabetes management strategy, but restricting total carbohydrates to less than 130 grams/day is not recommended (ADA, 2007b). In addition, saturated fat and dietary cholesterol should be limited because of the increased risk of cardiovascular disease from diabetes. If an adult with diabetes consumes alcohol, total intake should be limited to moderate amounts (i.e., one standard drink per day or less for women; two standard drinks per day or less for men). In addition, other health behaviors, including medication adherence, physical inactivity, and tobacco use can all affect blood glucose levels and the progression of diabetes.

In addition to health behaviors, patients with diabetes must monitor their feet, eyes, and renal function for complications related to the progression of the disease. Neuropathy and peripheral vascular disease place patients with diabetes at increased risk of ulcers and undetected wounds, particularly on their feet. Patients are asked to check their feet to identify cuts or sores that could become infected if they are not caught early. In addition, patients are instructed to always wear shoes that fit well, wash and dry their feet daily, maintain healthy nail care, and avoid skin removal. Diabetic retinopathy is the leading cause of blindness in patients 20 to 74 years of age. Damaged blood vessels associated with diabetic retinopathy can result in blood or fluid leakage in the eye, which can lead to impaired vision and blindness. Kidney functioning must also be regularly monitored for evidence of kidney disease. To accomplish all of these evaluations, patients with diabetes are often required to make multiple appointments with physicians.

Diabetes management may require patients to adhere to multiple and sometimes complex medication and insulin regimens. Medication and/or insulin (CDC, 2005) is prescribed for 85% of individuals with diabetes, but adherence to medication regimens is often poor (Donnan, MacDonald, & Morris, 2002) and depressive symptoms further impair adherence (Kilbourne et al., 2005). There is insufficient evidence to suggest that any particular intervention increases adherence to medication treatment recommendations in adults with Type 2 diabetes over the long term (Vermeire et al., 2005). Therefore, it is important for providers to regularly monitor adherence to diabetes medications and consider multiple strategies for improving adherence.

Environmental Factors

Social support is an important factor in the management of diabetes. Significant others in the patient's life may be overly critical or fail to support the patient in the multiple behavior changes necessary, particularly food choices. Job flexibility and finances may limit the patient's ability to attend appointments, buy appropriate foods, or purchase glucose monitoring equipment.

Management Demands

The complexity and duration of the physical, emotional, behavioral, and environmental factors of diabetes self-management can make it one of the most challenging chronic illnesses to manage (Glasgow &

Nutting, 2004). The amount of effort required to manage different components can vary considerably from patient to patient and within patients over time. Nonadherence is one of the most common reasons for which a patient is referred to a behavioral health provider (Glasgow & Nutting, 2004). However, nonadherence as a global patient trait may not be accurate, and the behavioral health provider often can have the greatest effect by focusing on specific lifestyle factors or management behaviors (Glasgow & Nutting, 2004). In addition, targeting problem-solving skills may help patients improve the management of their diabetes (Glasgow, Fisher, Skaff, Mullan, & Toobert, 2007).

SPECIALTY MENTAL HEALTH TREATMENT

Intensive lifestyle interventions that include dietary, physical activity, and behavioral interventions improve the management and decrease the risk of diabetes incidence in people identified with prediabetes (Diabetes Control and Complications Trial Research Group, 1993; Diabetes Prevention Program Research Group, 2002; Gillies et al., 2007; Norris et al., 2005). A review of heterogeneous interventions demonstrated that teaching self-management strategies can improve the health behaviors and physiological outcomes associated with diabetes over a 6-month period (Norris, Engelgau, & Narayan, 2001). Helping patients with diabetes make changes in their diet or lose weight is frequently a target of treatment. However, a review examining the effect of type of dietary advice (e.g., low fat, low glycemic index, low carbohydrate, low calorie, very low calorie) on diabetes outcomes concluded that there were not enough high quality studies on which to draw firm conclusions to guide practice (Nield et al., 2007). Thus, there is not one universally recommended diet with diabetic patients; rather, different primary care providers (PCPs) and dietitians recommend a variety of eating plans.

The Look AHEAD study, which is a multicenter, randomized controlled trial examining whether weight loss and increased physical activity in a sample of patients with Type 2 diabetes reduces their cardiovascular morbidity and mortality may provide additional information about the benefits of lifestyle changes and how to achieve and maintain those changes in specialty care settings (The Look AHEAD Research Group, 2006). However, in current practice, fewer than 50% of patients with diabetes attend diabetes education or behavioral change classes, and behavioral interventions have often not been integrated into diabetes care (Fisher & Glasgow, 2007). Integrating behavioral health consultants (BHCs) into primary care is one method for bringing behavioral interventions to more patients with diabetes.

BEHAVIORAL HEALTH IN PRIMARY CARE

Diabetes is the fifth most common diagnosis in outpatient medical settings (Hing, Cherry, & Woodwell, 2006). Medical management of Type 2 diabetes in primary care settings, even with the use of dietitians and diabetes educators, results in less than half of the patients with diabetes reaching targets for glycemic control (Spann et al., 2006). It is challenging for PCPs to meet the standards of care necessary for patients with diabetes (Parchman, Romero, & Pugh, 2006), particularly with regard to education and encouragement of self-management activities (Glasgow & Strycker, 2000).

Interventions for developing self-care behaviors can be adapted for the fast pace of primary care (Peyrot & Rubin, 2007). Integrating education and behavioral interventions for diabetes into primary care improves control of diabetes (Ridgeway et al., 1999). Also, the use of depression care managers and intensive primary care-based interventions for depression has been shown to decrease death rates in diabetes patients over a 5-year period (Bogner, Morales, Post, & Bruce, 2007) and are cost-effective (Katon et al., 2008; Simon et al., 2007). Diabetes interventions in primary care can be as effective as interventions provided in specialty mental health settings; however, primary care interventions affect more people and can be comparatively more cost-effective (Glasgow, Nelson, Strycker, & King, 2006). Overall, there is good evidence to suggest that the biopsychosocial factors that contribute to diabetes can be targeted effectively in primary care settings.

PRIMARY CARE ADAPTATION

BHCs can use evidence-based assessments and interventions to integrate behavioral science more effectively into primary care, as recommended by Fisher and Glasgow (2007). In addition, BHCs can facilitate ongoing contact with patients with diabetes to improve the long-term effectiveness of these interventions. We focus on how BHCs can help PCPs improve the management of physiological factors, reduce emotional distress, and facilitate health behaviors in their patients with diabetes.

Assess

Assessment of patients with diabetes should include questions regarding the key biopsychosocial factors relevant to diabetes, with a focus on modifiable risk factors. In addition, obtaining information regarding the patient's goals for change, as well as what the PCP believes the patient needs to change, helps guide the intervention process.

Modifiable Risk Factors

Physical factors. Potentially modifiable risk factors that are physical or biological in nature include the following:

- high blood pressure,
- problems with overweight or obesity,
- frequency of hyperglycemia and hypoglycemia, and
- HbA1c levels.

To assess these areas, we recommend initially reviewing the medical record for information regarding medical history, particularly high blood pressure, HbA1c test results, and any documentation related to problems with hypoglycemia. We then ask patients additional questions, such as the following:

- In a typical day, how many times do you measure your blood sugar level?
- In a typical week, how many times do your blood sugar levels run too high?
- In a typical week, how may times do your blood sugar levels get too low?
- Have you had any serious problems, such as car accidents or passing out because of low blood sugars?

- What medications are you taking? What difficulties are you having with your medications?

Emotional and cognitive factors. Assessing emotional and cognitive factors relevant to diabetes involves questioning the patient about the presence of problems with depression, anxiety, worry, stress, and anger. The Diabetes Distress Scale 2 (DDS2; Fisher, Glasgow, Mullan, Skaff, & Polonsky, 2008) is a two-item screening measure derived from the full-scale Diabetes Distress Scale 17 (DDS17; Polonsky et al., 2005) and is useful for screening for emotional distress in patients with diabetes. The DDS2 has a respectable .95 sensitivity and .87 specificity relative to the DDS17 classification of patients reporting low or high distress (Fisher et al., 2008).

In the assessment, we focus most attention on potential problems with depression, anxiety, and general distress because these emotional problems are most commonly associated with diabetes. In addition to gathering information about the presence of emotional problems, we ask questions to evaluate the effect these problems have on the management of diabetes. For example, we might ask the following:

> You described feeling quite a bit of sadness over the past few months. How has this affected your ability to stick with your plans to change your diet and to exercise more? How else has it affected your management of your diabetes or your weight?

Alternatively, for a patient with high levels of worry about the consequences of diabetes, we might say the following:

> You mentioned that you worry a lot about your diabetes and the possible health complications that you might develop in the future. Some people find that this kind of thinking helps keep them "on track" with managing their diabetes. Others find that worry about diabetes leads to difficulty managing their health. They may avoid checking blood sugars for fear that they are too high or not follow up with medical

appointments to avoid hearing bad news. How has worry affected your diabetes management?

Behavioral factors. Assessment of behavioral factors focuses on the following major areas: eating patterns (i.e., particularly carbohydrate intake patterns, saturated fat, and cholesterol), current and past strategies for managing weight, habits related to monitoring blood sugars (e.g., timing, frequency), response taken when blood sugar readings are too high or too low, medication adherence, physical activity, and use of tobacco and alcohol. In addition, we ask about adherence to recommendations regarding foot care and various medical appointments (e.g., eye checks). The Summary of Diabetes Self-Care Activities (SDSCA; Toobert, Hampson, & Glasgow, 2000), although a long measure to use consistently in a primary care environment, may be useful as a systematic tool to screen for diabetes-related health behaviors or to guide assessment questions.

Chapters 6 and 12 contain suggestions for assessing diet and weight, physical activity, and tobacco and alcohol use. The following are some examples of questions we might ask to assess other behavioral factors specific to diabetes management:

■ How often do you check your blood sugar level?

■ What times of day do you typically check your blood sugar?

■ What gets in the way of checking your blood sugar as often as your primary care provider recommends?

■ Have you noticed any patterns related to high or low blood sugar levels (e.g., time of day, physical activity, eating habits)?

■ What do you do when your blood sugar reading is too high?

■ What do you do when your blood sugar reading is too low?

■ Has your primary care provider or diabetes nurse educator recommended a specific eating plan for you? If so, can you describe it for me (i.e., carbohydrate counting, exchange diet, low-fat diet, low-calorie diet)?

■ When was the last time you checked your feet for cracks or sores?

■ When was your last diabetic eye exam?

■ What problems, if any, are you having with your medications? How difficult is it to take them as your primary care provider recommends?

Environmental factors. Environmental risk factor assessment largely focuses on the presence and quality of social support. We gather information about the patient's perception of the amount and quality of the support they receive from their partner and family. We might ask, for example, how family members support their efforts to change their eating patterns or whether they experience conflict over food issues (e.g., family member criticizing their eating behaviors, partner unhappy with the effects of meal changes on their own eating habits). We also inquire about whether the patient would be willing to involve their partner or another close family member in future medical or behavioral health appointments related to diabetes management in an effort to foster greater understanding of diabetes and the recommended lifestyle changes and perhaps to learn additional ways to support the patient in his or her diabetes management.

Goals for change. Finally, we want to understand the goals that the patient and the PCP have for better diabetes management. We review the PCP's referral question and, if possible, speak with the PCP about his or her primary goals for the patient (e.g., keeping HbA1c below 6%–7%, decreasing blood pressure, losing 5%–10% of body weight). We ask patients what they believe their PCP wants them to change to determine whether they have an accurate understanding of their PCP's recommendations. We then assess the patients' goals. What do they want to change? Do they want to feel less depressed or less anxious about health problems? Do they want increased energy and ability to engage in physical activities? Do they believe that better managing their diabetes will help improve their quality of life? These broad, goal-oriented questions lead well into discussions of recommended changes.

Advise

In shifting from assessment to advising, we begin with a summary of our understanding of the problem. Of particular relevance for many patients with diabetes is the large number of behavior changes required to best manage their illness, compared with some other chronic conditions. Therefore, if the patient has expressed feeling overwhelmed or discouraged by the multiple changes required for good management of diabetes, we reflect and validate this perception of multiple challenges inherent in the self-management of a chronic disease such as diabetes. Some of these changes may seem easy to the patient (e.g., checking feet daily) and others that may seem quite difficult (e.g., regular blood sugar monitoring, eating changes, exercise). We balance this, however, with statements reflecting hope. Diabetes is one chronic disease that is quite responsive to behavioral changes over which the patient can exert control. Although some factors in diabetes cannot be changed, many factors that affect the course of the disease are modifiable. We then make a clear statement identifying which biopsychosocial factors are modifiable and the expected benefits from making such changes. We often describe diabetes as being more like a marathon than a sprint and discuss the need to pace how many changes are made at one time. Finally, we check to make sure the patient understands the advice and the rationale for the recommendations. Such an interaction might sound as follows:

> It sounds like you're feeling a bit overwhelmed by all the changes you've been asked to make to better manage your diabetes. You've been told by your health care providers that you should take your medicine regularly, check your blood sugar more often, lose weight, exercise daily, manage your stress better, and decrease your use of alcohol. That is certainly a lot of change and it's not surprising that you feel overwhelmed at times. However, you're aware that not making changes can lead to some bad health complications in the future. One positive aspect is that many, if not most, of these negative outcomes can be prevented through changes in your behavior. Certainly, some aspects of diabetes are outside of your control. Nevertheless, there are many aspects that you can control—changes that you can make—that will help you stay

healthier longer. Sometimes it is easier to treat diabetes like a marathon, rather than a sprint, and to pace how you make these changes in your life.

> Because of what you've told me today and what your health care providers have shared with me, I have some specific suggestions for changes you could make that can improve your management of diabetes and your long-term health. Two suggestions in particular stand out at this point. One is to increase how often you are checking your blood sugar, as a first step toward getting it under better control. Knowing your blood sugar levels will allow you to take steps needed to keep your blood sugar from getting (or staying) so high. These steps could involve taking medicine, cutting back on your carbs, or going for an extra walk, for example. Over the long term, keeping your blood sugars in a healthier range will help prevent some of the medical problems associated with diabetes. A second suggestion is to increase your physical activity. Results from research suggest that if you begin and maintain regular physical activity, you will gain better control of your blood sugar. Again, this should help to prevent many of the long-term complications of diabetes. Do these two recommendations make sense to you? What questions do you have? Why do you think it might be important to focus on these areas?

Agree

The agree phase of the interaction involves a shift from providing advice regarding general recommendations for change (described previously) to collaboratively setting specific goals related to these recommendations. In working jointly with the patient to negotiate a specific goal, you should balance professional judgment with patient preference. It is often helpful to suggest several options and see whether the patient gravitates toward one. Although this is a standard approach helpful in working with patients with a variety of behavioral health or medical conditions, it may be especially important for patients with diabetes, who frequently feel overwhelmed by the large number of changes they have been told to make in a short period of time. As an example of coming to agreement on a specific plan for increasing physical activity, you could propose several options, including increased walking through the use of planned short bursts (e.g., walking for 10 minutes three times per day), a more sustained period (e.g., walking 30 minutes a day with a partner), or through lifestyle activity with the goal of specific increases in steps per day (i.e., measured by a pedometer).

As you and the patient develop the specifics of the goal, the chances of success will be enhanced if the patient believes the changes are important and feasible. Sensitivity to the patient's of level of motivation and efficacy may be especially important among patients with diabetes, given the high number of changes required to manage the illness well. Asking questions such as, "How likely is it, on a scale of 0% to 100%, that you will be able to make this change in the next month?" or "How confident are you that you can meet this goal?" can provide useful information for tailoring the difficulty level of the goal. Ultimately, you want the patient to leave with a specific behavior-change goal involving at least moderate degrees of self-efficacy and motivation to make the change. If the patient appears ambivalent about making the change, guiding a discussion about the advantages and disadvantages of making the change and of not making the change may help increase motivation (see chap. 3, this volume, on motivational enhancement for additional guidance).

Assist

Common interventions for better biopsychosocial management of diabetes include the following:

- addressing comorbid mental health problems (e.g., depression, anxiety, stress reactions),
- making health behavior changes (e.g., related to physical exercise, diet, medication use and adherence, blood sugar monitoring, response to high or low blood sugar readings, tobacco cessation, alcohol use reduction),

- assisting with building communication skills (i.e., particularly with health care providers and family members),
- performing interventions within the patient's primary support system (e.g., family, partner), and
- encouraging the use of community support organizations (e.g., religious organizations, local YMCA or community centers, national diabetes organizations).

Approaches for addressing a number of these interventions are described in detail in other chapters of this volume. Strategies for addressing depression, anxiety, and stress reactions can be found in chapters 3 and 5. Approaches for helping patients make health behavior changes such as modifying diet, exercise habits, and mediation compliance are addressed in chapters 3 and 6, respectively. Rather than revisit these approaches here, we refer the reader to the other relevant chapters and instead focus here on diabetes-specific issues that may arise when addressing these areas, as well as on interventions not covered elsewhere.

Blood sugar monitoring.   Regular monitoring of blood sugar levels is a cornerstone of diabetes management for many patients. Appropriate monitoring provides the patient with information needed to make daily decisions regarding eating, exercise, and medication use to help keep blood sugar levels within healthy ranges. Regular monitoring also provides the health care team with valuable information for tailoring recommendations regarding these key areas. Some newer glucose monitoring devices now store information regarding blood sugar levels that can be downloaded at the PCP's office. Although this information is helpful for the medical team, it does not provide the patient with much immediate information regarding trends in blood sugar levels and related variables. Therefore, we encourage many patients to keep a personal monitoring log and record blood sugar levels as well as key factors (e.g., time of day, exercise, carbohydrate intake, medication). See Figure 7.1 for an example of such a form. We modify this form for patients, as needed, because of their particular behavioral health needs (e.g., add columns for tracking fat or calorie intake, eliminate medication section if not relevant, alter the mood type that is monitored).

Diabetes Self-Monitoring Form

Date _____

Eating (carbohydrates):

Food	Time	Carb count
_____	_____	_____
_____	_____	_____
_____	_____	_____
_____	_____	_____
_____	_____	_____
_____	_____	_____
_____	_____	_____
_____	_____	_____
_____	_____	_____
_____	_____	_____
_____	_____	_____
_____	_____	_____

Medication:

Type	Amount	Time
_____	_____	_____
_____	_____	_____
_____	_____	_____
_____	_____	_____
_____	_____	_____
_____	_____	_____

Physical activity:

Type	Duration	
_____	_____	_____
_____	_____	_____
_____	_____	_____

Blood sugar readings:

Blood sugar	Time
_____	_____
_____	_____
_____	_____
_____	_____
_____	_____

Stress level today: (0 [*none*]–10 [*severe*] scale):
Rating: _____
Relevant Factors: _____

FIGURE 7.1. Diabetes self-monitoring form.

Assessment of barriers to blood sugar monitoring may reveal problematic beliefs or behaviors to target in intervention. For example, some patients feel embarrassed about checking blood sugars away from home (e.g., in a restaurant, during an afternoon of shopping, at a party). Cognitive interventions targeting thoughts contributing to embarrassment and subsequent avoidance of monitoring may then be indicated (see chap. 3, this volume). Some patients may see the needle prick as a significant barrier to regular monitoring of blood sugar and may avoid or limit monitoring as a result. Guiding the patient through brief exposure-based interventions (see chap. 5, this volume) can help increase comfort levels with drawing the small amount of blood, typically one drop, needed to check blood sugar.

Response to "highs" and "lows" in blood sugar. Patients need to take appropriate corrective action in response to blood sugar levels that are too high or too low. Recommendations about the specific actions that they should take must come from the patient's PCP or other medical provider. For hypoglycemia, the typical recommendation involves eating or drinking a product with high glucose content. For hyperglycemia, there tends to be greater variability in recommendations, depending on patient characteristics, medication regimen, degree of hyperglycemia, and time of day. PCP recommendations may range from altering medication amount or timing, engaging in an immediate bout of exercise, delaying food intake, or altering food intake. Close coordination among the PCP, BHC, and patient ensures that all parties understand the recommended actions. The BHC and the patient may then work together to develop a plan for improved adherence to the corrective action plan.

Physical activity. The addition of regular physical activity to dietary changes contributes to improvements in blood sugar control (Nield et al., 2007). The National Institutes of Health's Look AHEAD study encourages patients with diabetes to accumulate at least 175 minutes of moderately intense physical activity (e.g., brisk walking) per week and 10,000 steps per day through lifestyle activity (The Look AHEAD Research Group, 2006). These recommendations obviously need to be tailored to the individual, particularly in identifying an initial manageable goal. Before helping a patient plan an individualized activity plan, however, it is important to check with the PCP to determine whether there are any medical contraindications to increasing physical activity or engaging in exercise that is more vigorous. The suggestions presented in chapter 6 for helping patients increase physical activity are relevant for patients with diabetes.

Some additional considerations exist when working with this unique population. Given the risk of hypoglycemic episodes developing during the course of increased physical activity, patients should be advised to take several precautions (Callaghan,

Gregg, Ortega, & Berlin, 2005). Eating 1 or 2 hours before increased physical activity or exercise can help reduce the risk of hypoglycemia. The PCP can provide advice about whether a patient should have a snack before exercise and whether he or she should exercise when blood sugar is high. Patients should wear identification with their personal information, emergency contact, and medical alert (i.e., indicating that they have diabetes) when exercising away from home. Patients should know the relationship between eating, exercise, and blood sugar changes, and be vigilant in attending to any signs of hypoglycemia (e.g., shakiness, confusion, weakness, headache) that may develop during exercise. They should have quick access to sources of sugar (e.g., glucose tablets, hard candy, fruit juice, soft drink) when exercising. If exercising away from home, patients should carry these items with them. Patients may need to check their blood sugar levels more frequently during exercise to ensure that levels do not become too low during periods of activity. Finally, patients need to ensure they wear shoes and socks that fit well and check their feet for redness after exercise.

Eating habits. Given the lack of evidence supporting one type of dietary plan over another for patients with diabetes (e.g., low fat, low carbohydrate, low glycemic index, low calorie; Nield et al., 2007), it is crucial that the BHC work closely with the patient's medical team when implementing interventions related to dietary changes. Ideally, patients should have an individualized dietary plan developed in conjunction with a dietician and/or PCP. The BHC can then help the patient implement this plan more successfully. The ADA (http://www.diabetes.org) and the NIDDK (http://www2.niddk.nih.gov) have resources related to the various types of diets followed by patients with diabetes. We also recommend keeping a nutritional reference guide handy (e.g., Holzmeister, 2006; Warshaw & Kulkarni, 2004) to help estimate the carbohydrate, fat, and calorie content of common foods.

Depression, anxiety, and emotional distress. Helping patients with diabetes to decrease depression, anxiety, or stress is similar to helping nondiabetics develop these skills. Chapters 3 and 5 have more detailed discussions of working with these problem areas. One issue specific to diabetes, however, is the relationship between emotional functioning and blood glucose levels. The presence of depression or anxiety may interfere with healthy diabetes management behaviors through lowered motivation to eat healthy, exercise, and adhere to other recommendations. Therefore, in working with patients with diabetes who are also experiencing problems with mood management, we specifically assess and target health-related behaviors that are being negatively affected.

In addition to affecting diabetes-related health behaviors, emotional functioning can affect blood glucose directly. Many people with Type 2 diabetes find that emotional stress leads to higher blood sugars. Discussing this relationship between stress and blood glucose levels often provides additional incentive for patients to engage in stress- and mood-management strategies such as relaxation training or cognitive disputation (see chap. 3, this volume).

Social support.   As with many other chronic illnesses, social support may help patients with diabetes cope better with the disease and with the many recommended lifestyle changes. To this end, we strongly encourage patients to identify someone (e.g., a partner, another family member, friend) who might be willing to support them in their diabetes management. The patient may invite the support person to attend behavioral health, diabetes education, and other medical appointments. The BHC may work together with the patient and support person to increase helpful types of support (e.g., praising healthy food choices, joining the patient in exercise activities, agreeing on decisions regarding grocery shopping and restaurant choice) and to decrease unhelpful behaviors (e.g., overcontrol of food, excessive criticism of eating or exercise habits). The BHC may also work with the patient to improve skills in assertive communication to help the patient ask for what he or she needs from family, friends, or medical providers. Community resources (e.g., local YMCA, community centers, diabetes support groups) and national diabetes organizations (e.g., ADA) may provide additional sources of support. It is of note that the ADA Web site (http://www.diabetes.org) contains links to find local diabetes-related events. We recommend that BHCs become aware of local and national resources and encourage patients to use them.

Arrange

BHCs provide a key function in helping coordinate and arrange access to the numerous resources that may benefit patients with diabetes. For example, BHCs may be the first to identify a need for psychotropic medication evaluation, additional dietary guidance, education on how to use the blood glucose monitor correctly, or additional social support. Developing knowledge of available resources to meet these needs, along with a willingness to coordinate referrals to psychiatry, nutritional medicine, diabetes educators, and community resources, can help the BHC link patients with needed services.

We also recommend that BHCs develop explicit criteria with patients and medical providers about when the patient should revisit the BHC. For example, you might recommend that the PCP refer the patient to you again if his or her HbA1c level rises above 7. You could encourage a patient who has worked with you on weight loss to come back to see you if he or she has gained 5 pounds. Alternatively, you may decide that this patient needs to meet with someone on the medical team, including the BHC, at least once per month until the HbA1c level is at an acceptable level. Ultimately, the message to both medical providers and patients should emphasize that diabetes is a chronic disease requiring lifelong behavior changes; therefore, intermittent consultations with a BHC over the life span should be the norm for good diabetes care.

SUMMARY

Diabetes, a disease seen commonly in primary care environments, can often be managed with behavioral and cognitive changes. The chronic nature of diabetes requires that the primary care team remains involved with the patient. BHCs should be careful to screen for and help the PCP target, in addition to the health behavior changes that affect the course of diabetes, depressive, anxiety, and general distress symptoms. The BHC can play a vital role in helping the team develop the behavior and cognitive change plan that will work best for each patient and help to maintain the patient's involvement in the change plan.

CHAPTER 8

IRRITABLE BOWEL SYNDROME

Adult functional gastrointestinal disorders (FGID) are characterized by a set of recurrent or chronic symptoms related to the functioning of the digestive system (Drossman, 2006). Typical symptoms include pain, nausea, diarrhea, bloating, constipation, belching, and heartburn. A diagnosis of FGID is made when symptom-based diagnostic criteria are met and are not explained by other identifiable structural problem, infection, or abnormality (Drossman, 2006).

Irritable bowel syndrome (IBS) is one of the most common FGIDs, with estimated prevalence rates between 10% to 15% (Brandt et al., 2002). IBS affects between 19 million and 34 million Americans, with 250 million lost schooldays and workdays and $10 million spent in medical costs annually (Blanchard, 2001; Drossman et al., 1993; Talley, Zinsmeister, Van Dyke, & Melton, 1991). It is the most researched FGID with more data on the effects and treatment of psychosocial factors than any other FGID (Chang et al., 2006). A diagnosis of IBS is made when recurrent abdominal pain or discomfort has occurred at least 3 days per month in the last 3 months and is associated with two or more of the following symptoms: (a) improvement with defecation, (b) onset associated with a change in frequency of stool, and (c) onset associated with a change in form (i.e., appearance) of stool (Longstreth et al., 2006).

Given the prevalence and effects of IBS and the likelihood that primary care providers (PCPs) may lack the training, time, or interest in assessing and treating the psychosocial aspects of IBS (Williams, Budavari, Olden, & Jones, 2005), this chapter focuses on key components of an evidence-based biopsy-chosocial assessment and treatment of IBS within the primary care clinic.

SPECIALTY MENTAL HEALTH

In a meta-analysis of randomized controlled studies, Lackner, Mesmer, Morley, Dowzer, and Hamilton (2004) concluded that psychological treatments significantly reduced composite IBS symptom scores obtained from self-report daily diaries, reduced abdominal pain and bowel dysfunction, and were associated with reduced depression and anxiety symptoms. There were too few studies to meta-analytically assess the strength of one psychological treatment against another. Other reviews (e.g., Blanchard & Scharff, 2002; Brandt et al., 2002; Spanier, Howden, & Jones, 2003), which included additional studies that were not as methodologically strong as the ones included in the Lackner et al. (2004) review, found similar results. The reviews concluded that there were positive benefits from multiple psychological interventions, which included biofeedback, cognitive and behavioral treatments, brief psychodynamic therapy, hypnotherapy, and relaxation training. These strategies were found to be effective for reducing gastrointestinal symptoms, improving depressed mood, improving anxious mood, increasing adaptive functioning, enhancing quality of life, or some combination of improved outcomes.

It is important to emphasize that many of the studies in these reviews lacked adequate control participants and, therefore, did not control for the placebo effect of attention, support, and expected outcome (Blanchard & Scharff, 2002; Brandt et al., 2002; Spanier et al., 2003). The few studies that did include viable attention placebo control groups found no significant difference in outcome between treatment and control groups. Many studies had small subject numbers and were subject to selection bias through subject recruitment from the general population. Despite these limitations, a broad conclusion can be drawn that some treatment, or perception of treatment, appears to be better than no treatment.

BEHAVIORAL HEALTH IN PRIMARY CARE

To date, only one study has examined psychological treatment for IBS in a primary care clinic (Kennedy et al., 2005). This randomized controlled trial compared a group receiving a combination of medication and cognitive–behavioral therapy (CBT) delivered by trained primary care nurses with a group receiving medication only. CBT consisted of six 50-minute sessions, which included education, methods to decrease unhelpful thoughts, behavioral techniques aimed at improving bowel habits, and stress management. Combined CBT and drug therapy produced a significant decrease in IBS symptoms over medication alone. This co-located primary care behavioral health study suggests CBT can be delivered in primary care and produces a better outcome than medication alone.

PRIMARY CARE ADAPTATION

Drossman and Thompson (1992) presented a stepped-care treatment heuristic that takes into account increased levels of symptom severity and functional impact. They conceptually categorized patients with IBS into three categories with recommendations for different intensity levels of care for each group.

Mild Symptoms

About 70% of those seeking medical care for IBS fall into this group. Patients with mild symptoms have minimal distress or psychological disturbance, and their symptoms are transient and/or have only minimal effects on daily functioning. Recommendations typically include dietary changes (e.g., reduced fat,

lactose, caffeine, alcohol, sorbitol, gas-producing foods such as beans), using fiber supplements, reassurance that symptoms are not life threatening, and education about IBS and the factors that influence it. Intervention by a behavioral health provider is generally not required in these cases.

Moderate Symptoms

Patients with moderate symptoms are most likely to benefit from working with a behavioral health consultant (BHC). Approximately 25% of those seeking medical care for IBS fall into this group. These patients are more likely to experience the following:

- a moderate correlation between their symptoms and particular events,
- mild symptom consistency,
- mild disruption of activity,
- moderate health care use, and
- mild psychological distress.

Treatment might include symptom monitoring to identify and change or manage exacerbating factors. Dietary and behavioral modifications may be the primary areas of intervention (e.g., decreasing or eliminating certain foods, learning relaxation techniques, questioning or changing stressful or anxious thinking, pain management strategies, problem-solving). Pharmacotherapy may also be used alone or in conjunction with dietary and behavior change.

Severe Symptoms

About 5% of those seeking medical care for IBS have severe symptoms. They may experience the following:

- severe symptom consistency,
- severe activity disruption,
- high medical use, and
- severe psychiatric diagnosis.

Patients with severe symptoms often do not improve with typical treatments in the primary care setting and should be referred to a specialty mental health provider. A multicomponent treatment and management strategy is recommended that includes medication, behavioral intervention, and physician-initiated behavioral management strategies. Components include setting realistic management goals, shifting responsibility for treatment decisions to the individual after providing options, expressing a commitment to improving the individual's well-being, and having regular brief follow-up appointments to support adherence. It is common for these patients to be reluctant to accept a referral to a specialty mental health provider. Because they are likely to benefit from such a provider, particular attention must be paid to reassure them that the referral does not mean a dismissal of their physical symptoms or to imply that their symptoms are imaginary. If the PCP is uncomfortable with this discussion, the BHC can be brought in to help the individual better understand the link between biological, behavioral, and psychological factors and how a more intensive level of service can help.

Standard Procedure

Setting a standard clinical pathway can be helpful to ensure that all patients with moderate to severe symptoms and functional impairment are referred to the BHC for a targeted assessment, treatment, or assistance, with a specialty mental health referral as needed. Patients might be told the BHC appointment is a standard procedure and is done to ensure the best comprehensive individualized care.

Collaborative Relationship

A strong physician–patient relationship is important for successful management of IBS (Chang et al., 2006; Levy et al., 2006; Williams et al., 2005); we believe this same principle generalizes to the BHC. Drossman (1994) suggested guidelines for providers and health care workers treating FGID that facilitate a collaborative self-management approach between the individual and the primary care team. Those suggestions include the following:

- Acknowledge the individual's distress and disability from the illness by saying, "This has been hard for you, and you're just not sure how to make this better."
- Educate by saying, "Lets make sure we are both on the same page about what IBS is and is not. I have a handout, I'd like to review with you." (See Figure 8.1.)
- Actively listen and respond to the individual's agenda by saying, "What would you like to see changed or be different?"

- Reframe interactions to focus on what the individual is trying to say rather than focusing on items of disagreement.
- Do not look for a cure; instead, focus on the management of symptoms and improvement in function and quality of life.
- Encourage the individual to be actively involved in care.
- Offer tasks or responsibilities in a systematic fashion. You might say, "One of the first things we can do is have you monitor your symptoms for two weeks to make sure we have identified all the foods, environments, stressors, or any other factors that may be affecting your IBS symptoms."
- Begin by addressing psychological issues that the individual sees as being relevant to their IBS symptoms. The issues about which the individual has little understanding or recognition, can be addressed later. You might say, "It sounds like you have noticed that when you have a lot more demands at work your IBS symptoms worsen. We can discuss ways to manage those demands differently so that they don't affect your symptoms so severely."
- Be clear and honest with your beliefs. For example, when a PCP sets boundaries such as not prescribing medications or conducting additional tests he or she does not feel are needed, explain the rationale for those decisions with the patient.
- Be flexible.
- Be available for ongoing care.

Part of your job as a BHC may be to foster an appreciation for this approach with primary care team members who appear to be struggling with, or are frustrated with, their interactions with patients who have IBS. Highlighting that additional evidence-based ways of intervening and interacting with these patients and providing patient educational materials or suggestions on how to do things differently may help foster this approach for the struggling PCP. The more the team can promote a positive attitude and exchange of information, the more they can help patients understand the legitimacy of their disorder and the factors involved in its management. They may also empower and encourage patients to experiment with more effective coping behaviors and ongoing self-management. This approach may

---

What Is IBS?

Irritable bowel syndrome (IBS) is a pattern of symptoms that indicate an abnormal condition.

Common IBS Symptoms: Stomach pain, cramping or discomfort, gas, bloating, painful constipation and/or diarrhea, alternating constipation and diarrhea.

Causes: Feces are moved by muscles in your colon. Some nerve impulses speed up contractions whereas others slow them down. When these contractions are well balanced, normal bowel movements occur.

People with IBS have a colon that is more sensitive and reacts more easily to a variety of triggers that would not affect others as much. When your colon moves slowly or stops, more water than usual is absorbed, resulting in constipation. When your colon moves fast, not as much water is absorbed, resulting in diarrhea. Bloating, pain, and cramping can occur with a colon spasm and/or excessive gas.

Triggers: Some common triggers include the following:

- Diet. High fat foods, high calorie or large meals, milk products, alcohol, caffeine, and carbonated drinks can significantly increase colon contractions, producing cramps and diarrhea.
- Emotions. Stress can produce colon spasms. Many people with IBS are sometimes anxious and tense; have emotional ups and downs; may eat quickly; have hurried, unplanned meals; do not get enough sleep. These things may also worsen IBS symptoms.

Treatment: Once you know what things contributing to your symptoms, you can work with your health care team to design a plan for your unique situation. This plan may include the following:

- Diet. Your medical provider may suggest you modify what you eat in the following ways: (a) Avoid or reduce high fat foods and large quantities of food, (b) decrease fried foods, milk, and milk products, (c) avoid or decrease caffeinated drinks and alcohol, and (d) slowly increase foods containing fiber.
- Medication. If appropriate, your medical provider may prescribe medications for you. These may include the following:
  - Antispasmodics (e.g., dicyclomine) to help normalize colon contractions by regulating the chemicals that produce rhythm-controlling impulses.
  - Tranquilizers (e.g., lorazepam) to help calm you a little so unusual stresses are less likely to trigger an attack or make symptoms worse.
  - Serotonin-4 receptor 5HT4 agonists to activate 5HT4 receptors in your colon, normalizing impaired motility by stimulating colon secretion and inhibiting sensitivity.
- Psychophysiological and behavioral changes. Because stress, changing emotions, anxiety, worry, and depressed mood can contribute to initiating symptoms or making them worse, learning strategies to manage emotional distress through relaxation and/or questioning and/or changing unhelpful thoughts can be helpful to decrease the frequency and intensity of your IBS symptoms.

In addition, changing behaviors, such as increasing physical activity, getting quality sleep, eating meals at the same time each day at paced intervals, and minimizing or eliminating alcohol, caffeine, and/or tobacco, can have a positive effect.

FIGURE 8.1. What is IBS? handout.

be particularly useful when working with those who have had prior unsatisfactory medical encounters.

The following sections provide focused assessment, treatment, and management recommendations based on the research literature and clinical experience. The strategies are intended to reduce IBS symptoms, enhance functioning, decrease frequency and intensity of symptom exacerbation, and improve overall quality of life. The assessment must elicit quality information in a short time, while ensuring that the patient feels understood and respected.

Assess. Producing a focused assessment in a short period of time that identifies relevant problem areas can be a challenge. A functional psychosocial assessment can take several directions. To obtain a reasonable picture of the factors contributing to IBS, the assessment should include the following (Blanchard, 2001; Levy et al., 2006; Toner, Segal, Emmot, & Myran, 2000; Williams et al., 2005):

- a review of physical symptoms;
- exclusion of comorbid psychiatric diagnoses;
- identification of current stressors or stressful life events (e.g., abuse); and
- a review of health beliefs and a consideration of factors preceding symptoms and occurring after symptoms, such as thoughts, reactions of others, and patient behavior (i.e., antecedents and consequences).

An excellent example of a detailed specialty mental health clinic examination can be found in Blanchard (2001), but this history takes approximately 45 minutes, so it is not well-suited for a typical primary care setting. The following assessment approach covers the biopsychosocial spectrum, but it is considerably more focused and allows time to start an intervention during the first appointment.

Introduction and education. Similar to others (e.g., Blanchard, 2001; Chang et al., 2006; Toner et al., 2000), we believe a brief introduction, including information about who you are, your role in the primary care team and, specifically, your understanding and explanation of factors involved in IBS, is a critical factor in eliciting active individual participation and facilitating quality information collection in a short period of time. The introduction sets the stage for the appointment; our experience suggests that skipping this or doing it poorly can elicit a more guarded attitude by the patient resulting in a less interactive exchange and, therefore, a less productive assessment. Figure 8.2 is a sample script that might be used as an introduction that also includes educational information. We encourage you to adapt this script to your interaction style and then consistently use it with each patient with IBS you see.

Behavioral Health Consultant Introduction and IBS Explanation Script

Before we start today, let me explain to you a little bit about who I am and what I do in the clinic. I'm the behavioral health consultant for the clinic and a [state your profession] by training. I work with the primary care team in situations where good health care involves paying attention not only to physical health but also to habits, behaviors, emotional health, and how those things interact with each other.

As I understand it, Dr [doctor's name] wanted me to see you in regard to your IBS symptoms. Is that your understanding of why you're here? [Patient agrees.]

Before we go any further, there are some things I would like to share with you about IBS. IBS is a real disorder and the symptoms are not in your head. People with IBS have a colon that tends to be more sensitive and reacts more easily to a variety of triggers that would not affect others as much. We know IBS symptoms can decrease your quality of your life and interfere with a variety of activities. Research also suggests that IBS is not believed to cause any permanent harm to your intestines and does not lead to any serious disease, like cancer. We also know that symptoms can be influenced by many factors including food, hormones, activity, and stress. Although there is no one thing or specific medication that will cure IBS, there are many things, including medication, that can be used to help reduce the frequency and severity of your symptoms, improve your quality of life and daily functioning.

My job is to help you and your provider to be more successful at managing your IBS symptoms. To do this, I'm going to spend about [number] minutes with you in a consultation appointment to get a snapshot of your current difficulties: what's working well and what's not working so well. Before you leave today, we'll take the information you've given me, and together you and I will come up with a set of IBS management recommendations that seem attainable. Recommendations might include things you do on your own with continued follow-up with Dr [name]. Or, we may decide to have you come for follow-up visits with me if we think it would be best in helping you acquire specific management skills. We might also decide that you'd benefit from longer or more frequent specialty services. If that is the case, Dr [name] and I will work to get those services scheduled for you. The bottom line is that Dr [name], the rest of the primary care team, and I want to work together with you in a coordinated approach to get the best outcomes.

Do you have any questions about any of this before we begin?

FIGURE 8.2. Behavioral health consultant introduction and IBS explanation script.

Functional assessment. As discussed in chapter 2, we encourage you to use foundational questions and adapt them, as needed, to the specific presenting problem of the patient. Specifically, with those experiencing IBS, it can be helpful to ask questions about physiological symptoms first. If there have been delays in diagnosis or a history of unsatisfactory outcomes of medical treatment, some patients may feel they have been discounted and passed-off by the time you become involved in care. Focusing on their physical symptoms first gives you the opportunity to establish a collaborative interaction focused on what they may know best (i.e., their symptoms) and validate their concerns (Blanchard, 2001; Toner et al., 2000). This positive momentum can help you make the transition to the psychosocial part of the functional assessment. Additional IBS specific assessment questions are listed in Figure 8.3. The questions are geared toward giving you a focused glimpse of areas that may be significant so you can accurately decide which areas need further assessment for developing a tailored self-management plan.

Summary. At the conclusion of the assessment phase, a summary statement should be provided to ensure you have understood the patient correctly and to communicate that understanding. That summary might be stated as follows:

> I'd like to summarize my understanding of what you told me to make sure I have it right before I lay out recommendations for you to consider. It is important that you correct me if I've missed something or have something wrong, because my recommendations are going to be based on my understanding of your situation. It sounds like you become stressed at times when you are at work, and this stress response is related to how you think your boss and coworkers might judge your work and perceive your value as an employee. When this happens, your symptoms, particularly your pain, really increase. This affects your ability to be as productive at work as you could be and negatively influences how you interact with your family after work,

> because the pain makes it difficult to be the kind of spouse and parent you would like to be. You've also noticed that when you're stressed, you tend to not sleep as well and that perhaps some of the food you eat during times such as these may be upsetting your stomach; however, you're not sure what foods those are because they seem to vary. Do I have it right or did I miss something?

Sometimes, patients do not notice any association between their symptoms and emotional state. A weekly IBS symptom and stress monitoring diary is provided in Figure 8.4 to help you and the patient evaluate this relation. The symptom diary is also a good way to assess change over time; symptoms being monitored can be changed to depression, worry, anxiety or anger to help the individual examine the association between relevant emotional states and symptoms (Blanchard, 2001).

Advise. The next step is to advise the individual about their options for treatment and self-management. At some point in the initial appointment, we suggest you provide the individual with an IBS educational handout (see Figure 8.1). The PCP can provide this handout to the individual or you can provide it after the introduction or at the end of the initial appointment. It is common for patients to feel overwhelmed or confused by medical information. Yet, it is clear that those with IBS want, need, and deserve convincing, easy-to-understand explanations about the nature of their symptoms, factors involved in exacerbation, and options for self-management (Chang et al., 2006; Drossman, 2006; Longstreth et al., 2006; Williams et al., 2005). Most specialty mental health, multicomponent treatment packages include educational information (e.g., Blanchard, 2001; Toner et al., 2000). This information can help patients feel more comfortable about a collaborative self-management model of care. They should be encouraged to review the handout to identify factors they can influence or control that may help decrease symptoms and improve functioning (Chang et al., 2006; Drossman, 2006; Longstreth et al., 2006; Williams et al., 2005). As with many chronic

---

Additional Questions for a Focused IBS Assessment of Physical and Medical Factors

---

Frequency and Intensity of the Problem

- Symptoms of IBS can be different for different people. What are your IBS symptoms?
- Which of those symptoms bothers you the most?
- On a scale of 0 to 10, with 0 meaning the symptom is gone and 10 being [the most bothersome symptom] is the most bothersome or painful it has ever been, what would be the average number you would give to [the most bothersome symptom] over the last 2 weeks? What is the highest number? What is the lowest number?

Health Habits

- Do you use laxatives to manage your symptoms? If so, how often do you take the laxatives?

Diet

- Do you eat foods that are high in fat, such as red meat, ice cream, or cheese?
- How often do you drink milk or food products that contain milk? Is it lactose free? Do you look at labels carefully to see if food contains milk?
- How often do eat foods that produce gas, such as beans?
- Do you eat foods that are high in fiber, such as whole wheat bread, apples, pears, raisins, or bran flakes? Do you take fiber supplements?

Psychosocial Factors

<u>**Relationship With Significant Other**</u>

- Would you describe your relationship with your significant other as "Poor," "OK, but could be better," "Good," or "Excellent"?
- On a scale of 0 to 10, with 0 being not satisfied at all and 10 being the most satisfied you can imagine, what number would represent your satisfaction with this relationship?

<u>**How Others Respond to Symptoms**</u>

- How do members of your family, coworkers, or close friends respond to your symptoms?

<u>**Relations With Others**</u>

- Do you find it difficult to make decisions?
- Do you generally express what you feel?
- Can you be openly critical of others' ideas, opinions, or behaviors?
- Do you have difficulty refusing requests even if you don't want to do what is being asked?

<u>**Life Stress**</u> or <u>**Negative Life Event**</u>

- If you were to rate your average stress level over the last month on a scale of 0 to 10, with 0 being no stress and being completely relaxed and 10 being the most stressed you could imagine, what number would you give as your average stress level? What was your highest and lowest stress level during this time?
- Does anything seem to be associated with your stress level changing?
- Have you noticed any changes in your IBS symptoms as your stress level changes? [Sometimes people might not notice changes in their symptoms because of stress. If they say there has been no change, it might be helpful to have them rate IBS symptoms and stress level on the patient handout in Figure 8.4.]
- Is there anything unpleasant, bothersome, or distressing happening in your life right now, besides your IBS symptoms, that you would like to see be changed or different?
- Is there anything unpleasant, bothersome, or distressing that happened in your past (e.g., physical or sexual assault; physical, sexual, or emotional abuse; near death experience; or belief that you were going to die), besides your IBS symptoms, that is distressing or bothersome to you now?

FIGURE 8.3. Additional questions for a focused IBS assessment of physical and medical factors.

Weekly IBS Symptom and Stress Monitoring Diary

Use the rating scale below to rate how much of a problem these symptoms were for you during the day.

Rating scale: **0**   **1**   **2**   **3**   **4**   **5**   **6**   **7**   **8**   **9**   **10**

None   *Moderate*   *Extreme*

Symptoms	Sunday	Monday	Tuesday	Wednesday	Thursday	Friday	Saturday
Abdominal pain							
Abdominal tenderness							
Constipation							
Diarrhea							
Diarrhea (# of times)							
Bloating or fullness							
Nausea							
Flatulence							
Belching							
Did you avoid certain activities in response to these symptoms? (Y or N)							

Use the rating scale below to identify your average stress level for the day.

Rating scale: **0**   **1**   **2**   **3**   **4**   **5**   **6**   **7**   **8**   **9**   **10**

None   *Moderate*   *Extreme*

	Sunday	Monday	Tuesday	Wednesday	Thursday	Friday	Saturday
Average stress level							

FIGURE 8.4.   Weekly IBS symptom and stress monitoring diary.

conditions, self-care for chronic IBS is vital for effective coping and management (Chang et al., 2006; Drossman, 2006; Longstreth et al., 2006; Williams et al., 2006).

To target IBS symptoms, some strategies (e.g., relaxed breathing, PMR, cue-controlled relaxation; see chap. 3, this volume) may directly target a decrease in arousal, whereas others may be more focused on improving mood management (e.g.,

cognitive disputation, behavioral activation, increase physical activity; see chap. 3 and chap. 5, this volume) and/or decreasing or minimizing triggers (e.g., dietary changes, eating schedule, improved sleep; see chap. 5 and chap. 6, this volume). If the individual indicates significant distress related to past physical or sexual abuse, referral for outpatient specialty mental health treatment is likely the best recommendation, as treatment for these problems is not ideally suited to 30-minute consultation appointments.

When you start to introduce interventions, it is important to offer individualized advice about what might be most helpful. You can base this advice on the following:

- hypothesized trigger(s) for symptoms,
- what the individual believes is important,
- what the individual is ready to change,
- what may improve quality of life, and
- what the patient is motivated to try.

The following paragraph is an example of what you might say in the advise phase.

> One place we could start is to teach you how to relax yourself by changing your breathing. A relaxation skill such as deep breathing can help you manage your stress response at work. I like to start with breathing techniques, because I have found that many people can achieve their goals with this easier strategy. By changing your breathing pattern, you can help turn on your body's natural relaxation response and perhaps decrease the symptoms you notice when you increase your stress response. If the breathing techniques don't work, there are other relaxation strategies we can use, but they take more time and effort. We can set a plan so you can do this throughout the day. You can use this technique in a way that no one will know you are doing it so you will be able to relax yourself even if others are around.
>
> Another thing that might help with the stress cycle you described is to learn some ways to question what you are thinking and develop the skills to choose how you want to respond instead of just reacting to situations. This puts you in the driver's seat. You can't stop your mind from thinking, but you do have the ability to notice those thoughts, question how useful they are, and evaluate how consistent they are with your values. From there, you can make a decision on how you would like to think in that situation so you can respond in a way consistent with what you want to do.
>
> To examine how food is related to your symptoms, it would be helpful for you keep a food diary in which you write down all the things you eat, monitor changes in your symptoms, and see whether there is any association between your symptoms and what, when, or how fast you eat. Do you think you might want to try any or all of these things, or are there other targets for change that we haven't discussed that are more important to focus on at this time?

Agree. It is important to have the individual tell you what they are willing to try before launching into the active phase of intervention. Our experience suggests that when medical or behavioral health providers skip this step, the individual may not feel like they are part of a collaborative team, may have unvoiced concerns about the plan, and may be less motivated to follow through. This can leave the patient without an effective intervention and create frustration on the part of the patient and the medical team when symptoms and functioning do not change.

As suggested by the research, there are many strategies patients with IBS can use to decrease symptoms. The goal of this phase is to reach an agreement and establish a commitment to doing something differently. Many people are willing to try what you suggest if you have done a good job of associating your recommendations with their goals of decreasing or managing their symptoms. Sometimes, the individual may not be sure of what he or she wants to change or can be ambivalent about making changes. If this is the case, you might suggest trying only one or two things or recommend that he or she think about the options until a follow-up appointment for further review and discussion.

Assist. Once the patient has agreed to an intervention plan, the focus of the appointment should shift to a review of the strategies and discussion of what factors are needed to help him or her follow through with the plan. In general, the plan might be geared toward reducing the frequency and intensity of symptoms, better toleration of symptoms, and/or continuation of valuable functional activities if symptoms do not change. This might include a discussion of when and where patients will do an activity, identifying who in their life they might turn to for support, or helping them access local community resources (e.g., physical activity class, dietary education or cooking class at the local community center). Many concurrent and contributing mental health disorders, especially depression and anxiety conditions, can be managed in focused 30-minute primary care appointments. Patients frequently prefer to get these services within the primary care clinic because that is where they are being treated for the IBS. We encourage you to use a stepped approach with the interventions, starting with the easiest change first and then building as needed over time if the first step does not produce the desired results. This stepped approach frequently delivers desired outcomes. Because of the effect of stress on IBS and the co-occurrence of anxiety and depressive symptoms with IBS, we use interventions that we have discussed in chapters 3 and 4 to help patients manage IBS. Interventions might include the following:

- relaxation breathing and cue-controlled relaxation (see chap. 3, this volume),
- progressive muscle relaxation (see chap. 3, this volume),
- cognitive disputation (see chap. 3, this volume),
- anxiety or depression treatments (see chap. 5, this volume),
- assertiveness or communications skills training (see chap. 3, this volume),
- diet change (see Figure 8.5 for a dietary tracking form and a list of foods that commonly increase IBS symptoms), and
- pain management (see chap. 11, this volume).

Arrange. We recommend having the individual follow up with you, their PCP, or both in a scheduled manner in 2 to 4 weeks. This will facilitate ongoing assessment of intervention effectiveness, timelier treatment changes, and collaboration to help the patient maximize self-care. In addition, in light of research showing equal improvement for those receiving a credible attention placebo compared with an active treatment intervention, unidentified factors occurring within the scheduled follow-up appointments may be therapeutic. There is no specific guide as to when to suggest a referral for more intensive treatment in a specialty behavioral health setting. However, if symptoms and functional impairment are not changing in some way after three to four appointments, or if the individual is having difficulty following through on recommended changes, we suggest you consider recommending a referral for more intensive treatment in a specialty mental health setting.

SUMMARY

The treatment of IBS can be a challenge. Multiple cognitive and behavioral interventions appear to be effective for decreasing symptoms and improving function. During assessment, it is important to interact in a collaborative manner, in which you acknowledge the patient's distress, educate on IBS, ask questions related to physiological symptoms first, focus on symptoms management rather than a cure, engage the individual in a plan of self-care, and be available for ongoing follow-up assessment and intervention. It may be helpful as part of your ongoing assessment to have individuals monitor their symptoms to highlight associations between various mood and/or food intake associated with an increase in symptoms. Treatment can include a variety of approaches that match the symptom profile (e.g., relaxed breathing for increased stress response associated with symptoms); ongoing follow-up may be indicated even when symptoms are minimal.

IBS Diet Monitoring

It may be helpful for some patients to examine what, how much, when, and how fast they eat to determine whether these factors are contributing to symptoms. One way to do that is to keep a simple food diary and compare it with the symptom diary in Figure 8.4, make planned changes based on the data, and see what results the planned changes produce.

Personal Food Diary

Date or day: _____

Time of day	Food or beverage item	Serving size	Total time to finish	Fast food or restaurant food (Yes or no)	Comments (e.g., stressors, eating due to boredom or emotions)

Foods That Might Increase IBS Symptoms

Excessive amounts of: (a) grape, apple, or prune juice; (b) prunes, apples, bananas, or raisins; or (c) citrus fruits (e.g., oranges, grapefruit, pineapple).

Grain products, such as: wheat, rye, or bran.

Vegetables and legumes, such as: (a) Cabbage, cauliflower, or broccoli; (b) baked or boiled beans; or (c) onions, peas, radishes, or potatoes.

Dairy products, such as: (a) Cheese, milk, butter, or yogurt; or (b) ice cream, or sour cream.

Other items, such as: nuts, chocolate, eggs, high fat foods, alcohol, caffeine, carbonated drinks.

Other Resources

Many books are available that discuss dietary changes for IBS. Some examples include the following:

Peikin, S. R. (2004). *Gastrointestinal health: The proven nutritional program to prevent, cure, or alleviate irritable bowel syndrome (IBS), ulcers, gas, constipation, heartburn, and many other digestive disorders* (3rd ed.). New York: HarperCollins.

Magee, E. (2000). *Tell me what to eat if I have irritable bowel syndrome: Nutrition you can live with.* Franklin Lakes, NJ: Career Press.

Van Vorous, H. (2000). *Eating for IBS: 175 delicious, nutritious, low-fat, low-residue recipes to stabilize the touchiest tummy.* New York: Marlowe.

FIGURE 8.5.   IBS diet monitoring handout.

CHAPTER 9

CHRONIC OBSTRUCTIVE PULMONARY DISEASE AND ASTHMA

Pulmonary disease encompasses a wide range of diagnoses, including acute lower respiratory infections (e.g., pneumonia, influenza, acute bronchitis), chronic lower respiratory disease (e.g., chronic obstructive pulmonary disease [COPD], asthma, cystic fibrosis, bronchiectasis), adult respiratory distress syndrome, pulmonary edema, and interstitial lung diseases, among others. This chapter focuses on two pulmonary diseases frequently seen in primary care clinics: COPD and asthma. Because of the frequent presence of complicating behavioral and psychosocial factors in managing these diseases, they present unique challenges to primary care providers (PCPs) and behavioral health professionals working in primary care. Fortunately, individuals with COPD and asthma have responded to specialty mental health treatment, either alone or in a multidisciplinary context (e.g., Devine & Pearcy, 1996; Emery, Schein, Hauck, & MacIntyre, 1998; Takigawa et al., 2007) and may benefit from consultative behavioral health intervention in the primary care setting. This chapter focuses specifically on how to adapt and apply evidence-based behavioral assessment and interventions with a challenging population, primary care patients diagnosed with COPD and/or asthma.

CHRONIC OBSTRUCTIVE PULMONARY DISEASE

COPD, a chronic lower respiratory disease, includes emphysema and chronic bronchitis. Its pulmonary component is characterized by airflow limitations that are progressive and not fully reversible. COPD is a leading cause of morbidity and mortality in the United States, accounting for 8 million outpatient visits, 1.5 million emergency services visits, and 726,000 hospitalizations (Global Initiative for Chronic Obstructive Lung Disease [GOLD], 2006; Mannino, Homa, Akinbami, Ford, & Redd, 2002).

Prominent symptoms include dyspnea (i.e., airflow limitation), chronic cough, and chronic sputum production. The functional impact of COPD can range from mild to severely debilitating. In more advanced stages, COPD often results in significant decrements in functioning and quality of life, including limitations in physical activity, work, self-care, recreation, and family routines; alterations in mood and cognitive functioning; social isolation; physical deconditioning; weight loss; and economic status. The most common risk factor for development of COPD is cigarette smoking, although exposure to other air pollutants may also increase risk (GOLD, 2006).

Key Biopsychosocial Factors in COPD

Understanding the biopsychosocial factors associated with COPD is important to successful consultation with medical personnel. The following highlights those important areas.

Physical factors. The physiological changes responsible for the decreased lung function seen in COPD are considered largely irreversible and are generally the result of underlying irritation or inflammation (i.e., swelling) of lung tissue, most commonly resulting from a history of tobacco smoking. Biological factors that further increase COPD risk in smokers include genetic factors, respiratory infections, and airway hyperresponsiveness, all of which appear to be involved in COPD pathogenesis (Pauwels & Rabe, 2004). It is beyond the scope of this chapter to describe COPD pathophysiology in detail, but others have summarized it (e.g., Barnes, 2003; Doherty et al., 2006; GOLD, 2006).

Medical treatment of COPD primarily involves use of medications to decrease symptoms and complications. Medications have not been found to reverse the long-term decline in lung functioning. Practice guidelines recommend bronchodilator medications (i.e., β2-agonists such as Proventil, Ventolin, or Serevent; anticholinergics such as Atrovent or Spiriva; methylxanthines such as Phyllocontin or Uniphyl) used on a regular or as-needed basis to reduce symptoms, with the addition of inhaled glucocorticosteroids (e.g., Aristocort, Flovent) for symptomatic COPD patients with severe or very severe COPD (GOLD, 2006). Survival of individuals with chronic respiratory failure may be increased by long-term administration (i.e., more than 15 hours per day) of oxygen, which may be appropriate for patients with very severe COPD. Surgical treatments (e.g., lung transplantation, lung volume reduction) are not recommended as first-line or routine treatments for COPD, although there is some evidence from nonrandomized trials and observational studies that surgery may be appropriate for certain patients with advanced COPD (GOLD, 2006).

Low weight is an area of concern for many patients with COPD. A body mass index (BMI) of less than 25 in patients with COPD is an independent predictor of increased mortality, and treatment to increase weight is a predictor of survival (Schols, Slangen, Volovics, & Wouters, 1998). In addition to higher risk of death, underweight patients with COPD have a lower health-related quality of life compared with normal weight patients with COPD (Shoup et al., 1997).

Emotional and cognitive factors. Yohannes, Baldwin, and Connolly (2000), in their meta-analysis of depression and anxiety in older adult patients with COPD, reported a 40% prevalence rate of comorbid depression and a 36% prevalence of anxiety symptoms. Depression and anxiety may result from the decreased functioning, loss of roles, and decreased self-efficacy that can accompany the progression of COPD. The inactivity and anhedonia often seen in depressed individuals may lead to further physiological deconditioning, worsening the patient's ability to engage in physical activity. Anxiety symptoms may result from and compound the frightening symptom of dyspnea (i.e., shortness of breath) in an *anxiety–dyspnea* vicious cycle (e.g., dyspnea leading to decreased physical activity, leading to deconditioning, leading to worsening dyspnea on exertion, resulting in cognitive responses of alarming predictions, increasing anxiety and fear, leading to worsened dyspnea; see Figure 9.1). Some patients may avoid activity altogether because of anxiety-worsened dyspnea (Ries, 2005). Breaking this cycle may require cognitive interventions as well as breathing retraining and relaxation skills.

Behavioral factors. Nicotine use and physical inactivity are two primary behavioral factors exerting strong influence on the quality of life and symptom progression of those with COPD. Smoking cessation is critical in slowing the progression of COPD; practice guidelines (GOLD, 2006) recommend tobacco cessation counseling and pharmacotherapy for all tobacco users at risk of or diagnosed with COPD.

Individuals with COPD often reduce or eliminate physical exercise because of dyspnea. Unfortunately, lowered physical activity leads to physical deconditioning, and worsened dyspnea on later exertion. Functioning and quality of life gradually decrease as ability to engage in activity progressively declines. Thus, exercise training is considered a standard component of treatment for COPD (Nici et al., 2006).

Environmental factors. Although chronic exposure to tobacco smoke is the primary environmental risk factor for development of COPD, exposure to indoor air pollution and occupational hazards (e.g., dust, gases, fumes) may also increase risk (Pauwels & Rabe, 2004). If present, interventions to reduce any ongoing exposures are warranted.

Specialty Mental Health

Although physiological changes are largely responsible for COPD symptoms, treatment focused exclusively on modifying or addressing the biology of

---

Shortness of Breath Cycle for COPD and Asthma

Many people with COPD or asthma experience a *shortness of breath cycle*. In this cycle, shortness of breath from COPD or asthma leads to worry and panic, which in turn worsens shortness of breath. Here are the steps that often occur:

    Shortness of breath leads to . . .

- Worry (e.g., about breathing, passing out, dying), leading to . . .
- Anxiety or panic physical reaction, leading to . . .
- Increased breathing rate, leading to . . .
- Less effective (i.e., rapid, shallow) breathing, leading to . . .
- Increased oxygen use by, and less oxygen available for muscles, leading to . . .
- More shortness of breath . . .
- And the cycle continues.

You can stop the shortness of breath cycle by following these steps:

1. When you first notice shortness of breath, STOP your activity.
2. Rest. Sit down or lie down, if possible.
3. Relax. Use diaphragmatic breathing or pursed-lip breathing techniques.
4. Reassure yourself. Tell yourself reassuring thoughts about your symptoms.
5. Take medications, if appropriate, following your PCP's recommendations.
6. After your breathing improves, gradually resume activity, in a paced manner.

FIGURE 9.1. Shortness of breath cycle for COPD and asthma handout.

COPD is incomplete. The importance of nonpharmacological and nonmedical approaches to treatment of COPD, particularly through multidisciplinary pulmonary rehabilitation programs, is well-established (Nici et al., 2006; Ries et al., 2007).

Most specialty mental health interventions have been evaluated as components of multidisciplinary pulmonary rehabilitation programs, rather than as stand-alone psychological or behavioral interventions. These programs aim to increase functioning, reduce symptoms, and decrease costs of medical intervention (Nici et al., 2006). The psychosocial components of pulmonary rehabilitation often involve promotion of social support, self-management education, breathing strategies, anxiety and depression management, behavioral activation, and relaxation training (Devine & Pearcy, 1996; Guell et al., 2006; Hill, 2006; Nici et al., 2006).

The American College of Chest Physicians (ACCP) and the American Association of Cardiovascular and Pulmonary Rehabilitation (AACVPR) reviewed the literature on pulmonary rehabilitation and concluded that multidisciplinary pulmonary rehabilitation approaches lead to decreased dyspnea, improved health-related quality of life, decreased health care use, and improved exercise tolerance. They noted that although evidence for the effectiveness of stand-alone or short-term psychosocial interventions is lacking, expert opinion recommends including educational and psychosocial interventions in comprehensive treatment programs (ACCP–AACVPR Pulmonary Rehabilitation Guidelines Panel, 1997). Devine and Pearcy's (1996) meta-analysis of 65 evaluations of pulmonary rehabilitation programs found improvements in psychological well-being, endurance, functional status, VO$_2$ max (cardiovascular fitness), dyspnea, and treatment adherence. It is notable that they also found that interventions consisting of relaxation alone led to significant improvement in dyspnea and psychological well-being.

Behavioral Health in Primary Care

A review of the literature revealed no published studies of behavioral treatment of COPD in primary care settings by behavioral health professionals. However, results of a randomized controlled trial of a brief cognitive–behavioral (CBT) intervention (Kunik et al., 2001) appear promising and can inform practice in a primary care setting. The intervention consisted of a 2-hour CBT group intervention with components of education (i.e., role of anxiety and depression in chronic illness, role of thoughts and behaviors in emotion), relaxation training (i.e., diaphragmatic breathing, postural changes), cognitive interventions (i.e., thought stopping, self-instructional training), and graduated practice (i.e., education on role of exposure, practice in learning new coping skills). Participants received handouts and audiotapes that reviewed skills and provided practice exercises, and received brief weekly phone calls for 6 weeks after the primary intervention. Compared with a control group receiving a 2-hour COPD education class and weekly calls, the CBT group showed significant decreases in measures of depression and anxiety, although no difference in physical functioning.

Primary Care Adaptation

The results discussed in the previous section show promise for brief, stand-alone CBT interventions and use of guided self-help materials in the management of patients with COPD in primary care. Although Kunik et al.'s (2001) research was not conducted in a primary care setting, an intervention of similar intensity (i.e., 2 hours of CBT intervention) could certainly be consistent with primary care behavioral health practice. Furthermore, adapting other main psychosocial components of pulmonary rehabilitation programs (e.g., behavioral activation, depression management, promotion of social support) to primary care may also benefit patients. The following sections provide specific recommendations on putting such interventions into practice.

Assess. Perhaps the most important consideration to assess on referral of a patient with COPD is whether he or she smokes tobacco. Assessment and treatment of tobacco dependence in primary care is discussed more fully in chapter 6. If the patient is willing to quit, focused tobacco cessation interventions often take precedence over other behavioral health interventions for COPD, given the potential for slowing the rate of progression of the disease through tobacco cessation. In addition, you should evaluate other areas, including the following:

- peak flow (i.e., how fast air moves out of the lungs) and dyspnea symptoms;
- medications;
- effects of COPD on work, social, and family functioning;
- effects of COPD on emotional and cognitive functioning;
- health-related behaviors (e.g., smoking tobacco) affecting COPD; and
- behavioral interventions tried to date.

Figure 9.2 provides specific assessment questions that the behavioral health provider might ask about each domain.

Awareness of the overlap of COPD symptoms with certain psychological symptoms is necessary to avoid over-diagnosis of mental health disorders. For example, symptoms of weight loss, fatigue, decreased concentration, and lower energy in a patient with COPD may be the result of physiological changes resulting from COPD, rather than being indicative of depression. Similarly, chest pain, shortness of breath, and choking may be due to COPD itself, rather than because of an anxiety disorder (Labott, 2004). To distinguish between physical symptoms of COPD and depression or anxiety, pay particular attention to cognitions consistent with a psychological disorder (e.g., negative or anxious thinking) as well as the reported mood itself (e.g., feeling "down" or "worried").

Cognitive impairment may be present in patients with COPD because of hypoxemia and may negatively affect adherence to medical recommendations and quality of life. Administration of the Mini-Mental State Examination (Folstein, Folstein, & McHugh, 1975) can help determine whether referral for more thorough neuropsychological evaluation is warranted.

Advise. The results of the functional assessment guide the recommendations provided to the patient. Given the clinical complexity of COPD in most patients, there will likely be more than one identified problem area that could be targeted for intervention. Common areas include tobacco cessation, improved nutrition and weight gain, increasing physical activity and exercise, relaxation training, breathing strategies (e.g., pursed-lip breathing), mood management,

---

Sample Assessment Questions for COPD

Dyspnea and Peak Flow
- How often do you feel you can't get enough air?
- What kind of activity leads to feeling out of breath?
- What affects your breathing the most (e.g., physical activity, stress, emotions)?
- What is your baseline or average peak flow?
- What is your best and worst peak flow?

Medications
- What medications do you take, and when do you take them?
- What side effects do you notice when you take your medication (e.g., tremor, anxiety, nausea, headache, shortness of breath)?
- Have you ever taken medication for depression or anxiety?

Work, Social, and Family Factors
- How has COPD changed what you do at home? At work?

Functioning
- Are you having trouble getting things done around the house? How so?
- What has changed, if anything, about what you do for fun? With friends?
- Describe what you do in a typical day.
- How has your family responded to your COPD?

Emotional and Cognitive Factors
- What changes have you seen in your mood as your COPD functioning has gotten worse?
- How has your mood been lately? Have you been feeling more down or sad?
- How often do you feel worried or stressed?
- What goes through your mind when you have trouble catching your breath?
- What do you do when you feel you are having trouble getting enough air?
- Have you noticed any changes in your concentration or memory?

Health-Related Behaviors
- Do you smoke? What are your thoughts about quitting?
- What forms of exercise are you getting?
- [If patient appears underweight.] What is your height and weight? Have you lost weight recently? What do you eat in a typical day?
- To your knowledge, are you exposed to indoor air pollutants, at home or work?

Interventions to Date
- Do you practice any form of relaxation (e.g., visualization, diaphragmatic or pursed-lip breathing, guided imagery)?
- Have you ever participated in a pulmonary rehabilitation program?

FIGURE 9.2. Sample assessment questions for COPD.

or adherence to medical recommendations. The following example illustrates how you might advise a patient with COPD on options for change.

> It's great that you have already quit smoking. Congratulations! Staying tobacco-free is the number one thing you can do to help manage your COPD. On the basis of the other information you shared with me this morning, I think there are several more areas we could focus on that would help you feel and function better. One area is your physical activity. As you've had more trouble with your breathing symptoms, you've cut back on your physical activity. That makes sense in the short term because it doesn't feel good to be short of breath. Unfortunately, in the long term, the inactivity leads your body to

become more deconditioned and out of shape. This makes it even harder in the future to do activities you'd like to do, and worsens your breathing problems. Therefore, we could work with your medical providers to help you develop and stick with a plan for gradually increasing your physical activity levels.

A second area that really stood out in our discussion was your description of what happens when you notice your breathing symptoms worsening. You become worried that you won't be able to breathe and that you may pass out. This anxious thinking then worsens your breathing in a vicious cycle. I could teach you some breathing strategies to help control your breathing and promote relaxation. Are you interested in pursuing either or both of those options?

Agree. Often, patients select one of the areas that you have just discussed and recommended. However, they may not always choose to address an area that you believe is most in need of change. In this instance, it is often best to work with patients on goals that they have freely selected, with the hope that their motivation to make additional changes in other important areas will increase in the future as they experience success on initial goals. The following is an example of how a behavioral health consultant (BHC) might respond to a patient who appears to have a goal for treatment that differs from those recommended.

It sounds like you're not too interested at this point in working toward increasing your activity level or in making changes in how you manage your anxiety and breathing. You are concerned, though, about the conflicts you've been having with your husband over sharing the household responsibilities, as you've been able to do less around the house. We can certainly focus on this. Learning new ways to communicate and negotiate responsibilities that have changed because of your COPD sounds

important to you. Why don't we start there? Later, as your communication improves, you may find that you'd also like to focus on one of the other areas we discussed.

Assist. This section provides details on a number of frequently used interventions for patients with COPD, adapted for primary care. These include exercise training, breathing strategies, tobacco cessation strategies, strategies to increase weight, and strategies for the anxiety–dyspnea cycle.

Exercise training. You should closely coordinate with the patients' medical provider any plan to increase exercise in patients with COPD. Before working on increasing exercise, ensure the patient is medically cleared for home-based (i.e., rather than supervised) exercise and have received an exercise prescription. This may involve cardiopulmonary exercise testing to ensure that it is safe for the patient to exercise. You may assist the patient in goal setting, motivation, tracking progress, and relapse prevention to support the recommended exercise plan. Typical recommendations for exercise training in patients with COPD include strength and endurance training at least three times per week, with higher intensities achieving better physical outcomes than lower intensities. Although pulmonary rehabilitation programs may use cycling or treadmill walking, most patients initiating home-based exercise programs find walking programs easier. In addition, the exercise prescription may include upper extremity strength training, because many COPD patients may experience fatigue when performing daily living tasks with their hands and arms. Chapter 6 contains additional information on working with primary care patients on increasing physical activity.

Diaphragmatic breathing and pursed-lip breathing. Training in relaxation methods is standard in most behavioral components of pulmonary rehabilitation programs. This training may involve teaching diaphragmatic breathing, progressive muscle relaxation, or other forms of relaxation. The resources available in chapter 3 are certainly relevant for the patient with COPD who needs additional skills in relaxation. Several adjustments may need to be made for the patient with COPD because of the physiology of the disease. Patients with COPD have an obstructive airway disease, with trapped or residual air in the lungs worsening the feelings of breathlessness and dyspnea. For those with mild disease, standard training in diaphragmatic breathing may be appropriate to help manage physiological anxiety symptoms. For those patients with more advanced stages of COPD, however, a more controlled technique, pursed-lip breathing, can be an appropriate alternative. In pursed-lip breathing, patients more actively expel air from the lungs. The result is often similar to that of diaphragmatic breathing: lowered physiologic arousal and heightened awareness of body response. For a more detailed description of this exercise, see the handouts on pursed-lip breathing (Figure 9.3) and shortness of breath cycle (Figure 9.1).

An additional modification to standard relaxation training made for patients with COPD involves an expanded rationale for using breathing relaxation methods. Discussion with the patient that diaphragmatic breathing and pursed-lip breathing can increase oxygen saturation, decrease respiratory rate, and decrease dyspnea may help increase motivation to regularly use the techniques.

Tobacco cessation. Chapter 6 contains guidelines for helping individuals quit smoking in a primary care behavioral health consultative practice. These strategies are appropriate to use with patients with COPD in primary care. With this population, it may be particularly helpful to focus on the ways that the patient's COPD symptoms and prognosis are closely linked to his or her current smoking behavior. Using motivational enhancement strategies can help the patient identify discrepancies between goals and hopes (e.g., live longer, do more, feel better) and current behavior (i.e., continuing to smoke despite its role in worsening COPD symptoms).

Increasing body weight. As discussed previously, underweight patients with COPD have lower quality of life and increased mortality. The American Thoracic Society (ATS) recommends caloric supplementation in patients with COPD who meet one of the following criteria: a BMI of less than 21, a weight loss of greater than 5% in the previous month, or a weight loss of greater than 10% in the previous 6 months (Nici et al., 2006). You can serve as a resource to help these patients alter eating habits to support a gradual, modest weight gain. Weight gain

---

Pursed-Lip Breathing

Pursed-lip breathing is one of the simplest ways to control shortness of breath in COPD and asthma. It provides a quick and easy way to slow your pace of breathing, making each breath more effective.

What Does Pursed-Lip Breathing Do?
Pursed-lip breathing improves ventilation and releases trapped air in the lungs, decreasing the feeling of breathlessness. It helps keep the airways open for a longer time and prolongs exhalation to slow the breathing rate. It helps improve breathing patterns by moving old air out of the lungs and allowing new air to enter the lungs. It causes general relaxation and allows you to control your symptoms.

When Should I Use This Technique?
Use this technique during the difficult part of any activity like bending, lifting, or climbing stairs or when you are finding yourself anxious or breathless. Practice four to five times a day at first so you can get the correct breathing pattern.

Pursed-Lip Breathing Technique
- Relax your neck and shoulder muscles and breathe in (inhale) slowly through your nose for two counts, keeping your mouth closed. Don't take a deep breath; a normal breath will do. It may help to count to yourself, "Inhale, one, two."
- Pucker or purse your lips as if you were going to whistle or gently flicker the flame of a candle.
- Breathe out (exhale) slowly and gently through your pursed lips while counting to four. It may help to count to yourself, "Exhale, one, two, three, four."

FIGURE 9.3. **Pursed-lip breathing handout.**

efforts can focus on both modifying the patient's existing dietary habits and recommending the inclusion of energy-dense supplements available for purchase in the grocery store. In an initial assessment of eating habits, we typically ask individuals to describe their eating habits on a typical day or on the previous day, including types of foods, amounts, timing and location of eating. On the basis of this brief assessment, we help patients identify additional foods that they are willing to eat and develop a written plan for integrating these foods into their daily eating habits. Although we encourage patients to consider nutritious options, we recognize that the patients may better achieve their weight gain goals if they select foods they like, even if nutritional value is not ideal. We also encourage patients to keep a written record of their eating and their progress toward their eating goals (see Figure 6.3, for a food diary). If initial interventions at the primary care level are not successful, we discuss with the patient's PCP the possibility of a referral to a nutritional specialist for additional assistance.

Dealing with the anxiety–dyspnea cycle. For patients with COPD who demonstrate an anxiety–dyspnea cycle, described earlier, the first intervention involves education about the relationship between physiology, thoughts, and emotions. The shortness of breath cycle handout (see Figure 9.1) often proves helpful in illustrating the way that shortness of breath can lead to anxiety or panic, which ultimately worsens dyspnea. Once patients have an understanding of this cycle, interventions to stop the cycle can be introduced. These interventions may include stopping activity, resting, relaxing (e.g., diaphragmatic breathing, pursed-lip breathing), using reassuring thinking, taking medications if indicated, and ultimately resuming activity in a paced manner.

Arrange. Follow-up with the primary care BHC, if indicated, ideally should be arranged before the patient leaves the clinic. Many patients with COPD will be able to make positive behavioral changes within a small number of appointments (i.e., one–four). However, some patients would benefit from referral to a specialty mental health provider or to a multidisciplinary pulmonary rehabilitation program. These options may be considered if, on initial evalu-

ation, the patient's COPD is severe or, in more mild or stable cases, if the patient does not show adequate progress in making changes through primary care behavioral health intervention. Providers should ensure that patients are familiar with local resources for specialty mental health care and pulmonary rehabilitation programs.

ASTHMA

Asthma, another chronic lower respiratory disease, differs from COPD in a number of ways, including risk factors, pathophysiology, and response to corticosteroid treatment. In addition, although the airflow limitation in COPD is progressive, asthma is characterized by variable airflow obstruction that is typically reversible (Barnes, 2003).

The National Institutes of Health has adopted the following working definition of asthma (National Asthma Education and Prevention Program [NAEPP], 2007):

> Asthma is a chronic inflammatory disorder of the airways in which many cells and cellular elements play a role . . . In susceptible individuals, this inflammation causes recurrent episodes of wheezing, breathlessness, chest tightness, and coughing, particularly at night or in the early morning. These episodes are usually associated with widespread but variable airflow obstruction that is often reversible either spontaneously or with treatment. The inflammation also causes an associated increase in the existing bronchial hyperresponsiveness to a variety of stimuli. Reversibility of airflow limitation may be incomplete in some patients with asthma. (p. 14)

This document is available from the National Institutes of Health Web site (http://www.nhlbi.nih.gov/guidelines/asthma/asthgdln.pdf).

Asthma affects a large proportion of adults and children; 7.2% of adults and 8.9% of children in the United States currently have asthma (Bloom, Dey, & Freeman, 2006; Pleis & Lethbridge-Cejku, 2006). In addition, asthma poses a significant burden on the health care system. In 2004, in the United States alone, asthma accounted for 1.8 million emergency department visits (McCaig & Nawar, 2006), 1 million hospital outpatient visits (Middleton & Hing, 2006), and 13.6 million physician office visits (Hing, Cherry, & Woodwell, 2006).

Symptoms of asthma include cough, wheezing, shortness of breath, chest tightness, and sputum production. Symptoms may be present continuously or episodically and may vary from day to day. Aggravating or precipitating factors include viral respiratory infections, environmental allergens (i.e., indoor or outdoor), exercise, occupational allergens, environmental change, irritants (e.g., tobacco, air pollutions, aerosols), emotional expressions (e.g., hard crying, laughing), drugs (e.g., aspirin, beta-blocks, nonsteroidal anti-inflammatory drugs), cold air, and endocrine factors (e.g., pregnancy, menses). Severity of asthma is classified by clinical features and is categorized as intermittent, mild persistent, moderate persistent, or severe persistent. The severity category drives decisions regarding medical treatment (NAEPP, 2007).

The effects of asthma can range from minimal interference and near-normal functioning to high levels of impairment, including the need for frequent unscheduled medical care and emergency visits, missed workdays and schooldays, limitations on physical activity and exercise, and nighttime awakening because of symptoms. Treatment goals, as designated by the National Heart, Lung, and Blood Institute (NHLBI), include aims to normalize both physical and psychosocial functioning and are specified as follows:

- to be free from troublesome symptoms,
- to maintain "best" lung function,
- to be able to participate fully in activities of choice,
- to not miss work or school because of asthma symptoms,
- to have few or no urgent care visits or hospitalizations for asthma,
- to use medications to control asthma with as few side effects as possible, and
- to be satisfied with asthma care. (NAEPP, 2007, p. 131)

Key Biopsychosocial Factors in Asthma

As with COPD, BHCs should be knowledgeable of the biopsychosocial factors associated with asthma. This will help the BHC focus on appropriate assessment variables and effectively communicate with patients and providers.

Physical factors. The inflammation of airways causes the hallmark symptoms of asthma (e.g., chest tightness, wheezing, breathing difficulty) as well as hyperresponsiveness of the airways to a variety of stimuli. Obstruction of airflow is often variable and may be reversible with treatment or may remit spontaneously. An overview of the pathogenesis of asthma can be found in the NAEPP's (2007) "Expert Panel Report."

A primary physical factor routinely measured in asthma assessment and treatment is peak expiratory flow, commonly called *peak flow*. Peak flow is a measurement of how well patients can exhale air. As airways become narrowed, air becomes trapped in the lower segments of the lungs and peak flow values decline. Measurements of peak flow are not typically used for diagnosis, but rather for ongoing monitoring of changes in the severity of airflow obstruction. Peak flow monitoring can be accomplished at home with an inexpensive peak flow monitor. To assess peak flow, individuals inhale deeply, place their lips around the mouthpiece of the monitor, and exhale as quickly and forcefully as possible. NAEPP (2007) recommended that patients with moderate persistent or severe persistent asthma monitor their peak flow on a daily basis. A major benefit of daily monitoring is the ability to detect worsening of respiratory function before noticeable symptom changes, hence providing the opportunity to make alterations in medication administration early in an asthma exacerbation. Daily peak flow monitoring can also alert patients to how diligent they need to be regarding pacing physical activity, practicing stress reduction techniques, and reducing allergen exposure.

Medical treatment aimed at modifying physical factors related to asthma primarily involves prescription medication. Medications for asthma include those designed to be used daily for long-term prevention and control of inflammation and exacerbations and those that give quick relief of symptoms during asthma exacerbations. For optimal control of asthma, patients should be using both types of medications correctly. See NAEPP (2007) for a listing of commonly used long-term and short-acting medications for asthma.

To minimize overdiagnosis of mental health problems, you should be aware that some patients might experience medication side effects that overlap with symptoms of mental disorders. For example, systemic corticosteroids may lead to appetite changes, weight gain, and mood alteration; methylxanthines may lead to insomnia and gastrointestinal symptoms; and short-acting inhaled β_2-agonists may lead to tremor and heart rate changes (NAEPP, 2007).

Emotional and cognitive factors. As with COPD, the presence of co-occurring anxiety symptoms complicates the assessment and treatment of patients with asthma. Patients with asthma are at increased risk of having panic attacks compared with the general population of primary care patients (Goodwin et al., 2003). Anxiety or panic may further worsen respiratory symptoms through hyperventilation. There is evidence that some individuals with asthma may experience bronchoconstriction and worsening respiratory symptoms in response to psychological stress (Busse et al., 1995). In addition, anxiety symptoms may lead to overuse of quick relief asthma medications and are associated with more frequent treatment with steroid medications (Carr, 1998). Finally, health beliefs about asthma (e.g., "Asthma is not a serious illness") or asthma medications (e.g., "I don't need to take my inhaled corticosteroids if I'm not having symptoms") can affect patterns of medication use (Chambers, Markson, Diamond, Lasch, & Berger, 1999).

Behavioral factors. Certain behaviors may predispose the patient to asthma exacerbations. Smokers have poorer response to corticosteroids and poorer control of asthma symptoms (Chaudhuri et al., 2003; Thomson, Chaudhuri, & Livingston, 2004). Exercise-induced asthma symptoms also may be influenced by behavioral factors. Individuals who experience asthma symptoms during exercise may not engage in appropriate behaviors to manage these symptoms properly (e.g., lack of warm-up period,

failure to use appropriate medications prior to exercise). As a result, they may limit or avoid exercise or other physical activity as much as possible because of concerns about worsening symptoms. Other behavioral factors that may impair management of asthma include poor adherence to medical recommendations (e.g., failure to use daily peak flow monitoring or home-based action plans) or inappropriate use of medications (e.g., overuse of β_2-agonist).

Environmental factors. Exposure to certain factors in the physical environment may contribute to asthma exacerbations. These may include, among others, animals, mold, pollen, cold air, and airborne chemicals or dust. Social and family factors also may play a role in effective management, particularly in children (e.g., parental knowledge and beliefs, school environment, medication procedures).

Specialty Mental Health

Specialty psychoeducational intervention programs for patients with asthma lead to a variety of positive outcomes. Devine's (1996) meta-analysis of 31 studies of psychoeducational interventions found improvements in lung functioning (e.g., asthma attacks, peak expiratory flow rate, dynamic respiratory volume), adherence to medical treatment recommendations, and functional status; decreases in health care use; improved use of medications and inhaler use; and improved psychological well-being. Treatments typically included the following components: education; behavioral skill development, including relaxation training; cognitive therapy; and general psychosocial support.

Newman, Steed, and Mulligan (2004) reviewed 18 studies of self-management interventions for asthma. They found that treatment typically addressed recognizing and avoiding triggers of asthma, monitoring symptoms and adjusting medications, and increasing adherence to recommendations about medication. Interventions were delivered in group and individual formats and ranged from 1 to 12 hours in length. Improvements in lung functioning were found in 57% of studies. Of the studies that measured quality of life as an outcome, 50% found improvements. Decreased health care use was found in 64% of interventions, and behavior changes related to asthma management were found in 57% of the studies.

NHLBI guidelines reflect the recognition of the importance of self-management approaches in asthma treatment (NAEPP, 2007). Their recommendations for effective asthma management include the following four broad components: (a) assessment and monitoring of lung function, (b) control of factors contributing to asthma severity, (c) pharmacologic therapy (i.e., long-term control and quick relief medications), and (d) education for partnership in asthma care. Within these broad domains, BHCs may play a particularly useful role in helping patients to adhere to recommendations regarding daily self-monitoring of peak flow, to appropriately use written action plans developed between the patient and PCP for asthma exacerbations, to modify behaviors to reduce exposure to factors that worsen asthma, to reduce barriers to adherence to medication recommendations, and to use relaxation and stress management skills to remain calm during asthma exacerbations, potentially preventing some exacerbations.

Behavioral Health in Primary Care

No studies examining the effects of brief behavioral health consultation in primary care settings on asthma outcomes could be found in the current literature.

Primary Care Adaptation

The following recommendations regarding behavioral interventions for patients with asthma in primary care are based on adaptations of specialty behavioral health treatment for asthma and the clinical practice guidelines developed by NHLBI (NAEPP, 2007) described earlier.

Assess.   As with COPD, brief assessment of patients with asthma should include evaluation of symptoms and functioning. See Figure 9.4 for examples of assessment questions you might consider using for patients with asthma. Respiratory symptom and function questions focus more explicitly on peak flow and whether the patient is using regular peak flow monitoring to guide day-to-day decision making regarding home management of asthma.

Medication compliance proves difficult for many patients with asthma, so a close examination of medication use is warranted to determine whether they are either overusing or underusing medications. A common pattern is overuse of quick-relief medications and underuse of long-term control medications, often because of mistaken beliefs about the role of different types of medication. Medical data on the number of primary, urgent, or emergency care visits also should be obtained during the assessment to help determine adherence to current care plans. From these, the BHC can further assess whether current barriers to maintaining good health are the result of poor adherence to previously constructed care plans.

Assessment of emotional functioning should include brief screening questions for anxiety and panic, given the role that such symptoms may play in worsening the management of asthma, especially in an anxiety–dyspnea cycle. Health-related behaviors, particularly those related to exposure to factors that exacerbate asthma, may also be assessed. Close attention to tobacco use or exposure to secondhand smoke, dust mites, mold, and other environmental factors at home or work is warranted (see NAEPP, 2007, pp. 129–130 for additional details). Finally, obtaining information on what, if any, interventions the patient has tried can help guide decisions regarding future strategies.

Advise.   The next step is to advise the patient on specific recommendations for change. The recommendations may be based on what you believe is the most important aspect to address (e.g., smoking cessation, regular use of long-term management asthma medication as prescribed); what the PCP believes is the most important aspect, on the basis of the referral question or issue (e.g., "Patient is not following the home-based action plan. Please assist."); or what you believe the patient might be most motivated or willing to try.

As with other types of patients, when working with individuals who have asthma, ensure your advice does not overstep bounds of competence and stray into the practice of medicine. Rather than providing specific advice about medical interventions, BHCs provide consultation to the PCP and reinforce

---

Sample Assessment Questions for Asthma

Peak Flow
- Do you monitor your peak flow at home? How often?
- What is your baseline or average peak flow? What is your best and worst peak flow?
- Has your peak flow dropped below [80% of personal best] since your last medical visit? What did you do?
- How often do you notice symptoms of worsening asthma?
- What affects your breathing the most (e.g., physical activity, stress, emotions)?

Medications
- What medications do you take? When do you take them?
- How many inhalers have you gone through in the last month?
- What side effects do you notice when you take your medication (e.g., tremor, anxiety, nausea, headache)? Have you stopped taking any regular doses for any reason?

Medical System Use
- When was your last hospitalization? How many hospitalizations have you had?
- Estimate how many primary care visits have you made in the last year.
- How many visits to the emergency room have you made in the last year?

Work, Social, and Family Factors
- How has asthma changed what you do at home? At work?
- What has changed, if anything, about what you do for fun?
- How many days of work/school have you missed due to asthma in the last year?
- What would you like to do that you can't do now, or as well, because of your asthma?
- How has your family responded to your asthma?

Emotional and Cognitive Factors
- Describe how your mood has been lately.
- How often do you feel anxious or panicky? When does this occur?
- What goes through your mind when you have an asthma attack?
- What do you do when you feel you are having trouble getting enough air?

Health-Related Behaviors
- Do you smoke? What are your thoughts about quitting?
- What forms of exercise are you getting? Are your symptoms worsened by exercise?
- What factors have you found make your asthma worse (e.g., animals, mold, pollution, cold air, foods, occupational exposures)? Which ones do you have the most trouble avoiding?

Interventions to Date
- Are you monitoring your peak flow? How often?
- Do you have a written action plan? Can you describe it for me?
- What kinds of problems do you have with following the plan?
- Do you practice any form of relaxation (e.g., visualization, diaphragmatic breathing, guided imagery)?

FIGURE 9.4. Sample assessment questions for asthma.

the medical treatment plans that the PCP and patient have jointly developed. For example, optimal medical treatment of asthma integrates home-based action plans into the patient's care to promote regular monitoring of lung function, early identification of exacerbations, followed by appropriate decisions regarding medication use and accessing additional medical help. These plans need to be developed jointly between the patient and the PCP, not the BHC, because they involve specific recommendations about medication use and when to access urgent or emergency care. However, you should be familiar with the format and content of the action plans used to assist patients in adherence. The following is an example of how you might advise a patient with asthma on treatment options, without crossing over the line of inappropriately providing medical, rather than behavioral health, advice.

I'm concerned by a few things I heard you mention this morning. One is that you feel your asthma is getting worse. You've had more exacerbations and have been to the emergency room twice in the last two months. I'm also concerned that you feel you're not able to manage your asthma at home. You say that you have a peak flow meter at home, and your PCP has asked you to check your peak flow each morning before you take your medication. However, you're having difficulty remembering to do this. It also sounds like you're not quite sure how to adjust your medications at home when you do get a peak flow reading that seems low to you, or when you notice your asthma symptoms worsening.

We know that it takes a partnership between medical providers and patients with asthma, with active participation from both sides, to effectively manage asthma. You're doing a great job remembering to take your long-term control medications. However, some of the other aspects of your care have been difficult, such as peak flow monitoring. In addition, you don't have a written home action plan that would help you make decisions about what to do when your lung function gets worse.

I have a couple of recommendations. The first is that we set up an appointment for you with your primary care provider to develop a written home action plan, which is the form she uses with most of her patients with asthma [show blank action plan that has not been completed]. Your primary care provider will likely look at what your peak flow readings have been and use that information to set guidelines about when to take certain steps, such as taking additional medication or seeking medical care.

My second recommendation is that you and I work together to help you stay consistent with your daily peak flow monitoring, because your primary care provider really thinks it is important in getting your asthma under control. We can develop some ways to help you remember to do the monitoring each morning and tackle any other barriers that might be getting in the way. What do you think about these options?

Agree. Once you have discussed with the patient your recommendations for change, you and the patient need to come to agreement on the specific direction you will take. We typically recommend that the patient select just one, or two at the most, area(s) to change at a time with additional areas being targeted later after initial progress has been made, if needed. Some amount of artful negotiation may be needed to come to mutually agreed-on goals, as can be seen in the following example of a patient who is unwilling to monitor peak flow daily but wants to see improvements in her ability to be physically active with her children.

> Your primary care provider really wants you to monitor your peak flow every day. She and I both believe this is critical in helping keep you out of the emergency room, but it sounds like you really don't want to focus on this right now. You say you've done it before for a few weeks and didn't find it helpful and that you find it hard to remember to do it. What you're really concerned about is how your asthma has gotten in the way of being active and has restricted you from doing things such as riding bikes or playing tag with your kids. You'd like to be able to do these things you enjoy more often.
>
> In many ways, the two issues are linked. Regular monitoring of your peak flow can help you take your medications in a way that will minimize your asthma symptoms. This, in turn, will allow you to be more active. However, we certainly can begin by working on other strategies

that may help improve your ability to be physically active with your kids, even if you're not ready right now to go back to the daily peak flow monitoring. Then later, when you're ready, we can shift our focus back to the peak flow monitoring, perhaps coming up with some ideas on how to make it easier for you. How does that sound to you?

An additional issue in the agree phase arises when family is involved in the management of asthma, whether in adults, adolescents, or children. Often, the proposed plan involves cooperation or action on the part of the family of the patient with asthma. For example, a spouse might be asked to change her smoking behaviors in the home to minimize the amount of smoke exposure that her husband with asthma receives. Parents may be needed to assist with the complicated medication regimen for their child or with educating school personnel on actions to take if symptoms increase. Whenever possible, you should elicit the agreement of all relevant parties (i.e., spouse, parent, child) before moving on to the assist phase of the interaction.

Assist. Achieving the goals of good asthma management involves a number of complex choices and behaviors on the part of the patient. These range from monitoring lung functioning or symptoms, managing acute symptom exacerbations, and using medications appropriately, to identifying and modifying triggers (e.g., tobacco smoke, occupational exposures).

Monitor peak flow. In accordance with expert recommendations regarding management of asthma (NAEPP, 2007), many PCPs will want their patients with moderate persistent and severe persistent asthma, or those with severe exacerbations, to measure and record their peak flow on a daily basis. You can help patients achieve this goal by working to increase motivation for this behavior change. This may be done through psychoeducation regarding the role that peak flow measures can play in providing early warning of exacerbations, even before physical symptoms may be noticeable to the patient. It may also be achieved through motivational interviewing strategies, such as highlighting discrepan-

cies between the patient's overall asthma goals and current behavior or having the patient verbalize arguments for making the change, for example. You may also assist the patient in identifying and eliminating barriers to regular monitoring. Providing a monitoring form that is easy to use, and helping the patient identify cues to help remember to monitor, may also prove useful. The patient asthma diary (Figure 9.5) provides one example of a monitoring form that patients may find helpful in recording their peak flow, along with several other relevant variables (i.e., asthma symptoms, effects of symptoms on activity, and exposure to triggers).

Manage acute exacerbations. Many medical providers routinely use written asthma action plans for their patients with asthma to help them make appropriate decisions regarding medication use and seeking medical assistance during asthma exacerbations, in accordance with National Institutes of Health recommendations (NAEPP, 2007). If medical providers are not using a standard form, you might consult with your PCPs to create a form that meets their needs but also is easy for the patient to use (see NAEPP, 2007, pp. 117 and 119, for examples). BHCs then may play a large role in monitoring and assisting patients in understanding and following the action plan. Working with patients to identify and remove barriers to monitoring routinely falls within your scope of care. For example, you might help the patient plan a strategy to ensure that the action plan is available in various locations (e.g., work, car, home) through use of multiple copies, laminated copies, wallet cards, and so forth. Finally, you can assess whether psychological factors such as high anxiety are interfering with plan implementation when exacerbations occur. If so, assisting the patient in remaining calm during exacerbations may be indicated. This could take the form of teaching skills to rest, relax, and use reassuring thinking during exacerbations. The patient can learn and practice cognitive disputation skills, relaxed breathing, and perhaps enlist a significant other to help coach him or her in relaxed breathing. Information on the anxiety–dyspnea cycle (Figure 9.1), and the handout on pursed-lip breathing (Figure 9.3), discussed previously in the COPD section, may also be useful for these patients with asthma.

Patient Asthma Diary

Instructions. Please record your peak flow number(s) in the spaces provided for each date. Rate your asthma symptoms of coughing, wheezing, and shortness of breath (SOB) on a scale of 0 to 3 (0 = *no noticeable symptoms*, 1 = *mild*, 2 = *moderate*, 3 = *severe*). List any activities that you restricted because of your symptoms. List any exposure to potential triggers or factors that worsen your asthma. Finally, record the number of puffs of your quick-relief inhaler (bronchodilator) you used to control your symptoms.

Date	Peak flow a.m.	Peak flow p.m.	Symptoms (0–3) Cough	Symptoms (0–3) Wheeze	Symptoms (0–3) SOB	Activity restriction	Exposures	Inhaler puffs (quick relief)
‾‾	‾‾	‾‾	‾‾	‾‾	‾‾	‾‾‾‾	‾‾‾‾	‾‾‾‾
‾‾	‾‾	‾‾	‾‾	‾‾	‾‾	‾‾‾‾	‾‾‾‾	‾‾‾‾
‾‾	‾‾	‾‾	‾‾	‾‾	‾‾	‾‾‾‾	‾‾‾‾	‾‾‾‾
‾‾	‾‾	‾‾	‾‾	‾‾	‾‾	‾‾‾‾	‾‾‾‾	‾‾‾‾
‾‾	‾‾	‾‾	‾‾	‾‾	‾‾	‾‾‾‾	‾‾‾‾	‾‾‾‾
‾‾	‾‾	‾‾	‾‾	‾‾	‾‾	‾‾‾‾	‾‾‾‾	‾‾‾‾
‾‾	‾‾	‾‾	‾‾	‾‾	‾‾	‾‾‾‾	‾‾‾‾	‾‾‾‾

FIGURE 9.5. Patient asthma diary handout.

Use medications correctly. The referral question from a PCP may indicate concerns about medication use, such as, "Patient is not regularly using her budesonide inhaler. Seen in urgent care last week. Please assist," or, "Patient is using more than two canisters of albuterol a month. May be using for anxiety symptoms. Please evaluate." Alternatively, you may discover inappropriate medication use patterns in your initial assessment or on review of self-monitoring forms. After ensuring that you and the patient both know the type, dose, timing, and frequency recommended by the PCP, you should identify barriers to appropriate adherence. For the patient underusing his or her long-term control medications (e.g., budesonide inhaler), asking about his or her understanding and beliefs about the role of this medication in asthma control may reveal an incorrect belief that this medication only needs to be taken when he or she experiences symptoms. Effective interventions may include informing him or her that daily use of long-term control medications (e.g., anti-inflammatories) is the most effective way to control persistent asthma. In addition, it may be helpful to provide behavioral strategies to assist the patient to remember when to take medication as well as cognitive strategies for countering incorrect beliefs about the medication use.

Overuse of quick-relief medications may result from a number of factors. Some patients may not have their symptoms well controlled by their current long-term control medication or may not be effectively avoiding factors that exacerbate their asthma. These reasons could necessitate another appointment with the PCP to evaluate whether long-term control medication needs adjusting, or they may require renewed efforts by you to identify and modify potential triggers. Patients with anxiety symptoms, however, may overuse their quick-relief medications by using their inhaler in response to physical symptoms of anxiety (e.g., increased heart rate, rapid shallow breathing, tightness in chest) rather than to symptoms of an asthma exacerbation. If this is clearly the case, the patient may benefit from modifying symptom perception and learning anxiety management strategies (e.g., deep breathing, pursed-lip breathing, reassuring thinking).

Recognize and minimize triggers. Reducing exposure to factors that exacerbate asthma is a core asthma management strategy. Having the patient

---

Factors That May Worsen Asthma

Directions. The following is a list of irritants or allergens that may increase asthma symptoms in some people. Please check the boxes in front of factors that you believe you may be exposed to.

- Pets (type _____)
- Moistness or dampness in any room of the house (e.g., basement)
- Visible mold in the home
- Cockroaches in the home
- Use of a "swamp cooler" or humidifier
- Tobacco smoke (i.e., at home or work)
- Wood-burning stove or fireplace used at home
- Unvented stoves or heaters
- Sulfite sensitivity (i.e., symptoms after eating shrimp, dried fruit, beer, wine)
- Beta-blocker medication
- Aspirin or other nonsteroidal anti-inflammatory medications
- Pollens (e.g., trees, grass, weeds)
- Perfumes
- Cleaning agents
- Other _____

FIGURE 9.6.   Factors that may worsen asthma handout. From *Expert Panel Report 3: Guidelines for the Diagnosis and Management of Asthma* (pp. 129–130), by National Asthma Education and Prevention Program, 2007. Copyright 2007 by the National Institutes of Health. Adapted with permission.

complete a checklist of factors he or she may be exposed to can provide a starting point for developing a behavioral plan to minimize exposure. Figure 9.6 contains a sample checklist that may prove helpful. Alternatively, some patients benefit from 1 to 2 weeks of self-monitoring, tracking exposure to potential triggers along with changes in asthma symptoms or peak flow readings. If warning indications are discovered, you may then recommend that the PCP evaluate whether allergy testing is warranted to assess sensitivity to possible indoor allergens or whether other medical interventions for allergies are warranted. Once factors that exacerbate asthma have been identified, the BHC can work with the patient to develop strategies to reduce exposure. (see NAEPP, 2007, pp. 129–130, for additional details).

Stop smoking. Smoking worsens lung function in patients with asthma and decreases the effectiveness of many asthma medications. Therefore, quitting smoking may be the most important change that patients can make to improve their asthma management. For more information, see the discussion earlier in this chapter on smoking cessation for patients with COPD as well as the more detailed information on tobacco cessation in primary care found in chapter 6.

Minimize exercise-induced bronchospasm. Medical recommendations for minimizing exercise-induced bronchospasm include using medications, such as brochodilators, before exercise as well as engaging in an adequate warm-up period prior to exercise (Nici et al., 2006). Often, patients have already discussed this problem with their PCP and are aware of his or her recommendations regarding medication use. Many patients, however, are either not aware or do not follow recommendations regarding an adequate warm-up period. You can work with patients to regularly incorporate a 6- to 10-minute period of gradual warm-up, typically walking, before exercise that is more vigorous.

Arrange.   As with patients with COPD, some patients with asthma may show a rapid improvement in self-management behaviors within a few appointments. Others, however, will require referral for specialty mental health treatment. Need for a referral may be higher when there are significant mental health disorders affecting the self-management approach to asthma care. For example, patients with comorbid panic disorder may need a more intensive level of treatment.

SUMMARY

Pulmonary disorders, particularly COPD and asthma, are a major cause of disability and health care burden. These diseases often have a significant negative impact on physical functioning, psychosocial functioning, and quality of life. COPD and asthma are among the most common chronic illnesses seen at primary care medical clinics and are often difficult for PCPs to manage in the allotted 15- to 20-minute medical appointment because of the complex interaction between physical, behavioral, emotional, and environmental factors often seen in these patients. BHCs can assess and intervene with appropriate evidence-based strategies to address behavioral, emotional, cognitive, and environmental factors (e.g., smoking, anxiety or panic, physical inactivity, medical noncompliance, inappropriate use of medication) that may be making symptoms and functioning worse. BHCs can also assist the PCP in identifying which patients are not benefiting from intervention at the primary care level and can recommend referrals to specialty mental health providers when indicated. Overall, the hope is that through behavioral health consultation in primary care, patients with COPD and asthma will experience improved management of their disease, better functioning, and increased quality of life.

CHAPTER 10

CARDIOVASCULAR DISEASE

Cardiovascular disease (CVD) is an umbrella term that refers to diseases of the heart and blood vessels. Some of the more common conditions and diseases that fall under this umbrella include coronary artery disease, cardiomyopathy, valvular heart disease, pericardial disease, arteriosclerosis, atherosclerosis, aneurism, high blood pressure, stroke, and peripheral artery disease (see the Mayo Clinic Web site at http://www.mayoclinic.com/health/cardiovascular-disease/HB00032 for additional information). Since 1900, except for 1918, CVD has been the number one cause of death in the United States; approximately one person dies every 36 seconds from CVD (Rosamond et al., 2007). Over one third of the U.S. population has some form of CVD, contributing to an estimated $431.8 billion in direct and indirect costs (Rosamond et al., 2007).

Scheidt (1996), whose book serves as a useful resource for behavioral health professionals working with CVD, categorizes CVD into three major areas: (a) coronary heart disease, (b) valvular heart disease, and (c) cardiomyopathy. Coronary heart disease, also referred to as *coronary artery disease,* results from the buildup of fatty deposits (i.e., atherosclerosis) on the arterial walls that supply the heart with blood. It can result in transient chest discomfort (i.e., angina pectoris), heart attacks (i.e., acute myocardial infarctions), and sudden cardiac death. Valvular heart disease affects one or all four heart valves and results in insufficient blood flow or backward leakage through the heart valves. Valvular heart disease generally results from rheumatic heart disease, age-related degeneration, or congenital abnormalities. Cardiomyopathy refers to a weakening of the heart muscle and most commonly results in heart failure, an inability of the heart to pump sufficient amount of blood throughout body.

The development of CVD has been linked to a variety of biopsychosocial factors. Although certain risk factors, such as age, sex, race, and heritable risk, cannot be modified, the risk of developing CVD, particularly coronary heart disease, can be decreased by targeting physical, behavioral, and emotional risk factors. In this chapter, we discuss the factors that contribute to the development and progression of CVD. Familiarity with these factors can help you more effectively assess and facilitate change among patients with CVD. The interventions recommended in this chapter rely heavily on those described in chapters 3, 5, and 6.

PHYSICAL FACTORS ASSOCIATED WITH CARDIOVASCULAR DISEASE

The development and progression of CVD is often related to diabetes, high blood pressure, and hypercholesterolemia. Diabetes, which we discuss more extensively in chapter 7, is associated with the development of coronary heart disease, peripheral arterial disease, and, potentially, cardiomyopathy. Higher blood pressures are independent risk factors for developing CVDs, including coronary heart disease, strokes, and congestive heart failure (Kannel, 1996). Table 10.1 lists the classification of blood pressures. Among those 40 to 70 years old, the risk of CVD doubles for every 20 mm Hg increase in systolic blood pressure and 10 mm Hg increase in diastolic blood pressure starting at 115/75 mm Hg (Lewington, Clarke,

155

	TABLE 10.1	

Classification of Blood Pressure for Adults

Blood pressure classification	Systolic blood pressure (mm Hg)	Diastolic blood pressure (mm Hg)
Normal	<120	and < 80
Prehypertension	120–139	or 80–89
Stage 1 hypertension	140–159	or 90–99
Stage 2 hypertension	≥ 160	or ≥ 100

Note: From "Seventh Report of the Joint National Committee on Prevention, Detection, Evaluation, and Treatment of High Blood Pressure," by A. V. Chobanian, G. L. Bakris, H. R. Black, W. C. Cushman, I. A. Green, J. L. Izzo, Jr., et al., 2003, *Hypertension, 42,* pp. 1206–1252. Copyright 2003 by Lippincott Williams & Wilkins. Adapted with permission.

Qizilbash, Peto, & Collins, 2002). Individuals with prehypertensive blood pressures (i.e., systolic blood pressures between 120–139 mm Hg and/or diastolic blood pressures between 80–89 mm Hg) have a 90% greater risk of developing hypertension compared with individuals with lower blood pressures (Vasan et al., 2002). Essential hypertension is the most common primary diagnosis in the United States (U.S. Department of Health and Human Services [USDHHS], 2004a) and the most common diagnosis seen in primary care settings (Hing, Cherry, & Woodwell, 2006).

Cholesterol travels through our blood stream in two major forms of lipoproteins, *low-density lipoproteins* (LDL) and *high-density lipoproteins* (HDL). Excess LDL cholesterol, referred to as hypercholesterolemia, contributes to atherosclerosis (i.e., hardening of the arteries). Foods high in saturated fat, trans fat, and cholesterol increase levels of LDL. Low levels of HDL cholesterol are also related to increased risk of CVD. Table 10.2 shows the classification system used to identify high levels of cholesterol by the National Institutes of Health's National Cholesterol Education Program (2002). Overall, providers focus on the absolute value of LDL cholesterol as the primary target in lipid-lowering treatments (National Cholesterol Education Program, 2002).

HEALTH BEHAVIORS ASSOCIATED WITH CARDIOVASCULAR DISEASE

In addition to tobacco use (USDHHS, 2004b), overeating (Eckel & Krauss, 1998), and physical inactivity (Farrell et al., 1998; discussed in chap. 6,

this volume), dietary nutrient and alcohol consumption, as well as medication adherence affect the course of CVDs.

Dietary Nutrients

Individuals at risk of, or diagnosed with, CVDs are encouraged to modify the nutrient components of their diet. By following the *dietary approaches to stop hypertension* (DASH) eating plan, patients can reduce their blood pressure (Sacks et al., 2001) and risk for other cardiovascular events (Cook et al., 2007). The recommendations of the DASH eating plan are presented in Table 10.3. In addition, the American Heart Association recommends that individuals without coronary heart disease eat oily fish (e.g., canned light tuna, salmon, catfish), which have high concentrations of omega-3 polyunsaturated fatty acids, twice a week and those with coronary heart disease eat those fish or use supplements on a daily basis (Lichtenstein et al., 2006).

Alcohol Consumption

Alcohol consumption has a J-shaped curve relation with mortality. Individuals consuming a moderate amount of alcohol (i.e., daily consumption of one standard drink for women and two standard drinks for men) have a lower risk of death from all causes, including coronary heart disease, compared with individuals who do not drink alcohol and individuals who consume three or more drinks a day (Camargo et al., 1997; Di Castelnuovo, Rotondo, Iacoviello, Donati, & de Gaetano, 2002; Gronbaek et al., 1995). However, beyond moderate intake,

TABLE 10.2

Classification of Cholesterol for Adults

Cholesterol classification	9–12 hour fasting lipoprotein levels (mg/dl)
Total cholesterol	
Desirable	<200
Borderline high	200–239
High	≥240
Low-density lipoprotein cholesterol (LDL)	
Optimal	<100
Near optimal/above optimal	100–129
Borderline High	130–159
High	≥160
High-density lipoprotein cholesterol (HDL)	
Low (increased risk for CVD)	<40 (men); <50 (premenopausal women)
High (decreased risk for CVD)	≥60
Triglycerides	
Normal	<150
Borderline high	150–199
High	200–499
Very high	≥500

Note: CVD = cardiovascular disease. From "Third Report on Detection, Evaluation, and Treatment of High Blood Cholesterol in Adults (Adult Treatment Panel III)" (NIH Publication No. 02-5215), by the National Cholesterol Education Program, 2002. Retrieved January 6, 2007, from http://www.nhlbi.nih.gov/guidelines/cholesterol/atp3_rpt.htm. In the public domain.

alcohol begins to have a negative impact on cardiovascular health.

Medication Adherence

Among individuals with CVD, adherence to lifestyle and medication recommendations is a significant problem. For example, 70% of hypertensive patients fail to adhere to a recommended treatment regimen (Sherbourne, Hays, Ordway, DiMatteo, & Kravitz, 1992). Poor adherence to medication regimens among patients with CVDs may be affected by multiple factors that predict decreased adherence, including emotional difficulties (e.g., depression), asymptomatic conditions, and negative side effects of the medication (Osterberg & Blaschke, 2005). To improve

TABLE 10.3.

Components of the DASH Eating Plan (Based on a 2,100 kcal Diet)

Total fat	27% of calories	Sodium	2,300 mg[a]
Saturated fat	6% of calories	Potassium	4,700 mg
Protein	18% of calories	Calcium	1,250 mg
Carbohydrate	55% of calories	Magnesium	500 mg
Cholesterol	150 mg	Fiber	30 g

Note: From "Your Guide to Lowering Your Blood Pressure With DASH" (NIH Publication No. 06-4082) by the U.S. Department of Health and Human Services, 2006. Retrieved January 6, 2007, from http://www.nhlbi.nih.gov/health/public/heart/hbp/dash/new_dash.pdf. In the public domain.
[a]1,500 mg sodium was found to be more effective for lowering blood pressure, particularly among middle-aged and older adults, African Americans, and those diagnosed with high blood pressure.

adherence, researchers have focused on developing educational, behavioral, and organizational approaches (Johnson & Carlson, 2004). Helping patients establish readiness for self-care, setting specific goals, self-monitoring, and using cues are some of the behavioral strategies that could be incorporated into a primary care environment to assist patients with adherence. However, no method reliably increases adherence to medication regimens over the long-term in individuals with chronic medical conditions (Haynes et al., 2005). Therefore, it is important to recommend to PCPs that they regularly assess and target adherence to medications.

EMOTIONAL FACTORS ASSOCIATED WITH CARDIOVASCULAR DISEASE

Emotionally, stressors, depression, anxiety, and anger or hostility have been related to the development of CVDs. Both acute (e.g., bereavement, natural disasters, terrorist activities) and chronic stressors (e.g., work-related, marital, caregiving stress) have been linked to the development of CVD and hypertension (Larkin, 2005; Rozanski, Blumenthal, & Kaplan, 1999). In addition, individual differences in cardiovascular reactivity, the level of cardiac responses to a stressor, may serve as an independent risk factor for CVD (Manuck, 1994). Interventions that reduce stress responses have demonstrated short-term benefits for reducing physiological activity, but there is not well-established evidence that decreasing stress independently reduces risk for CVD (Rozanski et al., 1999).

Depression is associated with a variety of CVDs, including coronary heart disease (Musselman, Evans, & Nemeroff, 1998), coronary artery disease (Kop, 1999; Lesperance & Frasure-Smith, 2000), and heart failure (Havranek, 2006). Cardiac patients more commonly demonstrate depressive symptoms of tiredness, lack of energy, and irritability rather than the more common negative mood, guilty feelings, or low self-esteem symptoms (Kop, 1999; Kop & Ader, 2006; Lesperance & Frasure-Smith, 2000). These differences in symptom presentation likely contribute to the underdiagnosing of, and subse-

quent failure to treat, depression in cardiac patients (Freedland, Lustman, Carney, & Hong, 1992). Therefore, it is particularly important to carefully screen for depressive symptoms in patients with CVD. Treating depressive symptoms has not been shown to effectively reduce risk for future cardiac events (Berkman et al., 2003); therefore, the primary outcome is a reduction in depressive symptoms and an improved quality of life.

Anxiety symptoms are a chronic problem in 20% to 25% of individuals diagnosed with coronary heart disease (Januzzi, Stern, Pasternak, & DeSanctis, 2000) and may be present in 70% to 80% of individuals following an acute cardiac event (Trumper & Appleby, 2001). Anxiety disorders have been associated with increased risk of sudden cardiac death (Rozanski et al., 1999). Although not necessarily a significant contributor to the development of CVD, anxiety symptoms can be a significant consequence of CVD and its associated treatments (Sears, Todaro, Lewis, Sotile, & Conti, 1999).

Although data have shown that a Type A behavior pattern, first described by Friedman and Rosenman (1959), is not significantly related to coronary artery disease (Rozanski et al., 1999), research has turned to examining hostility, defined as anger, cynicism, and mistrust, as the primary factor of the Type A behavior pattern that is related to the development of coronary artery disease. The relation between hostility and coronary heart disease or atherosclerosis has been mixed (Bunker et al., 2003; Rozanski et al., 1999). Some individuals are examining whether the time urgency component of Type A behavior is a better predictor of CVD (Cole et al., 2001).

ENVIRONMENTAL FACTORS ASSOCIATED WITH CARDIOVASCULAR DISEASE

Environmental factors including social support and socioeconomic status affect CVDs. Small social support networks, low levels of perceived support, and social isolation are associated with increased risk of developing coronary heart disease, independent of other risk factors (Lett et al., 2005; Rozanski et al., 1999). Although there is some evidence that social support interventions improve a variety of problems (e.g., cancer, weight loss, surgery, birth preparation; Hogan, Linden, & Najarian, 2002), this research is often conceptually and methodologically flawed (Hogan et al., 2002), and efforts to improve social support do not reduce the frequency of coronary heart disease events (Lett et al., 2005). Similar to social support, low socioeconomic status is related to the development and progression of coronary heart disease. This holds true whether socioeconomic status is measured by education, income, or occupation (Rozanski et al., 1999).

SPECIALTY MENTAL HEALTH

Providers in outpatient clinical health psychology settings often see patients following a significant cardiac event (e.g., myocardial infarction) or a cardiac surgery (e.g., bypass surgery, placement of a stent). Providers may participate in comprehensive cardiac rehabilitation programs, which have been found to reduce subsequent cardiac mortality and risk factors (e.g., blood pressure, smoking, weight; Dusseldorp, van Elderen, Maes, Meulman, & Kraaij, 1999). Multiple studies, such as the PREMIER study (Elmer et al., 2006), have demonstrated that high intensity treatments for changing health behaviors can have an impact on physical factors that are risk factors for disease. Iestra et al. (2005) assessed the effect of changing health behaviors on mortality. The results of their study estimated mortality reductions for those with CVD to be 35% with smoking cessation, 25% with increased physical activity, 20% with moderate alcohol use, and 45% with dietary changes. These risk reductions are similar or greater than the risk reduction associated with preventive medication interventions (e.g., low dose aspirin, statins, β-blockers, ACE inhibitors; Iestra et al., 2005). Large trials such as Sertraline Antidepressant Heart Attack (SADHEART) (Glassman et al., 2002) and Enhancing Recovery in Coronary Heart Disease (ENRICHD) Patients (Berkman et al., 2003) have shown that although depressive symptoms can be reduced through medications or cognitive behavioral therapy in individuals at risk of CVD, there is no substantial evidence that the morbidity and mortality of CVD are reduced (Joynt & O'Conner, 2005).

BEHAVIORAL HEALTH IN PRIMARY CARE

In chapter 6, we discussed the data supporting interventions in primary care for the three most important health behaviors related to CVD: tobacco use, overeating, and physical inactivity. We do not know much about the effectiveness of trying to target multiple CVD health behaviors simultaneously in primary care settings (Goldstein, Whitlock, & DePue, 2004). Similarly, although we discussed the effectiveness of emotional management strategies in primary care in chapter 5, we do not have extensive data that tell us whether these interventions work for patients with CVD in primary care. Therefore, in our primary care clinical practice, we adapt our assessments and interventions on the basis of the available evidence to target the behaviors, thoughts, and emotions we know affect, and are affected, by CVD.

PRIMARY CARE ADAPTATION

Working in the primary care clinic places behavioral health consultant (BHC) on the front lines of CVD prevention and treatment. The American Heart Association considers diet and lifestyle changes "critical components" of the strategies to prevent CVD (Lichtenstein et al., 2006), and leaders in CVD treatment have called for increased emphasis on lifestyle interventions (Eckel, 2006). Target areas may include achieving a healthy weight (i.e., a body mass index <25 kg/m^2), being physically active, and avoiding tobacco, which are discussed in chapter 6. The American Heart Association also recommends that individuals maintain recommended levels of cholesterol, triglycerides, and blood pressure (Lichtenstein et al., 2006). Even small reductions in blood pressure in the population (e.g., a 5 mm Hg reduction of systolic blood pressure [SBP]) are believed to reduce mortality that is caused by coronary heart disease by 9% and all-cause mortality by 7% (Whelton et al., 2002).

Common medications used in the treatment of CVD can be found on the National Heart, Lung and Blood Institute Web site at http://www.nhlbi.nih.gov/actintime/HDM/HDM.htm. BHCs need to be familiar with these medications and their effects to effectively communicate and assess primary care patients with CVD. When assessing adherence to these medical treatments, it is helpful to be familiar with their side effects (e.g., increased urination with diuretics) to help patients adhere to their medical regimens.

In primary care, you are likely to start seeing a patient because he or she has been diagnosed with some physical condition associated with CVD, such as high blood pressure, hypercholesterolemia, or diabetes. As you conduct your assessment and develop interventions, it is important to be mindful of how these factors affect patients' physical condition and long-term risk of CVD.

Assess

CVDs are complex; therefore, before accepting these consults, understand the basic underlying pathology and the factors that may contribute to the presenting problems. Assessments of primary care patients at risk of, or diagnosed with, a CVD should include an evaluation of the following:

- their knowledge of their current condition,
- health behaviors that could potentially affect their cardiovascular system, and

- cognitive and emotional functioning and environmental factors known to influence CVD.

No assessment should occur unless the individual has been evaluated medically and the medical provider is requesting assistance with managing the patient's CVD.

As we have emphasized throughout this volume, it is important to select the questions most pertinent to the referral problem. If someone is referred for assistance with management of hypertension, it may be more important to focus on the sodium content of their food compared with someone referred for assistance with managing hypercholesterolemia, who would benefit most from limiting the amount of fats in their diet. Figure 10.1 presents the broad range of questions to consider asking. In addition to evaluating the factors that affect and are affected by CVD, motivation for change is especially important to assess. Someone who has undergone a surgery or had a heart attack may be more motivated to change their behaviors than someone diagnosed with hypertension or hypercholesterolemia because those diagnosed with the latter conditions often do not feel sick.

Assessment Questions for Patients With Cardiovascular Disease

The following questions represent a guide for the assessment of those referred for the reduction of risk or management of cardiovascular disease. Depending on the responses of the patient, you may want to ask questions that are more detailed.

Health Behaviors
- Do you use tobacco? How much? How often do you use it?
- What is your current weight? Height? [Determine BMI.]
- Describe what you typically have for breakfast, lunch, dinner, and snacks.
- How often do you eat red meat? How often do you eat out? Where do you usually eat?
- Do you monitor the amount of sodium and fat in the food you eat? How much do you typically eat in a day?
- How much alcohol do you drink each day? Each week?

Emotional Responses
- How stressed would you generally rate yourself, if 0 is no stress and 10 is the most stressed you could imagine?
- Have you had any recent major life changes, such as beginning or ending a relationship, moving, or changes in your financial status?
- Are the demands of your job difficult to manage? Would you describe your relationships as stressful?
- How do you manage stress? Who do you lean on for support? Do you easily loose your cool? Do you get frustrated quickly?

FIGURE 10.1. Assessment questions for patients with cardiovascular disease.

Physical factors. The patient's experience with physical symptoms will vary significantly depending on his or her CVD. Questions associated with physical factors should focus on assessing the patient's experience with physical symptoms, medications and side effects, surgical procedures and interventions, and the patient's understanding of his or her medical condition. If the patient has been diagnosed with a physical precursor to CVD, consider asking the following:

- What physical symptoms, if any, have you noticed associated with your condition?
- What medications have you been prescribed? What side effects have you noticed since starting that medication? Has your medication affected how you live your life?
- Have you noticed changes in your sleep?

If the individual has had a surgical procedure or significant cardiac event (e.g., a heart attack), consider asking the following:

- What physical symptoms do you notice that affect your daily living?
- Are you experiencing pain? If so, what does your pain keep you from doing?
- Do you tire more easily? Have you participated in a cardiac rehabilitation program?
- What is your plan for becoming more active?

Health factors. Health behaviors are some of the most important areas to assess because of their independent and direct effects on the cardiovascular system and because of the benefits associated with changing these behaviors. We cover some of the relevant health behaviors, including tobacco use, weight, and physical inactivity in chapter 6, and alcohol use in chapter 12. In addition to assessing these behaviors, we recommend you spend time evaluating whether the patient consumes high sodium and/or high fat foods and is taking medications as they are prescribed.

Unlike assessments associated with weight, when the primary focus is on calories, assessing sodium and fat intake is important for those referred for consultation related to CVD. If highly detailed analyses of their food is necessary, they should be referred to a specialist in nutrition. The intent of the

assessment is to identify foods that may be high in sodium or fat that could be decreased in the patient's diet. Significant sources of sodium are processed foods and condiments. Saturated fats are most commonly found in dairy, red meat, butter, and some vegetable oils. On the other hand, patients should generally increase their consumption of potassium, which is found in potatoes, spinach, bananas, and legumes (e.g., soybeans, lentils, kidney beans). Examples of questions you could ask to assess the patient's consumption of sodium and fat are as follows:

- What foods do you typically eat for breakfast, lunch, and dinner?
- How often do you eat red meat? How often do you eat out? Where do you usually eat?
- Do you monitor the amount of salt and fat in the food you eat? How much sodium do you typically eat in a day? Do you add salt to your foods? How much?
- How often do you eat processed or luncheon meats (e.g., turkey, ham)? Canned meats, fish, vegetables, or soups? Processed cheese? Frozen dinners or entrees? Mexican food? Foods with soy sauce? Salted snacks such as pretzels, chips, crackers, or popcorn?

In addition to food consumption, it is important to assess how patients are taking their medications. To assess medication adherence consider asking the following:

- How many medications are you taking? Do you take them as prescribed? How often do you miss taking a medication?
- What side effects concern you? Do you feel overwhelmed by the number of medications that you are taking?

Emotional factors. The patient with CVD will be at risk for some form of negative mood. Therefore, it is particularly important to screen these patients for depression, anxiety, anger, hostility, and stress, while also recognizing that targeting these emotional responses may improve their quality of life but that there is no consistent evidence that reducing these symptoms will necessarily reduce their risk of CVD. Chapters 3 and 5 provide descriptions of methods for assessing and targeting these emotions that are more detailed. If the patient experienced a particular cardiac event, such as a myocardial infarction, or if there have been invasive treatments, such as an implanted cardioverter defibrillator, you should spend some time asking how the patient's functioning has changed since that event. Collaborate with the physician to determine what are reasonable limitations on functioning. Negative mood may be assessed as follows:

■ Since your heart attack, what has changed in your daily functioning?
■ Do you feel down more often?
■ What activities have you taken out of your life? Are you interested in restarting them?

In addition, pain, particularly chest pain, may be a trigger for increased anxiety symptoms. Assess how their thoughts about pain affect their functioning, as follows:

■ Do you worry when you experience pain? Do you think it is a sign of a heart attack?
■ Because of your worry, do you avoid activities that might increase pain?
■ How would you tell the difference between cardiac-related pain and other pain?

Often patients hear of links between stress and CVD but may be less familiar with how other emotions relate to their cardiovascular problem. Similarly, obesity and sedentary behaviors are commonly cited as causes of heart disease, but individuals may be less familiar with the relation between tobacco use and heart disease. On the basis of the assessment, you can offer patients a menu of choices of which behaviors or emotions they would be most interested in targeting. An example might sound like the following:

> On the basis of what you've told me, it sounds like you may be experiencing a more negative mood, and may be depressed at times. The more depressed you are, the less you feel like doing physical activity and the more you eat as a way to comfort yourself. You find that you get yourself much more

stressed at work than you would like to be, and, recently, you've started smoking again as a way to manage stress. Is my understanding of your current situation accurate or have I missed something important?

The patient may be interested in targeting multiple behaviors, or just one. Focus on what the patient is interested in changing, but be realistic about the effects of the changes. Decreasing depressive symptoms may not significantly lower blood pressure, but doing so may improve the patient's daily functioning and motivation to make other changes in the future.

Advise

Quitting tobacco, losing weight, changing eating habits, and adhering to medication regimens are often the most important lifestyle changes for patients referred for CVD-related concerns. Following the assessment, you can list the possible areas that could be targeted. We have developed a handout that could be used with patients with high blood pressure to guide this discussion (see Figure 10.2). It is of interest that one review of randomized controlled trials that used counseling or educational interventions and/or medications targeting multiple cardiovascular risk factors (e.g., blood pressure, smoking, physical activity) and examining the effects on mortality, blood pressure and cholesterol changes, and smoking status, found limited or no significant changes in outcome measures (Ebrahim, Beswick, Burke, & Davey Smith, 2006). These data may suggest that it is most beneficial to individually target behaviors or problems rather than try to change multiple behaviors simultaneously. Review the possible areas that could be targeted while advising the patient about which areas would be most beneficial to target for his or her present condition. For example, you could say the following:

> Your weight is high enough that it may be affecting your blood pressure, and you are relatively sedentary. Decreasing your stress response, reducing your weight by 10%, increasing your physical activity, or stopping your smoking may

High Blood Pressure

Blood pressure is defined by two numbers, your systolic blood pressure and your diastolic blood pressure. Your *systolic blood pressure* is the pressure in your arteries when your heart is squeezing blood out to your body. The systolic blood pressure is represented by the top number of your blood pressure reading. Your *diastolic blood pressure* is the pressure in your arteries when your heart is relaxed; it is represented by the bottom number of your blood pressure reading.

What was your last blood pressure reading? Systolic = _____ Diastolic = _____

Often, you don't feel sick when you have high blood pressure. Except for the numbers on the blood pressure monitor, there may not be any other indication your blood pressure is high. Below is a table we can use to classify your blood pressure. How would you classify your blood pressure?

Blood pressure classification	SBP mm Hg	DBP mm Hg
Normal	<120	and <80
Prehypertension	120–139	or 80–89
Stage 1 hypertension	140–159	or 90–99
Stage 2 hypertension	≥160	or ≥100

SBP = systolic blood pressure; DBP = diastolic blood pressure.

Making Changes

Many different factors affect your blood pressure. Some of these factors you may be able to change; other factors you can't change. By making changes where you can, you can lower your blood pressure. The following is a listing of some of the factors that you can change.

How important is it to you to make these changes? If it doesn't apply or if it is not important, rate it a 0. If it is important, what steps can you take to make changes?

Tobacco Use

Quitting tobacco use is one of the most important health behavior changes you can make. If you are a non-smoker, great! If you currently smoke, have you considered quitting?

How important to you is it to quit smoking?

0———1———2———3———4———5———6———7———8———9———10

Not important   *Most important*

If tobacco cessation is important to you, what is your plan to quit tobacco?

_____

_____

Weight Loss

If you are overweight or obese, even small reductions in your weight (e.g., 10 pounds) can have a significant impact on your blood pressure. Weight loss requires a reduction in the number of calories you eat or drink and an increase in your physical activity.

How important is it to you to lose weight?

0———1———2———3———4———5———6———7———8———9———10

Not important   *Most important*

If weight loss is important to you, what can you do to start making changes in your eating, drinking, and physical activity habits?

_____

_____

FIGURE 10.2.   High blood pressure handout. (*Continued*)

Dietary Changes

Beyond weight loss, it is important to consider changing what you eat to reduce your blood pressure. A special diet called the DASH diet is often encouraged for individuals with high blood pressure. The DASH diet encourages you to decrease the amount of salt and fat in your diet while increasing the amount of potassium and fiber you consume. Often these changes require simple substitutions in your diet, such as replacing salt with other spices and choosing lower fat alternatives to your typical foods.

How important is it for you to change your diet?

0———1———2———3———4———5———6———7———8———9———10

Not important   *Most important*

If dietary changes are important to you, what are some of the foods that you are willing to substitute or eliminate from your diet?

_____

_____

Physical Activity

To improve cardiovascular health, it is recommended that you engage in 30 minutes of moderate intensity activity at least 5 days a week or vigorous intensity activity for 20 minutes at least 3 days a week.

How important is it for you to meet these activity recommendations?

0———1———2———3———4———5———6———7———8———9———10

Not important   *Most important*

If physical activity changes are important to you, how can you incorporate moderate or vigorous activities into your daily life?

_____

_____

Medication Adherence

If your blood pressure is in the hypertensive range, you may have been prescribed a medication to help you lower your blood pressure. However, the effectiveness of the medications depends on individuals taking them as they were prescribed.

How important is it for you to change the way you take your medications?

0———1———2———3———4———5———6———7———8———9———10

Not important   *Most important*

If medication adherence is important to you, what are some of the techniques you can use to manage your medications more effectively?

_____

_____

Stress Management

The stressors that you experience can contribute to higher blood pressure levels. You can manage stressors differently by changing the way you think or what you do and by using relaxation techniques.

How important is it for you manage your stress response?

0———1———2———3———4———5———6———7———8———9———10

Not important   *Most important*

If stress management is important to you, what are some of the techniques you can use to manage stressors more effectively?

_____

_____

FIGURE 10.2.   (*Continued*) High blood pressure handout.

help to reduce your blood pressure, whereas targeting your depressed mood may help you to enjoy more aspects of your life and improve your life satisfaction. Which of these things are you most interested in targeting?

Agree

Once you have advised patients on what they could possibly change, elicit from them what it is they want to change. Despite the known effect of tobacco cessation and weight loss on the risk and progression of CVD, patients may not be motivated to make the necessary changes at the time of the referral. Determine which behavior changes patients are motivated to make and develop a set of recommendations that reflect their current goals, and provide direction for continuing to assess their interest in making additional changes. For example, a patient diagnosed with hypertension who is overweight and who smokes one pack of cigarettes per day may agree to focus on medication adherence and fail to demonstrate interest in changing other health behaviors. The following are examples of recommendations you could make for the patient:

- Buy a pillbox that includes separate day and time slots.
- On Sunday evening, place medications in the appropriate time slot for each day.
- Take your medications each day.
- Consider quitting tobacco use.
- Consider implementing a weight loss plan.

The following are example recommendations for the primary care provider:

- Continue to assess whether the patient is motivated to quit tobacco or change eating habits.
- Consider asking whether the patient is ready to change, or ask the patient to rate the importance of each change on a scale of 0 (*not important*) to 10 (*very important*). For example, the patient may rate the importance of quitting tobacco use as a 3 and changing diet as a 4.

Assist

Knowing the relative effect of health behaviors and emotional responses on CVD will help guide appro-

priate behavior change recommendations. Obviously, the form of CVD alters the interventions that would be offered to patients. Given that hypertension is the most frequently encountered diagnosis, we focus on possible interventions for high blood pressure. In the primary care environment, many of these same interventions could be applied to patients with other forms of CVD, but modified in intensity or frequency.

Health factors. To assess whether the patient is moving in the right direction, it is important for the patient and all members of the health care team to set specific goals for any behavior change.

Tobacco use. We discuss methods for targeting tobacco use in chapter 6. It can be useful to spend some time discussing the effects of tobacco use on cardiovascular risk. It may even be helpful to demonstrate the impact that smoking has on blood pressure by comparing blood pressure values immediately after smoking with those after a couple of hours of abstinence. Assuming that the patient is motivated to quit, it is important to develop a plan that includes a quit date, how the patient will prepare before their quit date, medications and/or nicotine replacements, and methods for dealing with cravings and high-risk situations.

Excess weight. Methods for reducing weight are also discussed in chapter 6. As mentioned earlier, a 10-pound weight loss can significantly reduce risk of CVD and can result in lowered blood pressure, cholesterol, and improved diabetes management. Some individuals may find it overwhelming to monitor calories and make significant dietary changes. For individuals interested in losing weight, you can relate their cardiovascular health to reductions in their weight. As we discussed in chapter 6, you should establish a specific plan for how to reduce calories. Consider obtaining pre- and postintervention blood pressure and cholesterol readings to help the patient and medical team see the changes that weight loss can have on objective measures of cardiovascular risk.

Diet. Changing the content of patients' diets will require collaboration to identify foods that they could substitute for their typical diets. Use a handout such as the one in Figure 10.3 to help patients

Diet Change

To help reduce blood pressure, it is recommended that individuals reduce their sodium content to 2,300 mg or 1,500 mg. Below are alternatives to high-sodium and high-fat foods.

Reducing Salt Content

Foods high in salt (sodium)	Low-salt alternatives
▪ smoked, cured, salted, and canned meat, fish, poultry	▪ unsalted fresh or frozen beef, lamb, pork, fish, poultry
▪ regular hard and processed cheese	▪ low-sodium cheese
▪ regular peanut butter	▪ low-sodium peanut butter
▪ crackers with salted tops	▪ unsalted crackers
▪ regular canned and dehydrated soups	▪ low-sodium soups, broths, bouillons
▪ regular canned vegetables	▪ fresh and frozen vegetables
▪ salted snack foods	▪ unsalted snack foods

Reducing Fat Content

Food category	Foods high in fat	Lower fat alternatives
Dairy	▪ whole milk	▪ skim, 1%, 2% milk
	▪ ice cream	▪ sorbet, sherbert, frozen yogurt
	▪ cheese	▪ low- or reduced-fat cheese
Pasta	▪ ramen noodles	▪ rice
	▪ pasta with cream sauce	▪ pasta with tomato sauce
	▪ granola	▪ reduced fat granola
Meat, fish, poultry	▪ ground beef	▪ low-fat, extra-lean meats,
	▪ chicken or turkey with skin	▪ skinless chicken or turkey
	▪ hot dogs	▪ low-fat hot dog
	▪ bacon sausage	▪ turkey bacon
	▪ oil packed tuna	▪ water-packed tuna
	▪ whole eggs	▪ egg whites, egg substitute
Baked goods	▪ croissants	▪ hard rolls, English muffins
	▪ donuts	▪ bagels
	▪ muffins,	▪ reduced fat muffins
	▪ party crackers	▪ low-fat crackers
	▪ cake, cookies	▪ angel food cake
Snacks and sweets	▪ nuts	▪ popcorn, fruits, vegetables
	▪ ice cream	▪ frozen yogurt, pudding bars
Fats, oils, and salad dressings	▪ butter, margarine	▪ light margarine
	▪ mayonnaise	▪ light mayonnaise, mustard
	▪ salad dressings	▪ fat free salad dressing
	▪ oils, shortening, lard	▪ nonstick cooking spray

What are the changes that you plan to make in your diet?

Reduce salt by:_____

Reduce saturated fat by:_____

FIGURE 10.3.   Diet change handout. Reducing salt content data from "Alternatives to High-Sodium Foods," by the U.S. Food and Drug Administration, n.d. Retrieved January 9, 2007, from http://www.fda.gov/fdac/foodlabel/sodtabl.html. Reducing fat content data from "The Practical Guide: Identification, Evaluation and Treatment of Overweight and Obesity in Adults" (NIH Publication No. 00-4084), by the National Institutes of Health, 2000. Retrieved January 9, 2007, from http://www.nhlbi.nih.gov/guidelines/obesity/prctgd_c.pdf.

consider and identify diet alternatives. It may be necessary to briefly educate the patient about how to read a nutrition label and discuss the areas on the nutrition label to focus on. The most important changes will likely be reductions in salt and fat. Often patients are not aware of the salt and fat content in the foods they consume and how much they should be eating. As you develop a specific plan with the patient, assess what foods he or she could eliminate or substitute to make the necessary changes. For example, patients may not realize how much salt can be contained in canned soups. Discussing alternatives (e.g., low sodium soups), or decreasing the amount of canned soup they consume, could represent a significant change in their sodium intake.

Physical activity. Physical activity changes are also discussed in chapter 6. Specific goals to increase activity or to start exercise programs will increase the likelihood that patients will follow through with the plan. Particularly with exercise plans, it is important to collaborate with the patient's medical provider to make decisions about the intensity and duration of their exercise program. Discuss with the patient ways that he or she can increase physical activity. For reducing the risks associated with CVD, it is recommended that individuals engage in at least 30 minutes of moderate intensity activity most, if not all, days of the week. Help the patient define moderate intensity activities (e.g., brisk walking). We find that simply prescribing a change is less likely to work than spending some time figuring out what physical activity changes will fit into the patient's life (e.g., walking during work, taking the stairs, playing with children).

Alcohol. We address ways to target excess alcohol use in chapter 12. If patients are medically cleared to consume alcohol, and there is no concern or risk of alcohol abuse (e.g., a substance abuse history), then individuals should not be discouraged from drinking one (for women) to two (for men) "standard" (see chap. 12, this volume) alcohol containing drinks per day.

Medication adherence. To improve medication adherence, identify the barriers that interfere with taking medications as prescribed. Sometimes the regimen of medications is overly complex, and discussing a simpler regimen with the patient's medical provider may improve adherence. Simple tools, such as a medication box or organizer, with days and times during the week for each medication, can be used to organize pills according to the time of day that they should be taken. Consider using some external cue to remind patients to take their medications. There are multiple consumer products, including pill timers, clocks, pagers, and computer software that can be used to provide external prompts. Consider ways of enlisting the support of other individuals (e.g., spouse, significant other) to help improve adherence. Discuss situations that could lead to lapses in their medication regimen (e.g., traveling) and how the patient could plan to reduce the chances of nonadherence to the medication. If the patient is not motivated to take the medications (e.g., concerned about side effects), then consider methods of improving motivation, such as those presented in chapter 3.

Emotional factors. Patients diagnosed with a CVD often report some emotional distress. Identifying and targeting this distress can improve the patient's functioning.

Stress. If the individual struggles with stress management, consider teaching brief relaxation strategies (e.g., deep breathing, progressive muscle relaxation, guided imagery) and methods to change stressful thinking, as described in chapter 3. It may be useful to take blood pressure readings before and after the relaxation exercise to demonstrate the effect the relaxation has on their blood pressure. If patients are taking medications that lower blood pressure, relaxation exercises may result in some difficulty with blood pressures becoming so low that they experience difficulty moving from a seated to standing position. Therefore, carefully monitor such individuals as they make such changes and ask about lightheadedness. It is of interest that we have often found that individuals with CVD do not perceive themselves as being stressed. Therefore, consider using other terms for stress, such as distress, frustration, or being overwhelmed.

Depression. Interventions for depression and anxiety are usually not different for this population than for others, so the strategies in chapter 5 should be helpful with these patients. It is often useful to relate the changes to their cardiovascular functioning when appropriate. However, it would not be appropriate to state. "By decreasing your depressive symptoms, we will reduce your risk for having a heart attack." Instead, place the focus on improving their functioning by saying, "By decreasing your depressive symptoms, we can help you live your life more the way that you want to."

Incorporate behavioral activation with other potentially beneficial activities, such as increasing social support and physical activity can be helpful in reducing depressed mood. Patients may have depressive thoughts focused on how their CVD has changed their life or their outlook on life. Again, moving thoughts to focus on current functioning and methods of improving that functioning may help to decrease negative thinking related to their disease.

Anxiety. Although the physical aspects of anxiety may not be different among patients with CVD, the content of the thoughts may be unique. Individuals who have faced life-threatening situations (e.g., a heart attack) may have a fear of death associated with pain, which can be difficult to distinguish from benign pain. Schwartz, Trask, and Ketterer (1999) provide a table that helps to distinguish between cardiac-related chest pain and other sources of pain. For example, sensations of heaviness, pressure, tightness, jaw pain, and pain that radiates down the arm are unique sensations to angina compared with other sources of chest pain. Teaching relaxation strategies, targeting negative thinking by developing alternative reassuring thoughts, or using acceptance-based techniques (Hayes & Strosahl, 2004; Hayes, Strosahl, & Wilson, 1999) may help to reduce anxiety symptoms.

Anger and hostility. Managing anger and hostility requires individuals to change how they perceive situations and considering alternative responses. Providing brief assertiveness training (see chap. 3,

this volume) to distinguish between reacting to situations in an angry manner and using assertive language and responses may help to decrease the intensity of emotional responses. Brief relaxation methods, such as cue-controlled relaxation and diaphragmatic breathing (see chap. 3, this volume), may also be helpful skills for decreasing the intensity of the responses. Cognitively, using more reassuring thinking and decreasing alarming thinking may decrease the frequency that patients perceive situations as threatening.

Environmental factors. Social support is an important factor to consider in assisting patients with CVDs. To improve social support, examine how people found support in the past. Consider encouraging patients to spend more time with family, plan outings with friends, join a social club or group that has a shared interest (e.g., running groups), become more active with a religious organization, or join a volunteer organization. Exercise is such an important aspect of decreasing risk of CVD that it may be possible to combine exercise and social support interventions. Often, patients may demonstrate a reluctance to engage in an activity that is designed to facilitate enjoyment, but relating the activity to their functioning and to helping them live a more enjoyable life may improve the likelihood that patients will participate in the activity.

Arrange

The frequency of follow-up appointments will be dependent on the behaviors that are targeted. Just as with other patient populations discussed throughout this volume, you will find most patients require a small number of appointments (i.e., one–two) to begin making behavior changes in their lives. It is important to be aware of specialty groups or clinics that may be a resource for helping those patients who have a more difficult time initiating behavior changes. Knowing nutritionists, exercise physiologists, cardiac rehabilitation services, diabetes care clinics, and clinical health psychology specialty clinics can provide necessary support to the medical team for helping to manage patients with CVDs.

SUMMARY

Primary care environments offer unique opportunities to work with patients across the spectrum of CVDs. BHCs can have a tremendous effect on cardiovascular risk factors, particularly health behaviors. Simply targeting patients who have blood pressures in the prehypertensive or hypertensive range or cholesterol levels that are in hypercholesterolemia range, BHCs could fill their entire schedule. Working with these patients usually does not require specialized skills because the behavior changes or emotional responses are not different from many other patient populations. However, taking the time to develop a more in-depth knowledge of the cardiovascular system and how behavior, thoughts, and emotions affect and are affected by changes in the cardiovascular system, will contribute to more effective assessments and interventions for these populations.

CHAPTER 11

PAIN DISORDERS

Pain is one of the most prevalent complaints seen in general medical settings, accounting for over 80% of all physician visits (Gatchel & Turk, 1996). Low-back pain alone is reported by 5.6% of the adult population, with a lifetime prevalence of 60% to 70%. As many as 25% to 30% of people with low-back pain seek medical care (Kincade, 2007). Other common pain complaints seen in primary care include migraine and tension headaches, arthritis pain, and fibromyalgia.

The assessment and treatment of pain have changed over the past decades. The traditional medical model viewed pain from a purely physiological standpoint. The objective in pain assessment was to identify its biological cause. Treatment could then be accomplished by eliminating or blocking that cause. From this perspective, when a physical cause could not be identified, the pain was assumed to be psychologically generated; this was known as *psychogenic pain.* This model is no longer widely accepted. Newer understandings of pain and pain management have recognized the role that a variety of other factors, beyond physiology, play in pain. The gate-control theory of pain (Melzack & Wall, 1965) and the biopsychosocial model (Engle, 1977) have provided important frameworks for better understanding pain to help those who are experiencing pain to find ways of improving their quality of life.

With these new understandings, the role of behavioral health professionals in the assessment and treatment of pain conditions has expanded. In the old model, the role of the psychiatrist or psychologist was relegated to conditions in which the problem was judged to be imaginary or psychogenic. Now mental health providers collaborate with physicians to address multiple contributing and restorative factors; these include physical activity, emotional distress, beliefs about pain, physiological stress and relaxation, environmental demands, and general coping.

CLASSIFICATION OF PAIN DISORDERS

The *Diagnostic and Statistical Manual of Mental Disorders, Fourth Edition, Text Revision (DSM–IV–TR;* American Psychiatric Association [APA], 2000) provides a useful classification system regarding the interaction of psychological factors in pain conditions. Pain-related diagnoses fall mostly in the categories of *psychological factors affecting physical condition* and *somatoform disorders.* The primary distinction between the two categories is whether a general medical condition exists that fully accounts for the physical symptoms. In psychological factors affecting physical condition, a general medical condition accounts for the physical symptoms; however, psychological factors such as a mental disorder, emotional distress, or behavioral and lifestyle issues are determined to be affecting the medical problem. The result may be an exacerbation of symptoms, interference with treatment, a negative change in the course of the disease, or an additional health risk to the patient.

According to the *DSM–IV–TR,* somatoform disorders involve the "presence of physical symptoms that suggest a general medical condition (hence, the term somatoform) and are not fully explained by a general medical condition, by the direct effects of a substance, or by another mental disorder" (APA, 2000, p. 485). With these conditions, psychological factors play a role in the etiology of the physical symptoms. These include somatization disorder, undifferentiated somatoform disorder, and pain disorder.

Another useful classification differentiates between acute pain, recurrent pain, and chronic pain. Specific definitions for each vary in the literature; however, they are distinguished by the duration of time over which the pain occurs. Acute pain generally occurs with an injury or illness and resolves with healing or resolution of the illness. Recurrent pain is episodic, such as with migraine. Chronic pain is a persistent pain, lasting longer than 6 months.

SPECIALTY MENTAL HEALTH

Behavioral and cognitive–behavioral interventions are essential to successful treatment of chronic pain and are typically integrated into multidisciplinary chronic pain treatment programs. Cognitive–behavioral treatments alone have also been shown to result in significant changes in measures such as pain experience, cognitive coping and appraisal, and reduced behavioral expression of pain. A meta-analysis of research studies on cognitive–behavioral interventions by Morley, Eccleston, and Williams (1999) illustrates the success of these treatments.

BEHAVIORAL HEALTH IN PRIMARY CARE

Primary care-based treatment for pain disorders has been found to be helpful for reducing dysfunction and improving quality of life. Intervention consisting of telephone contact by primary care nurses resulted in decreased bodily pain, improved role functioning from a physical and emotional standpoint, and improved vitality (Ahles et al., 2006). In addition, a program to reduce fear and increase activity levels resulted in reductions in pain-related fear, average pain, and activity limitations resulting from back pain (Von Korff et al., 2005).

PRIMARY CARE ADAPTATION

The following section reviews how to adapt behavioral and psychological assessment and intervention for pain complaints in the primary care setting. Scripts are provided as suggested ways of discussing pain related topic areas with patients. The handouts

can be used to facilitate your assessment and interventions. It must be noted here that behavioral health interventions for pain should be done only in collaboration with a medical workup. Because pain can be a symptom of serious illness or injury requiring medical intervention, a thorough evaluation by a physician should be obtained before proceeding with assessments and interventions from a behavioral health perspective.

Assess

A functional assessment of a pain problem can help identify factors that contribute to initiation, exacerbation, or maintenance of pain, as well as identify factors that lead to excessive suffering from nociceptive pain. Key areas for assessment include

- variability in pain and factors that contribute to increases or decreases;
- functional impact of pain on daily activities;
- adaptive coping in response to pain, including emotional distress, cognitions, and behaviors; and
- the effects of social and environmental contingencies.

Evaluation by a specialty trained clinical health psychologist or similar specialist may be necessary for significantly impaired chronic pain patients, and a referral to a chronic pain rehabilitation program can be beneficial. For less impaired patients, a more focused pain assessment can be useful; this level is appropriate for the primary care setting.

The following questions are recommended for primary care assessment of chronic pain:

- general description of the pain: "Where is the pain located and what is its quality (e.g., aching, shooting, stabbing, binding, pinching, squeezing, throbbing)?";
- onset of pain: "When did the pain start? What was going on when the pain started?";
- frequency of the pain: "How many times per day, week, or month does it occur?"; and
- duration of the pain: "How long does the pain last when it occurs?"

A number of methods can be used to determine the intensity of the pain; however, the most common is a numerical rating of 1 to 10 with 1 representing *very mild pain* and 10 representing *excruciating pain*.

Obtain ratings for the pain at its worst, least, and most common, as follows:

- On a scale of 1 to 10, 1 being mild pain and 10 being excruciating pain, what is your pain level right now? Where is it on that scale at its worst? When is it at its best?
- What can you do to decrease the pain?
- What makes the pain worse?
- Why do you think you are experiencing pain? What has your physician told you about the cause of the pain?
- Describe a typical day, including home, work, and leisure time activities.
- How does the pain limit you? What would you be doing differently if you didn't have pain?
- How has the pain affected you emotionally? [Assess depression, anxiety, and anger.]
- How have others responded to the pain? Family? Friends? Coworkers?
- How would you like others to respond?
- What have you done to help deal with the pain? [Include medical treatments, procedures, and self-management strategies. Assess for inappropriate medication use, alcohol or drug abuse (see chap. 12, this volume), and excessive sleep or inactivity.]
- In what other ways has the pain affected your life?

Advise

Popular understandings of pain that are based in mind–body dualism, in which pain is viewed exclusively as either a physical problem or a psychological problem, continue to be prevalent. Therefore, a primary goal of the advise phase is to help patients understand the interaction of biopsychosocial domains in their pain problem and to increase motivation to address components such as emotions, thoughts, behaviors, and interpersonal issues as part of their approach to more effectively manage pain.

Providing the patient with a framework for understanding the role of psychological factors in pain may be helpful. The following script is one way of describing this framework:

> Pain is a complex problem; medical science is finding this to be more true all the time. Our old understanding of pain

such as yours was that pain was a direct reflection of an injury or disease and that the only way to address pain was to identify the physiological cause and remove it or block it. The problem with that model is that it didn't account for pain very well. In other words, sometimes there is a great deal of physical abnormality with little pain, and, at other times, there can be minimal or no physical disease but significant pain.

Let me give you a couple examples of how physical injury and the experience of pain don't always correspond well. One is the phenomenon of pain blocking. Take as an example a soldier who, in the midst of a battle, might fight bravely and assist his injured buddy get to a helicopter for medical evacuation. Only after his buddy is safe, does the soldier realize that he too has been injured. Because of situational demands, mental distraction, and the flow of adrenalin, he didn't recognize his own injury or feel the pain. In this situation, these other factors played more of a role in pain and perception of pain than did the actual physical injury.

Another example is a phenomenon called phantom pain, which sometimes occurs when people undergo amputation of a limb. These individuals sometimes feel pain in the location of the amputated limb even though that limb is no longer there. If pain was purely a physiological issue, phantom pain could not occur. These are just a couple of examples that show the role of psychological factors in pain perception. Let me be clear, this does not mean people make up their pain or that it is not real. Pain is real, as you know. Understanding and targeting these other factors, however, gives people more control over their pain.

One helpful way in which scientists have thought about how these nonphysical factors contribute to pain is that there is something like a "gate" [see

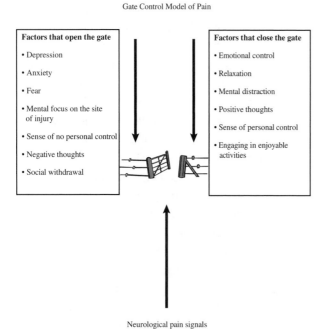

Gate Control Model of Pain

Factors that open the gate	Factors that close the gate
• Depression	• Emotional control
• Anxiety	• Relaxation
• Fear	• Mental distraction
• Mental focus on the site of injury	• Positive thoughts
• Sense of no personal control	• Sense of personal control
• Negative thoughts	• Engaging in enjoyable activities
• Social withdrawal	

Neurological pain signals

FIGURE 11.1.   Gate control model of pain handout.

Figure 11.1 for handout to use for this discussion] between the location of a physical injury and the brain. This gate affects the flow of the pain signals up and down your spinal cord. If the gate is wide open, pain signals flow freely and the brain will register more pain. If, however, the gate is slightly closed, the pain signals will be blocked and less pain will be perceived. Numerous factors contribute to how open the gate is. Negative emotion is one factor that can open the gate. People feel more pain when they are depressed, angry, or anxious. Reducing the intensity of these emotions can help close the gate and reduce pain. This is important, because chronic pain and its effect on one's life can contribute to feelings of depression, helplessness, anxiety, or frustration.

Negative thinking is also a factor that can open the gate. Often people will feel pain more at times when they are focused on the pain than they do when they are distracted from it. Parents use this with children; if a child is distressed over falling and skinning his knee, they will

kiss it to make it better and send the child off to play. The kiss did not heal the injury but it changed the child's mental focus, which reduced the pain. Because the sensation of pain automatically draws one's mental focus, it can require real skill to successfully distract oneself.

There are also behavioral and physical factors that open and close the gate. For example, if a person is overly inactive because it hurts to walk or exercise, their muscles will become weak, which, in turn, adds to pain. Lack of involvement in enjoyable activities contributes to depression and frustration, boredom, and more focus on the pain, which in turn opens the gate for pain signals.

Another helpful concept is the distinction between pain and suffering. Pain is the sensation caused by neurological signals from the site of an injury or disease to the brain; suffering is the sum total of the emotional, mental, behavioral, social, occupational, and lifestyle effects of the pain. As a behavioral health provider, there is not a lot I can do to help you with injury in your body; that's the role of your primary care provider. However, I can work with you and your primary care provider on some of those other components that play a role in how much you suffer from the pain. In other words, I can help you learn to take more control of your life so you are living more as you would like to rather than letting the pain have so much control in your life. That may or may not result in less pain; however, many patients report a better quality of life after this kind of treatment. Is that something you would be interested in working on together?"

From here, it would be important to discuss the skills and changes that you can use to help the patient learn, and describe how those changes would directly affect symptoms, functioning, and suffering. You might want to use a handout such as the one in Figure 11.2 to facilitate this discussion. The discussion might transpire as follows:

> One thing that seems to increase your pain is your stress level. One way to help you manage that would be to help you learn how to turn on your body's natural relaxation response by learning how to use slow, relaxed breathing. Another thing we might do is to help you learn how to question your thoughts. You said that sometimes you have a variety of unhelpful thoughts that run through your mind and, in reaction to those, you choose not to do things you enjoy, you withdraw from others, and you notice your pain more. By not reacting to those thoughts, by stepping back and questioning those thoughts, you can choose how you want to respond to the situation, which can make it easier to choose to do the things you enjoy and not make your pain intensity increase.

Agree

Behavioral health approaches to pain management are based on a self-management model of care. Improvements in pain management will not be the result of a procedure done by the provider on the patients but will come through changes patients make themselves. This requires a shift in thinking for many pain patients who want to be cured. The agree phase is important so that both the patient and provider have a common framework for moving forward.

Agreement should be reached in several areas before moving on to treatment. The first area is whether the patient desires a behavioral approach to treatment. If the patient's only agenda is to obtain pain medications, more exploration and education may be necessary before moving on. If agreement on this cannot be reached, you may conclude that the patient is not a good candidate for a behavioral pain management approach. A second area for agreement is the goals of treatment. Effort should be made to ensure the patient understands that the likely outcome of many pain management approaches is enhanced function, decreased distress, and improved quality of life rather an a cure for their pain disorder.

Understanding Chronic Pain

Chronic pain is best understood as an interaction of numerous factors. Many aspects of these factors can be addressed to help manage chronic pain conditions.

Factor	What you can do to improve pain management
Physical	▪ Keep muscles toned through physical activity. ▪ Take prescribed pain medication. ▪ Use relaxation techniques to relax muscles and control the stress response.
Emotional	▪ Use relaxation to control anxiety. ▪ Stay involved with relationships and enjoyable activities to protect against depression and other negative moods.
Cognitive	▪ Recognize unhealthy thinking patterns that interfere with adaptive coping with pain. ▪ Challenge faulty thinking and replace it with healthy thoughts.
Behavior	▪ Stay physically active. ▪ Pace your activities; avoid a cycle of overactivity and underactivity. ▪ Adhere to medical recommendations (including medications and physical therapy).
Social	▪ Discuss what you find helpful and not helpful with family and others who are close to you. ▪ Stay socially involved.

FIGURE 11.2. Understanding chronic pain handout.

It is important to clarify that this may not include freedom from pain. Further discussion of goal setting can be found in chapter 3 of this volume. Third, the provider and the patient should agree on the practical aspects of care. This may include homework assignments, frequent visits, commitment to self-monitoring, and involvement of family members.

Assist

Von Korff (1999) suggested a stepped-care framework for addressing low back pain in the primary care setting. This same framework, in fact, can be applied to a variety of pain conditions and symptoms (Gatchel & Oordt, 2003). In each step, assistance is given to help the patient understand pain and make changes to improve adaptive functioning. If lower levels of intervention are not effective, care can be advanced to the next level. It is not necessary to progress stepwise through the each level. Treatment should be tailored to each patient's needs; some patients will present to the primary care setting already in need of higher-level specialty care.

Step 1 is the lowest level of intervention and generally consists of education and advice about the importance of returning to daily activities as soon as possible. Avoidance behaviors and fears that physical activity will cause further damage can be addressed. Specific recommendations for increasing activities are generally helpful.

Step 2 involves intervention that is more intensive and may be appropriate for patients who have continued to experience pain for 6 to 8 weeks after initial onset and who continue to have significant limitations in their functioning because of their pain. This level of care may include using interventions to address beliefs about pain and controllability, self-efficacy issues, cognitive errors, and coping strategies (Turk & Monarch, 2002). Other interventions might include relaxation training, a structured exercise program, and/or self-monitoring to work on pacing of activities.

Step 3 is multidisciplinary chronic pain rehabilitation. This level of care is appropriate for patients who do not respond to less intense interventions and who are at risk of permanent disability. A broad range of complicating factors can be addressed, including psychiatric co-morbidity, family dynamics, and substance abuse.

According to this framework, steps 1 and 2 can be performed in the primary care setting. The level of care in step 3 is beyond the scope of primary care, and a referral will be necessary. The following are some suggested approaches to working with pain issues during an office visit.

Challenging unhealthy beliefs about pain.   In the course of an assessment, patients will often reveal attitudes and beliefs about pain that are unrealistic, unhealthy, and may contribute to disability and distress. Bringing these beliefs to patients' attention and helping them, through education and information, to develop more accurate and realistic beliefs and thought can be beneficial. Figure 11.3 is a patient education handout you can use to help patients question faulty beliefs.

Pacing activities.   Individuals with chronic pain often will fall into an unhealthy cycle of overactivity and underactivity. They get frustrated because their activities are limited by pain; therefore, when pain decreases sufficiently, they engage in physical behaviors as if they did not have a pain problem. This overuse, in turn, makes the pain worse again, resulting in another period of prolonged inactivity. This cycle not only increases pain severity but also significantly interferes with maximal functioning. The following script presents one way of discussing this with patients and offers a strategy for better pacing activities:

> People without chronic pain have an alarm system to tell them when something is wrong. If they feel pain, it can be taken as a signal to stop doing whatever they are doing as they might be harming themselves, such as walking on a sprained ankle. When you have chronic pain, however, this alarm system no longer works well. Because you have pain frequently or constantly, it no longer reliably serves to help you tell the difference between harm and hurt. If you stop doing everything when you feel pain, you will end up doing nothing. The fact that the pain is no longer a symptom of harm means that stopping activity is not indicated.

TRUE or FALSE? Common Pain Beliefs

- "Pain must be a sign of serious physiological disease or injury."
  FALSE. Pain is a neurological event that is not highly related to severity of harm. The best intervention for pain is rest and inactivity. For acute injuries, a short period of rest to allow healing to occur is helpful. When pain lasts beyond a normal healing period, it is best to be active to build strength and maintain full use of your body.
- "Other people must understand how much I hurt."
  FALSE. Making a point to ensure everyone around you knows how much you hurt and expecting them to really understand is likely to keep you focused on your pain and may lead you to feel disappointed, angry, resentful, and unsupported. It may be better to let a few key individuals know, those who can support you in coping adaptively with your condition, and let the others in your life continue to be unaware.
- "Having chronic pain means I am broken and a flawed human being."
  FALSE. Thinking about yourself in unrealistic, negative terms will likely make coping more difficult. It is best to find ways to live life with meaning, grace, and dignity, and to find ways to adapt to the pain.
- "Pain is ruining my life and will ruin my future."
  FALSE. Pain is a difficulty you have in your life; however, whether it ruins your life or your future is up to you.
- "I can't be happy as long as I have pain."
  FALSE. Pain can certainly affect your mood but it doesn't control it. Happiness is a choice and mindset.
- "If my doctor is recommending nonmedical intervention for my chronic pain, it must mean she does not believe me or thinks I'm exaggerating my pain."
  FALSE. The state-of-the-art treatment for chronic pain is to use a multidisciplinary approach that combines the expertise of many medical specialties to address multiple factors contributing to pain, such as emotions, thoughts, behaviors, social interactions, learning, and environment. This gives you the best chance of improvement.
- "The only worthwhile goal is to be pain free."
  FALSE. Although it is desirable to eliminate the pain, this may be an unrealistic goal. There are other worthwhile goals for improving your quality of life without eliminating the pain.

FIGURE 11.3. True or false? Common pain beliefs handout.

Because the "pain equals harm" message is well engrained in most of us, people with chronic pain often needlessly continue to use pain as a signal in this manner. As a result, they remain inactive, sitting or lying for extended periods. Because pain tends to fluctuate in a natural cycle, the pain will typically decrease. Being tired, bored, and frustrated with not having been doing anything, people often will become active, trying to make up for lost time and engaging in activities they could not do while they were experiencing higher levels of pain. As a result, these individuals frequently will be overly active, resulting in an increase of their pain. This cycle of underactivity and overactivity continues as a pattern.

Learning to pace your activities can break this pattern. Pacing involves doing a reasonable level of physical activity for a period of time you have determined to be appropriate, followed by a period of rest or sedentary activity that is long enough to allow you to be active again shortly. By deliberately pacing yourself, you can become more functional while avoiding the consequences of being overly active or inactive.

One pacing strategy I encourage you to use involves a 10-point rating scale to monitor your pain when you are active. If your pain level increases by two points above your normal level, it's time to take a break. Engage in a relaxation exercise or do something sedentary until your pain drops to its original level. Go back to your activity and continue in this cycle. For example, you are vacuuming and your pain is at a level 5 on the 1 to 10 scale. After vacuuming for 10 minutes, your pain increases to a level 7. You sit and read for a while. After about 15 minutes of reading, your pain has dropped back to a level 5. You begin vacuuming again. If this pattern continues, you now know that a cycle of 10 minutes of activity and 15 minutes of rest works for you when vacuuming. Different types of activity may stress your body differently, and, therefore, the rate of cycling can be adjusted for various activities. By planning your activities in this way, you can maintain your function and improve your satisfaction each day.

Relaxing for pain control. Muscle tension can contribute to pain in several ways. First, muscle tension is a direct contributor to some pain conditions. Examples include tension headaches and some forms of temporomandibular disorder. Second, people with chronic pain sometimes develop habits of muscle overuse in response to pain, which includes bracing behaviors in anticipation of pain or to protect injured areas. It also may include overuse of certain muscles to compensate for weak or painful muscles. Third, generalized tension in response to pain can further exacerbate the pain condition.

A variety of relaxation techniques can be used for managing chronic pain, including deep breathing, progressive muscle relaxation, and visual imagery. These techniques are reviewed in chapter 3. It is recommended that patients use relaxation both on a routine basis to prevent development of cumulative tension as well as in response to the onset or exacerbation of pain.

Coping with intense pain episodes. For patients who experience acute episodes of intense pain, learning strategies for coping with pain can improve quality of life. These strategies will not alleviate the pain but can help increase a sense of personal control and mitigate distress. A five-step model for teaching management of intense pain episodes is recommended (see Figure 11.4 for patient handout).

Managing your thinking. The thoughts related to pain that patients have can contribute to how well the pain is tolerated and can affect the consequences of the pain. Coach patients to recognize thoughts that work for or against them during pain episodes by using the following steps:

- Assess your self-talk before, during, and after the pain episode.
- Evaluate whether your self-talk was helpful or unhelpful (see Figure 11.4).
- Practice replacing unhealthy thinking with more helpful thoughts.

Staying as relaxed as possible. During an intense pain episode, people are likely to become tense as a way of bracing against the pain. Efforts to relax during pain episodes will often help increase the person's sense of self-efficacy, reduce emotional distress, and sometimes mitigate the pain intensity. Deep breathing (see chap. 3) can be a useful strategy. Recommend patients use deep breathing when they first feel an increase in pain. The technique should be used throughout the pain episode. The goal of the breathing exercise should not be to reduce or eliminate the pain. If patients perceive this as the goal, they are likely to discontinue its use as the pain increases. Instead, discuss relaxation as a strategy for distraction and for coping with, and successfully enduring, the pain episode.

Using imagery or distraction. Individuals with pain tend to suffer more when they are focusing on their pain than when they are distracted. Helping patients learn to distract themselves effectively by identifying and practicing specific activities or stimuli can be helpful. Examples include mental imagery of relaxing scenes, watching television, listening to music, playing video games, or performing mentally challenging activities, such as puzzles or games (e.g., Sudoku, crossword).

Using pain medications. Effective use of pain medications is also helpful for staying relaxed during intense pain episodes. Encourage the patient to discuss optimal management of pain medication with his or her physician. Some patients will wait until the pain episode is severe before taking prescribed medications. Sometimes this is because they want to minimize drug use; other times it is because they have

---

Five Steps for Managing Intense Pain Episodes

---

1. Manage your thinking. What do you think before pain episodes? What do you think during pain episodes? What do you think following pain episodes? Which of these thoughts are helpful in managing your pain? Which are unhelpful? How can you alter your thinking to make it more helpful?

Unhelpful self-talk	Helpful self-talk
I can't stand this pain. (Underestimating ability.)	I've dealt with it before; I can get through it again. (Acknowledging ability to tolerate pain.)
This pain is horrible, awful, terrible. (Emotional evaluations.)	This pain is an 8 on a scale of 1 to 10. (Concrete, unemotional evaluation method.)
This pain is ruining my life. (Global assessment.)	This is a difficult time for me. (Specific assessment.)
I can't do anything to make this stop. (All or nothing thinking.)	There are things I can do to get through this. (Avoiding all or nothing thinking.)

2. Stay as relaxed as possible. Use deep breathing when you first feel an increase in pain; continue using deep breathing throughout the pain episode.
3. Use imagery and distraction. Use relaxing imagery, watch television, listen to music, do a mentally challenging puzzle or game.
4. Use medications effectively. Recognize early warning signs of increased pain. Take medication early to help manage pain episodes better.
5. Use your support network. Talk with your family members or others about what they can do or say to help during a pain episode. Let them know what is not helpful during a pain episode.

FIGURE 11.4.   Five steps for managing intense pain episodes handout.

habituated to the pain and are not aware of the early signs of a severe pain episode. Recognizing early warning signs and taking medication at that point may help the patient manage pain episodes better.

Using your support network. Often people will withdraw from others during pain episodes and, in doing so, do not receive the benefits that their support network can give. One of these benefits is moral support and encouragement for getting through the pain episode. Supportive words from a significant other can encourage adaptive coping, discourage catastrophic thinking, and decrease distress. We frequently hear from patients just how helpful a significant other was in helping them deal with an intense pain episode. Furthermore, family members or friends who understand principles of coping with pain can help patients mentally distract themselves and effectively pace activities. This kind of support often requires education and training for the support person. Encourage patients with pain to bring their spouse or other supporters to their medical visits to receive this education. Patients should be encouraged to identify what type of support does and does not help; they can then be encouraged to share that information with significant others. It is best to share this information when the patient is at a baseline level of pain, and not during an acute pain episode.

Arrange

Many patients with acute, recurrent, and chronic pain have never been exposed to behavioral or cognitive pain management principles and approaches; therefore, stepped-care models integrating these principles into primary care is an important technique to use to manage patients experiencing pain. It might be helpful to have patients monitor their pain and their responses to their pain as a way to determine the effects of the interventions. A pain monitoring form such as the one in Figure 11.5 could be used for this purpose. Follow-up consultation appointments over 1 to 4 weeks to assess effects of the interventions and resolve problems will likely be warranted.

Monitoring Pain

Date, time	Pain Intensity 1 = mild, 10 = excruciating	Duration (hrs/mins)	Precipitating factors	Thoughts related to pain	Emotional reactions	Pain behaviors

FIGURE 11.5.   Monitoring pain handout.

For those who do benefit from the intervention, it is important to discuss when further medical evaluation or care for pain is indicated. Generally, this would occur when there is new pain or significant changes to the nature of the pain, location of the pain, or the intensity or character of the pain. Those who do not benefit from these primary care approaches and who display significant functional impairment may need to be referred on to higher level care. Referral to a specialty-trained clinical health psychologist may be useful to address complicating issues such as coexisting mental disorders, substance abuse, family conflict, secondary gain, and so forth. Many patients and family members will benefit from a chronic pain support group with a focus on enhancing coping and increasing function. Referral to a multidisciplinary chronic pain program will be helpful for others.

SUMMARY

Pain is one of the most common problems in primary care. Behavioral health assessment and interventions are now recognized to be essential components for helping patients manage pain, especially when it is chronic or when there is significant functional impairment. Key areas for assessment include pain variability, what increases or decreases pain, effect of pain on activities, how an individual copes in response to pain, and how social interactions and environment affect the individual. It will be important to provide the individual with a framework with which to understand various psychosocial factors and their effects on pain perception and functioning. Encouraging the individual to shift from pursuing a cure to focusing on management is important. Primary treatment may involve having them return to daily activities as soon as possible or increasing physical activity. Questioning unhelpful thoughts, using relaxation techniques and imagery, and social support can be effective components of a primary care pain management intervention. Integrated behavioral health providers in the primary care setting have a rich opportunity to help the primary care providers and their patients use effective nonpharmacological pain management strategies that can improve functioning and quality of life.

CHAPTER 12

ALCOHOL AND PRESCRIPTION MEDICATION MISUSE

ALCOHOL MISUSE

Alcohol misuse includes risky or hazardous drinking, defined as 8 or more drinks per week or 4 or more drinks per occasion for women and 15 or more drinks per week and 5 or more drinks per occasion for men (U.S. Preventive Services Task Force [USPSTF], 2004). Misuse also includes *harmful drinking*, defined as physical, social, or psychological harm as a result of alcohol consumption but not meeting criteria for alcohol dependence (i.e., difficulty limiting drinking, difficulty cutting down or stopping, tolerance, signs of withdrawal, continued drinking despite problems, a lot of time spent drinking, spending less time on other matters because of drinking; USPSTF). Approximately 30% of the adults in the United States drink at elevated risk levels (National Institute on Alcohol Abuse and Alcoholism [NIAAA], 2007a), meaning they drink at a level that leads them to have a greater chance of developing depression, sleep problems, liver disease, cancer, hypertension, gastrointestinal bleeding, and stroke (Rehm et al., 2003). Epidemiological data also suggest that those who engage in risky, hazardous, or harmful drinking are at increased risk of alcohol related problems (Dawson, Grant, & Li, 2005) such as violence and trauma-related injury (NIAAA, 2000).

Specialty Mental Health

A great deal of research has been conducted regarding mental health treatment for alcohol misuse, abuse, and dependence in specialty mental health and addictions treatment settings. In sum, a variety of strategies have been found effective, including brief interventions, social skills training, community reinforcement, behavior contracting, behavioral marital therapy, case management, and pharmacotherapy. See Miller and Wilbourne (2002) and Miller, Zweben, and Johnson (2005) for details of approaches and effectiveness.

Primary Care Adaptation

It is common for primary care providers (PCPs) to see individuals who engage in risky, hazardous, or harmful levels of drinking. Prevalence estimates from a variety of primary care settings and populations suggest that 4% to 29% of individuals are risky drinkers and 0.3% to 10% are harmful drinkers (Reid, Fiellin, & O'Connor, 1999). Whitlock, Polen, Green, Orleans, and Klein (2004) found that brief behavioral counseling in primary care for risky, hazardous, or harmful drinking was effective. After reviewing four "good quality trials," (i.e., good internal validity; see Whitlock et al., 2004 for specific criteria), they concluded that brief (i.e., ≤ 5-minute–45-minute) multiple contact (i.e., two–five contacts) interventions significantly reduced risky and harmful alcohol use. In addition, 10% to 19% more of the intervention participants achieved recommended drinking levels in comparison with control group participants. Individuals who received intervention also had a 13% to 34% greater reduction in total number of drinks in comparison to control groups. Effective interventions typically included feedback, advice, goal setting, and additional contact for support and assistance and were consistent with the USPSTF's 5A's (2004;

i.e., assess, advise, agree, assist, arrange) approach to effective behavioral counseling interventions in primary care.

PCPs have been encouraged to identify and treat those who are engaging in risky, hazardous, and harmful drinking; they have been provided with specific tools, strategies, and recommendations for doing so effectively (Fleming & Manwell, 1999; NIAAA, 2007a; Reid et al., 1999). Despite this, few PCPs use recommended screening or treatment protocols or even offer any other kind of treatment intervention within primary care (Friedmann, McCullough, Chin, & Saitz, 2000). Working in primary care as a behavioral health consultant (BHC), you have the ability to change how PCPs screen, assess, and intervene with alcohol misuse by changing their behaviors through education and training or by providing support assessment and intervention within primary care.

The updated NIAAA (2007a) publication "Helping Patients Who Drink Too Much: A Clinician's Guide" is an excellent source of information and contains useful clinical tools to help assess, treat, and refer individuals in the primary care setting who engage in risky, hazardous, harmful, abusive, or dependent drinking patterns. We encourage you to download this guide from http://pubs.niaaa. nih.gov/publications/Practitioner/CliniciansGuide 2005/clinicians_guide.htm. There, you will find downloadable pocket guides, online training, and PowerPoint presentations you can use to help teach other medical professionals to effectively screen for alcohol problems and assess and intervene for risky, hazardous, and harmful drinking. The following sections draw selected pieces from this guide as well as adapted evidenced-based strategies we use in our own clinical work.

Assess.   Regarding the assess phase, BHCs should develop methods for screening and diagnosing patients who may have difficulties with alcohol use. BHCs may also want to introduce these methods to other medical staff to enhance the identification of patients with alcohol problems.

Screening.   There is good evidence that screening can accurately identify individuals who are drinking in a risky, hazardous, or harmful manner (USPSTF,

2004). As such, the USPSTF (2004) and NIAAA (2007a) recommended incorporating alcohol screening into standard practice. The NIAAA (2007a) recommended two screening questions during medical interviews:

1. Do you sometimes drink beer, wine, or other alcoholic beverages? If yes, then ask the following:
2. How many times in the past year have you had five or more drinks in a day (for men)/four or more drinks in a day (for women)?

If individuals endorse that they have had at least four or five drinks in a day, then determine their weekly average by asking, "On average, how many days a week do you have an alcoholic drink? On a typical drinking day, how many drinks do you have?" Multiply the number of days a week by number of typical drinks to calculate the weekly average (e.g., 4 days per week × 5 drinks per day = 20 drinks per week). From here, conduct further assessment to make a differential diagnosis (see decision tree, NIAAA, 2007a, p. 4).

The Alcohol Use Disorders Identification Test (AUDIT; provided in Figure 12.1) and a short-form version of the Alcohol Use Disorders Identification Test-Consumption (AUDIT-C) are among the most widely recommended screening tools for alcohol problems. Consistent with literature recommendations, we suggest you consider using the AUDIT or the AUDIT-C, which consists of the first three questions of the AUDIT, as a pre-assessment or standard screening measure. The AUDIT-C, with a score of 4 or more, has performed better than the AUDIT, with a positive screening score of 8 or more, in identifying individuals as heavy drinkers (i.e., risky, hazardous, or harmful) who might benefit from brief primary care interventions (Bush, Kivlahan, McDonell, Fihn, & Bradley, 1998). A score on the AUDIT-C of 4 or more for women and 6 or more for men is considered a positive screen for risky, hazardous, or harmful drinking (NIAAA, 2007a). Furthermore, the AUDIT and AUDIT-C have been shown to be equal in identifying patients with heavy drinking, alcohol abuse, or dependence (Bush et al., 1998). Therefore, the AUDIT or the AUDIT-C can be used as effective screening mea-

---

Alcohol Use Disorders Identification Test (AUDIT)

Because alcohol use can affect your health and can interfere with certain medications and treatments, it is important that we ask some questions about your use of alcohol. Your answers will remain confidential, so please be honest.

Place an X in one box that best describes your answer to each question.

Questions	0	1	2	3	4
1. How often do you have a drink containing alcohol?	Never	Monthly or less	2 to 4 times a month	2 to 3 times a week	4 or more times a week
2. How many drinks containing alcohol do you have on a typical day when you are drinking?	1 or 2	3 or 4	5 or 6	7 to 9	10 or more
3. How often do you have 5 or more drinks on one occasion?	Never	Less than monthly	Monthly	Weekly	Daily or almost daily
4. How often during the last year have you found that you were not able to stop drinking once you had started?	Never	Less than monthly	Monthly	Weekly	Daily or almost daily
5. How often during the last year have you failed to do what was normally expected of you because of drinking?	Never	Less than monthly	Monthly	Weekly	Daily or almost daily
6. How often during the last year have you needed a first drink in the morning to get yourself going after a heavy drinking session?	Never	Less than monthly	Monthly	Weekly	Daily or almost daily
7. How often during the last year have you had a feeling of guilt or remorse after drinking?	Never	Less than monthly	Monthly	Weekly	Daily or almost daily
8. How often during the last year have you been unable to remember what happened the night before because of your drinking?	Never	Less than monthly	Monthly	Weekly	Daily or almost daily
9. Have you or someone else been injured because of your drinking?	No		Yes, but not in the last year		Yes, during the last year
10. Has a relative, friend, doctor, or other health care worker been concerned about your drinking or suggested you cut down?	No		Yes, but not in the last year		Yes, during the last year
					Total

FIGURE 12.1. Alcohol Use Disorders Identification Test (AUDIT). This questionnaire is reprinted with permission from the World Health Organization. To reflect standard drink sizes in the United States, the number of drinks in question 3 was changed from 6 to 5.

sures. Physicians are often taught to use the CAGE (Cut down, Annoyed by criticism, Guilty about drinking, needing an Eye-opener in the morning) as a way to screen for alcohol related problems. The CAGE is good for detecting alcohol abuse and dependence, but it is not as sensitive as the AUDIT in detecting alcohol misuse and would not identify a large number of individuals that might benefit from decreasing or stopping their alcohol use. Ultimately, the screening tools used should fit the clinic population and setting. For additional information on a variety of screening measures, see the NIAAA Web site at http://pubs.niaaa.nih.gov/publications/Assesing%20Alcohol/selfreport.htm.

If time limitations and individual burden are a concern, as they are in most clinics, we recommend using the AUDIT-C. If the individual's AUDIT-C or AUDIT score meets or exceeds a positive screening score, consider further assessment to determine whether abuse or dependence diagnostic criteria are met. We discuss this in the section on differential diagnosis.

Differential diagnosis. To help determine the best treatment course, it is important to determine whether patients meet criteria for alcohol abuse or dependence. Different courses of action are recommended for the individual who has an abuse or dependence diagnosis.

To assess *alcohol abuse,* you could ask, "In the past 12 months has your drinking repeatedly caused or contributed to any of the following?"

- Risk of bodily harm (e.g., drinking and driving, operating machinery, swimming).
- Relationship trouble (e.g., with family or friends).
- Role failure (e.g., interference with home, work, or school obligations).
- Trouble with the law (e.g., arrests, other legal problems).

If the individual answers yes to one or more of the questions, he or she meets criteria for alcohol abuse. Assess for dependence.

Alcohol dependence can be assessed by asking, "In the past 12 months have you experienced any of the following?"

- Not been able to stick to drinking limits (i.e., repeatedly gone over them).
- Not been able to cut down or stop (i.e., repeated failed attempts).
- Shown tolerance (i.e., needed to drink a lot more to get the same effect).
- Shown signs of withdrawal (i.e., tremors, sweating, nausea, or insomnia when trying to quit or cut down).
- Kept drinking despite problems (i.e., recurrent physical or psychological problems).

- Spent a lot of time drinking (i.e., or anticipating or recovering from drinking).
- Spent less time on other matters because of drinking (e.g., activities that had been important or pleasurable).

If the individual answers yes to three or more of the questions, he or she meets criteria for alcohol dependence. (See decision tree, NIAAA, 2007a, p. 5.)

Additional questions. There are several other areas you should assess, because the patient's answers will influence treatment recommendations and skill building during the advise and assist phases of the appointment.

- "What are the benefits of consuming alcohol?"
  For example, to relax, wind down, forget, provide distraction; because it feels good, helps sleep, and decreases anxiety.
  Intervention. Consider starting other activities that can provide similar benefits. See chapters 3 and 5 for examples of interventions to teach these skills.
- "Is there anything associated with an increase or decrease in use?"
  For example, drinking more with friends versus alone, drinking less or more when out of town.
  Intervention. Set a plan to minimize thoughts, behaviors, and environments associated with increased drinking and set a plan to increase thoughts, behaviors, and environments associated with decreased drinking.
- "How do others respond with increased or decreased use?"
  For example, "Friends say I am not as fun when I don't drink or drink less," "My husband says I am easier to be around when I drink more," "My children say they like me better when I don't drink beer."
  Intervention. Use these responses to evaluate patient's motivation to decrease drinking.

Advise. The goal of this phase is to inform individuals that their drinking rate places them at increased risk of medical problems and to show them how their current drinking pattern compares with other individuals in the United States You may want to use the patient education material on pages 24 and

25 of the NIAAA (2007a) publication "Helping Patients Who Drink Too Much: A Clinician's Guide" to assist with this. The following is an example of providing advice:

> On the basis of your current drinking pattern, you're drinking at a level that is higher than what we consider to be medically and behaviorally safe. This is putting you at increased risk for death, specifically through fatal injury, cancer, stroke, and high blood pressure. It could also lead to driving under the influence of alcohol or other risky or unsafe behaviors you might not engage in if you were drinking at a different level. If it's OK with you, I'd like to take just a moment to review with you what a "standard" drink is and how your current alcohol consumption compares with people in the United States. After that, I'd like to discuss whether now is a good time to commit to changing your alcohol intake. If you decide that it is a good time, we can review your options and design an individual plan for you that will meet your needs and lifestyle.

This may serve as a good time to gauge the individual's receptivity to change, and it might also be a good time to discuss common mistakes and assumptions people have about alcohol consumption. See Figure 12.2 for a handout you can use to dispel any misconceptions the patient might have regarding alcohol consumption.

Agree. Before moving to the assist phase with a specific plan to change alcohol consumption, it is important to determine whether the patient agrees that a change is necessary. One way to do this is to gauge readiness to change. If the individual seems ambivalent about changing, consider using motivational interviewing (MI) strategies to decrease ambivalence and increase willingness and motivation to change. See chapter 3 for MI strategies on reviewing risks and benefits of change, importance of change, and confidence in being able to change. The following are some specific questions using an MI approach that might be helpful in enhancing motivation to change.

> On a scale of 0 to 10, with 0 being *not important at all to alter drinking rate* and 10 being *extremely important to alter drinking rate,* how important is it to you to alter your drinking rate? How confident are you that you can alter

---

Common Mistakes and Assumptions About Alcohol

Drinking beer is safer than other drinks, so I only drink beer.
The belief that beer and wine are less intoxicating and safer and that hard liquor is more dangerous is false. It may take longer to get intoxicated because of the volume that has to be consumed, but the percentage of alcohol per volume from beer and wine will make someone as intoxicated as the same percentage of alcohol per volume of a drink that contains hard liquor.

Drinking with others is safer, so I never drink alone.
The belief that people who drink alone are the only individuals who may have problems is false. Drinking alone or with others does not determine intoxication level or problems associated with alcohol consumption.

Mixing types of drinks will increase intoxication, so I stick to drinking the same thing.
The belief that sticking with one type of drink will decrease intoxication is false. Mixing types of drinks has no differential impact on intoxication; intoxication is related to total amount of alcohol consumed.

Eating a meal before drinking is helpful in not getting as drunk, so I never drink on an empty stomach.
The belief that eating prior to drinking will keep an individual from getting intoxicated is false. Eating will slow down the absorption rate of the alcohol into the bloodstream, but not stop it.

FIGURE 12.2. Common mistakes and assumptions about alcohol handout.

your drinking habits, with 0 being *not at all confident* and 10 being *extremely confident?*

If the answer is less than 7 on importance or confidence, ask what the patient would have to change or what would need to be different to move the importance to a 7 or higher. If the answer is 7 or higher, ask what factors led them to have that much confidence or for it to be that important.

Once you have assessed importance and confidence, you should gauge the patient's willingness to change. You might then ask, "Are you willing to commit to changing your drinking pattern at this point in time?" If patients answer yes, discuss options for helping them to change. If they answer no, ask patients about major barriers to change and deal with these as you are able. If they are still not willing to change, let them know that you are available to assist with change when they decide they are ready.

Advise.   It is important to review options for change. You might provide the following change options for patients who are ready:

- reduce the number of drinks consumed (e.g., daily, weekly, in high-risk situations such as driving) or
- abstain from drinking for a particular period of time.

It may be helpful to have the individual tell you what the pros and cons are of reducing or abstaining before choosing a goal.

Assist.   The ways in which you can assist patients with reducing or stopping their drinking will vary depending on their goal and the individual factors involved in their alcohol consumption. To this end, we list a variety of options that you might use, as follows.

Reducing alcohol consumption. Educate on what a standard drink is, focusing on the type of drink the patient typically consumes.

Determine their drinking goal. As a way to reduce their risk of alcohol-related problems, we recommend encouraging patients to stay within moderate drinking limits: no more than two drinks a day for a man and one drink a day for a woman (NIAAA, 2007b). If

this is not acceptable, work with individuals to set some type of a decrease from their current level. Set a plan for the days they want to drink and how many drinks they will have on those days.

Keep track of the number of drinks consumed. Pick whatever is easiest for the individual. He or she could use a small spiral notebook, a Post-It note, calendar, personal data assistant, or Excel spread sheet, for example. Another method involves having a list of drinks per day that can be consumed and having the individual mark each drink off the list before it is consumed. It might look like this for a given 2-day period for a man: Monday. 1, 2; Tuesday. 1, 2.

We recommend that you give some suggestions on how individuals might track consumption and then ask whether any of those would work or whether they have additional ideas.

1. Review ways to pace drinking.
   - Put glass or bottle down between drinks (i.e., do not hold it in your hand).
   - After you've finished half your drink, wait 5 minutes before you take another sip.
   - Drink a nonalcoholic drink between your alcoholic drinks.
   - Have no more than one drink per hour.
   - Delay when drinking starts (e.g., wait 1.5 hours after getting home to have a drink).
2. Review ways to avoid or manage situations in which it may be a challenge for the individual to stay within his or her goals. See the four A's handout in Figure 12.3 to help plan for difficult situations. We recommend using this in an interactive fashion, with you filling in the form. Our experience suggests that the individual is able to solve problems more effectively and be more collaborative if you are the one writing things down through this process.
3. Review assertive communication skills to be able to refuse drinks when appropriate (see chap. 3, this volume).
4. Review stress and anxiety management skills to take the place of drinking for relaxation (see chaps. 3 and 5, this volume).

Stopping alcohol consumption. If stopping all alcohol consumption is the goal, then focus on avoiding or managing situations, assertive commu-

---

Four A's for Managing Alcohol Consumption

AVOID. What are the highly tempting situations in which you might drink more than your plan? Avoid these situations if possible over the next month.

1. _____
2. _____

ALTER. For situations you can't avoid, how can you alter them to make them easier?

1. _____
2. _____

ALTERNATIVES. What can you do with your mouth and hands when you want to drink and it is a day you are not drinking or have already reached your limit?

1. _____
2. _____

ACTION. When you get the urge to drink and it does not fit with your drinking plan, what can you do to be active or busy until the urge passes?

1. _____
2. _____

Are there situations in which it will be a challenge to stay within your drinking limits? If so, list them and what you will do to effectively manage those situations.

1. _____

Plan _____

2. _____

Plan _____

FIGURE 12.3. Four A's for managing alcohol consumption handout.

nication, and stress and anxiety management skills in the same manner as for those reducing consumption. Because alcohol consumption is a pleasurable activity for most drinkers, we recommend setting a plan to incorporate alternative pleasurable activities into the days and periods when individuals typically consume alcohol. See chapter 3 for instructions on goal setting to help produce a plan to increase enjoyable activities.

Arrange. For those cutting down as well as those who are stopping, we suggest the following:

1. A follow-up appointment can be made to assess adherence to the plan.
2. Support and encourage the individual to continue with the plan if it is working well. Ask whether there has been anything that has occurred that the individual sees as a future problem, and determine whether the plan can be modified to adapt to change. Collaboratively determine whether additional plans for follow-up would be helpful or whether checking on the plan at the next medical appointment might be the best option.
3. If the patients do not meet their goal, encourage them to learn from this experience (i.e., what went well, what didn't, how they might plan differently for the future).
   - Suggest that change can be difficult and may take a while.
   - Encourage and support any change that was made.

- Deal with barriers to the plan.
- Consider engaging the patient's social network for assistance.
- If unable to abstain or cut down, reassess for alcohol use disorder.
- Negotiate a follow-up appointment to assess the plan and resolve difficulties.

Alcohol Abuse and Dependence

The general recommendation is that those with abuse and dependence diagnoses are candidates for specialty substance abuse treatment and that they should follow-up with an addictions specialist for assessment and/or treatment (NIAAA, 2007a; Whitlock et al., 2004). However, patients may not be willing to go to a specialist. If not, you might engage in treatments in much the same way as for risky, hazardous, or harmful drinking with the following additions.

- The drinking goal recommendation should be abstinence for most, but if the patient is unwilling to abstain, negotiating a reduction may be helpful. It can reduce resistance to change and open the door for consideration of abstinence. It can also be a good way to work with individuals who do not want to stop drinking but want to avoid some of the consequences (e.g., being caught for driving under the influence, having trouble at work). These early steps in high-risk situations are usually more beneficial than an all-or-nothing approach with patients who are reluctant to change.
- Recommend a helping group or agency (e.g., Alcoholics Anonymous).
- For those with dependence, include medical management of withdrawal (see NIAAA, 2007a, for more guidance).

Summary

Alcohol misuse has numerous health and social consequences. With roughly one third of the individuals in primary care engaged in drinking patterns that increase their risk for physical and social consequences, primary care is ripe for alcohol misuse screening and intervention. Despite the data supporting the effectiveness of screening and brief

interventions for risky, hazardous, or harmful drinking, few PCPs use recommended screening or treatment protocols or offer any other kind of treatment within primary care. You can help to change this practice. We have provided information on how to access "Helping Patients Who Drink Too Much: A Clinician's Guide" and have discussed how you might apply this information along with other strategies within the 5A's framework.

Increasing screening using the AUDIT or AUDIT-C, comparing the individual's drinking rate with U.S. drinking norms, tailoring interventions to the patient's goals, and arranging for appropriate follow-up care will help you to effectively help PCPs and their patients manage risky, hazardous, and harmful alcohol consumption.

PRESCRIPTION MEDICATION MISUSE

The non-medical use, or abuse, of prescription drugs is a growing problem in the United States (National Institute on Drug Abuse [NIDA], 2005) with 6.4 million Americans age 12 years and older reporting the use of prescription medication for nonmedical purposes in 2005 (Substance Abuse and Mental Health Services Administration, 2006). The most commonly misused prescriptions are opioids, which are normally used to treat pain (e.g., oxycodone [OxyContin], combined hydrocodone and acetaminophen [Vicodin]); central nervous system depressants, which are frequently used to treat anxiety and sleep problems (e.g., diazepam [Valium], alprazolam [Xanax]); and stimulants, which are commonly used to increase attention, energy and alertness (e.g., methylphenidate [Ritalin], dextramphetamine [Dexedrine]; NIDA, 2006). Common consequences of prescription misuse or abuse might include addiction, dependence, respiratory depression, seizure, irregular heartbeat, and cardiovascular failure.

There is no common definition of the word *abuse* when examining inappropriate use of prescription medication (NIDA, 2005). In addition, the word abuse as used in various studies is not consistent with the *Diagnostic and Statistical Manual of Mental Disorders, Fourth Edition, Text Revision* (*DSM–IV–TR*; American Psychiatric Association, 2000) definition of abuse and can lead to confusion (NIDA, 2005). As such, we will focus on the more encompassing *prescription misuse,* which is the use of a prescription medication in a manner other than that intended by the prescribing PCP (Isaacson, 2000; Isaacson, Hopper, Alford, & Parran, 2005; NIDA, 2001). This might include using the medication in greater amounts, more frequently, for other symptoms, or with different administration routes, all of which might lead to adverse consequences (Isaacson, 2000; Isaacson et al., 2005; NIDA, 2001).

Your Role With Medication Misuse

There are a number of diagnostic (e.g., abuse, dependence) and intervention (e.g., pain management strategies) services the PCP may request from the BHC when dealing with suspected medication misuse. You may be involved with helping individuals learn specific skills to manage symptoms and/or tolerate distress more effectively so they use less medication. You might also help devise a plan and a schedule of medications to evaluate the individual's use when symptoms are more aggressively managed to help determine whether reporting of symptoms and medication use continues to escalate. Our experience suggests that BHCs may be relied on in the following ways:

- As an informal consultant for the PCP.
- To help the PCP and patient improve communication, and work out an agreed on solution for appropriate use of medication to continue receiving medication. This may be especially relevant if the individual is hoarding medication because symptoms such as pain or anxiety are not being adequately treated, and he or she is concerned about running out of medication when it is needed most.
- To support the PCP with his or her stance on stopping a prescription that is no longer medically needed.

We believe the following information is important, particularly for effectively informing and assisting the PCPs in your clinic with screening, recognition, and intervention information, and guidance in dealing with prescription misuse. We think helping the PCP to be aware of the potential for prescription misuse and to assess and intervene effec-tively improves the chances of preventing misuse or catching it early and may enhance the opportunity for better care and better satisfaction with care for both the patient and the PCP.

Assess. The general consensus by addiction medicine specialists is that physicians should avoid prescribing addictive, controlled medications to individuals who have current or past drug or alcohol abuse or dependence problems (Longo, Parran, Johnson, & Kinsey, 2000). It is optimal for initial screenings and documentations to include assessments of current or past abuse or dependence problems for all patients; however, this may not be appropriate or feasible for all settings. Therefore, we recommend the use of the following as a brief screen before commonly misused drugs are prescribed.

CAGE questions Adapted to Include Drugs (CAGE-AID; Brown, Leonard, Saunders, & Papasouliotis, 1998; Brown & Rounds, 1995) is one screening method. CAGE-AID has demonstrated good sensitivity (70%) and specificity (85%) for those answering one or more affirmative responses, identifying 78% of those who meet or have met criteria for a drug or alcohol abuse or dependence diagnosis (Brown & Rounds, 1995). Initial questions for CAGE-AID are:

1. Do you drink alcohol?
2. Have you ever experimented with drugs?

If the patient answers, "Yes," to both, ask the following questions using both the alcohol and drug questions. If the patient answers, "Yes," to just the drug question, ask the CAGE-AID questions only (i.e., including just the words in boldface and eliminating the words in italics). If the patient answers, "Yes," to just the alcohol question, ask the CAGE questions only (i.e., including just the words in italics and eliminating the words in boldface).

In the last year,
1. Have you ever felt you ought to cut down on your *drinking*/**drug use**?
2. Have people annoyed you by criticizing your *drinking*/**drug use**?
3. Have you ever felt bad or guilty about your *drinking*/**drug use**?

4. Have you ever had a *drink*/**used drugs** first thing in the morning to steady your nerves or to get rid of a hangover?

One positive answer indicates a possible problem and two positive answers indicate a probable problem. If a patient endorses one or more positives, we suggest asking specific *DSM–IV–TR* abuse and or dependence criteria questions, as discussed earlier in the chapter, to determine whether an ongoing alcohol or drug abuse or dependence problem exists or whether there was a problem in the past (see Figure 12.4 for the CAGE-AID clinician document).

A past abuse or dependence problem would not preclude an individual from receiving potentially addictive medication, but the problem should be noted and the following should be considered in concert with the patient and PCP.

- Discuss the pros and cons of using potentially addictive medications.
- Develop an agreement or plan that might include things such as taking medication on a schedule or following up with the PCP monthly to refill

the prescription and to minimize abuse or dependence risk.

A current substance abuse or dependence problem may warrant a referral to an addiction specialist for additional assessment and treatment. Furthermore, this should preclude the prescription of a potentially addictive controlled medication. If possible, treatment of the presenting problems should focus on other evidence-based procedures that minimize physical and emotional symptoms (e.g., questioning thoughts, relaxation, increasing valuable activities) and the use of efficacious non-addictive medications.

You can play an important role in helping PCPs develop management strategies for addictive medications. Some examples include the following (Isaacson, 2000; Isaacson et al., 2005; Longo et al., 2000):

- Develop a group practice policy for after hours prescriptions.
- Inform individuals about the prescription regimen and the refill policy before giving medication.

CAGE-AID

Initial questions for CAGE-AID (Cut down, Annoyed by criticism, Guilty about drinking, needing an Eye-opener in the morning-Adapted to Include Drugs).

1. Do you drink alcohol?	Yes	No
2. Have you ever experimented with drugs?	Yes	No

If yes to both, ask the following questions using both the alcohol and drug words. If yes to just the drug question, ask the CAGE-AID questions (i.e., include the words in boldface and eliminate those in italics). If yes to just the alcohol question, ask the CAGE questions (i.e., include the words in italics and eliminate those in boldface).

In the last year,

1. Have you ever felt you ought to cut down on your *drinking*/**drug use**?	Yes	No
2. Have people annoyed you by criticizing your *drinking*/**drug use**?	Yes	No
3. Have you ever felt bad or guilty about your *drinking*/**drug use**?	Yes	No
4. Have you ever had a *drink*/**used drugs** first thing in the morning to steady your nerves or to get rid of a hangover?	Yes	No

One positive answer indicates a possible problem and two positive answers indicates a probable problem. If there are one or more positives, we suggest asking specific *DSM–IV* abuse and/or dependence criteria questions to determine whether an ongoing alcohol or drug abuse or dependence problem exists.

FIGURE 12.4. CAGE-AID.

- Carefully document the diagnosis, the reason for using medication, the prescription policy, and individual education.
- Consult with other medical personnel.
- Carefully consider when prescribing multiple substances the benefit and risk of prescribing more than one controlled substance at a time.
- Maintain a refill flow chart for easy access to prescription refill history.
- Consider, recommend, and document nonaddictive medication and other treatment modalities. Use contracts to specify the PCP and patient role and the consequences of breaching the agreement. Highlight that the relationship is consensual and that there is room for negotiation (Fishman & Kreis, 2002). For an example of an opioid contract see the following Web site: http://www.painmed. org/pdf/controlled_substances_sample_agrmt.pdf.
- Know the signs of misuse, including,
  - losing medication;
  - running out of medication earlier than expected based on number prescribed and dose per day;
  - ongoing complaints of acute pain syndromes such as headache or toothache, particularly with a new PCP;
  - stating that he or she is new to the area, going to the emergency room for a prescription refill;
  - seeking new or multiple physicians, calling the clinic for a refill when the PCP is not in the clinic;
  - reporting multiple medical sensitivities or that nonaddictive medications do not work;
  - reporting they have a high tolerance to medication;
  - showing more concern about obtaining medication than the comprehensive management of the problem;
  - refusing additional diagnostic tests or referrals to specialists;
  - having extensive knowledge of a medication, how it works, and why it is needed;
  - manipulating the situation by playing one PCP's opinion against another;
  - threatening to get medication from a more caring or knowledgeable PCP; and
  - claiming that the PCP is the only one who can help by providing the prescription.

Assist. The following are strategies the BHC can suggest to the PCP for when and how to implement treatment (Isaacson, 2000; Isaacson et al., 2005; Longo et al., 2000).

- Provide specific instructions about how to take the medication and emphasize that it is to be used only for the problem for which it was prescribed.
- Remain empathic and direct concern in a nonjudgmental way. The following is an example for a patient with chronic pain:

  > I understand that you are concerned about the treatment and management of your pain. I want to work with you so that we can manage it in the best way possible. At the same time, I'm concerned about the way you are using your medication and that you are having difficulty taking it in the way in which it is designed to be used. I'm concerned about the short and long-term consequences of that type of use, which can include addiction, liver problems, and tolerance to the medications so that it no longer works for you.

- Consider further assessment by the BHC or by other professionals for assessment of abuse or dependence, and/or the development of additional skills to manage their condition.
- When a potentially addictive medication is not indicated, communicate this in a straightforward manner, explaining to the individual why this is the case and what the options are. If the patient is pressuring the PCP to fill the prescription, the patient should be told the medication cannot be prescribed. It can be useful for the PCP to express to the patient that it feels like he or she is being pressured to write a prescription that is not medically indicated. This could then be used by the PCP as a segue to discuss concerns about the patient's medication use and the potential misuse pattern that might be starting.

Summary

Millions of individuals in the United States misuse prescription medication. PCPs are under pressure by an ever-increasingly informed public to prescribe a variety of medications that relieve symptoms and decrease suffering. However, these medications can be misused in a manner that negatively affects health care and can lead to addiction. In addition to the skills you can offer, which can help manage a variety of problems that may lead to the discontinuation or reduction in medication use, you can proactively help PCPs be aware of, assess, and intervene effectively with prescription misuse.

Assisting your clinic in setting standards for screening and assessment with the CAGE-AID (see Figure 12.4) and/or differential diagnosis of abuse or dependence may be a significant role for the BHC. We have listed many prevention and management strategies and signs of potential medication misuse for you to watch for when helping a PCP assess a potential misuse situation. When intervening with misuse, we suggest recommending specific instructions on how to take the medication, remaining empathic and nonjudgmental, and helping the PCP be assertive in not prescribing or limiting medications, while at the same time working to provide symptom relief through other medication or therapies, including direct consultation with the BHC for symptom management.

CHAPTER 13

SEXUAL DYSFUNCTIONS

Sexual dysfunctions involve disruption in the sexual response cycle (i.e., desire, excitement, orgasm, resolution) or pain during sexual intercourse. They may be lifelong or acquired, generalized or limited to specific situations or partners, and may be the result of psychological factors, substance use, a general medical condition, or a combination of psychological and medical factors (American Psychiatric Association [APA], 2000). Men and women with sexual dysfunctions often experience decreased quality of life (Laumann, Paik, & Rosen, 1999), lowered self-confidence, and increased concerns about relationships (Symonds, Roblin, Hart, & Althof, 2003). This chapter focuses specifically on three of the more common sexual dysfunctions: male erectile disorder (ED), premature ejaculation (PE), and female orgasmic disorder (OD). Evidence-based specialty mental health interventions exist for each disorder; less is known about behavioral health interventions offered within the primary care setting.

ERECTILE DISORDER

Erectile disorder is defined as "persistent or recurrent inability to attain, or to maintain until completion of the sexual activity, an adequate erection" that causes distress or impairment in interpersonal relationships and is not due to a psychiatric disorder, medical condition, drug, or medication (APA, 2000, p. 547). This definition emphasizes the distinction between organic and psychogenic etiology. However, much of the more recent literature notes the frequent co-occurrence and reciprocal influence of biology and psychology in the etiology of ED, with few cases

being purely organic or psychogenic (e.g., Millner & Ullery, 2002; Riley & Riley, 1999; Rosen, Leiblum, & Spector, 1994).

ED affects 15 million to 30 million men in the United States, and rates increase with age (National Kidney and Urologic Diseases Information Clearinghouse [NKUDIC], 2005). The National Health and Social Life Survey found 5% prevalence of erectile dysfunction in men age 18 to 59 (Laumann et al., 1999). Rates are higher in primary care clinics (0.4%–37%) and in samples of older men (20%–52%; Simons & Carey, 2001).

Key Biopsychosocial Factors in Erectile Dysfunction

Understanding the biopsychosocial factors in erectile dysfunction is important if the behavioral health consultant (BHC) is going to conduct an effective assessment and intervention. The following are areas of particular importance.

Physical factors. Up to 90% of men with ED have at least one organic risk factor (Carrier, Brock, Kour, & Lue, 1993). These factors include age, certain medications (e.g., blood pressure medications, antidepressants, tranquilizers, antihistamines), medical conditions (e.g., cardiovascular disease, diabetes, multiple sclerosis), and injury (Lewis et al., 2004; NKUDIC, 2005). For a summary of the effects of medications on sexual health, see Finger (2007).

Medical treatments for ED have become increasingly available in recent years. Treatment options now include medication (e.g., Viagra), surgical prostheses or implants, penile injection therapy (i.e., using vasoactive drugs), and external vacuum pump devices and construction rings (Rosen & Leiblum, 1995). Figure 13.1 contains information in more detail regarding medical treatments for ED.

Emotional and cognitive factors.   In some individuals, emotional or cognitive factors may be primary causes of ED. In many others, thoughts and emotions serve as perpetuating factors, once ED has developed for other reasons. Anxiety, negative affect, stress-related symptoms, and other psychological problems, as well as attentional and perceptual processes including distracting or interfering

thoughts and performance-related anxiety or fears may all serve to precipitate or perpetuate ED (Carey, Wincze, & Meisler, 1993; Laumann et al., 1999; Rosen & Leiblum, 1995).

Behavioral factors.   Lifestyle behaviors, particularly use of substances, may play a role in ED. Tobacco use is an independent risk factor for ED (Lewis et al., 2004). Risk of ED also is higher in individuals with chronic alcohol consumption and use of certain illegal drugs such as heroin or methadone (Carey et al., 1993).

Treatments for Erectile Dysfunction

There are a variety of treatments available for erectile dysfunction (ED), including behavioral therapy or psychotherapy, drug therapy, vacuum devices, and surgery. You and your medical provider together can decide which treatments might be best for you.

Behavior Therapy or Psychotherapy
If ED is caused or worsened by anxiety or other psychological or behavioral factors, experts often advise using techniques that decrease the anxiety associated with intercourse. Your partner can help with the techniques, which include gradual development of intimacy and stimulation. Such techniques also can help relieve anxiety when ED from physical causes is being treated.

Drug Therapy
Drugs for treating ED can be taken orally, injected directly into the penis, or inserted into the urethra at the tip of the penis. In March 1998, the Food and Drug Administration approved sildenafil citrate (Viagra), the first pill to treat ED. Since that time, vardenafil hydrochloride (Levitra) and tadalafil (Cialis) have also been approved.

Viagra, Levitra, and Cialis work by enhancing the effects of nitric oxide, a chemical that relaxes smooth muscles in the penis during sexual stimulation and allows increased blood flow. Although these oral medicines improve the response to sexual stimulation, they do not trigger an automatic erection as injections do. Some men should not take these medicines because of possible interactions with other medications, such as nitrate-based drugs for heart problems.

Oral testosterone can reduce ED in some men with low levels of natural testosterone, but it is often ineffective and may cause liver damage. Patients also have claimed that other oral drugs, including yohimbine hydrochloride, dopamine and serotonin agonists, and trazodone, are effective, but the results of scientific studies to substantiate these claims have been inconsistent.

Many men achieve stronger erections by injecting drugs into the penis, causing it to become engorged with blood. Drugs such as papaverine hydrochloride, phentolamine, and alprostadil widen blood vessels. These drugs may create unwanted side effects, however, including persistent erection and scarring. Nitroglycerin, a muscle relaxant, can sometimes enhance erection when rubbed on the penis.

A system for inserting a pellet of alprostadil into the urethra is marketed as Muse. An erection will begin within 8 to 10 minutes and may last 30 to 60 minutes. The most common side effects are aching in the penis, testicles, and area between the penis and rectum; warmth or burning sensation in the urethra; redness from increased blood flow to the penis; and minor urethral bleeding or spotting.

FIGURE 13.1.   Treatments for erectile dysfunction handout. From *Erectile Dysfunction* (National Institutes of Health Publication No. 06-3923, pp. 3–5), by the National Kidney and Urologic Diseases Information Clearinghouse, 2005, Bethesda, MD: National Institutes of Health. Copyright 2005 by the National Institutes of Health. In the public domain. (*Continued*)

Vacuum Devices

Mechanical vacuum devices cause erection by creating a partial vacuum, which draws blood into the penis, engorging and expanding it. An elastic band is placed around the base of the penis to maintain the erection after the vacuum device is removed and during intercourse by preventing blood from flowing back into the body.

Surgery

Surgery usually has one of three goals:

- to implant a device that can cause the penis to become erect,
- to reconstruct arteries to increase blood flow to the penis, or
- to block off veins that allow blood to leak from the penile tissues.

Implanted devices, known as prostheses, can restore erection in many men with ED. Possible problems with implants include mechanical breakdown and infection, although mechanical problems have diminished in recent years because of technological advances. Implants may be malleable or inflatable.

Surgery to repair arteries can reduce ED caused by obstructions that block the flow of blood. The best candidates for such surgery are young men with discrete blockage of an artery because of an injury. The procedure is less successful in older men with widespread blockage.

Surgery to veins that allow blood to leave the penis usually involves an opposite procedure: intentional blockage. However, experts have raised questions about the long-term effectiveness of this procedure and it is rarely done.

For More Information

American Urological Association (AUA): 1-866-746-4282; http://www.auanet.org
American Diabetes Association (ADA): 1-800-342-2383; http://www.diabetes.org
American Association of Sex Educators, Counselors, and Therapists (AASECT): 1-804-752-0026;
   http://www.aasect.org

FIGURE 13.1. *(Continued)* Treatments for erectile dysfunction handout. From *Erectile Dysfunction* (National Institutes of Health Publication No. 06-3923, pp. 3–5), by the National Kidney and Urologic Diseases Information Clearinghouse, 2005, Bethesda, MD: National Institutes of Health. Copyright 2005 by the National Institutes of Health. In the public domain.

Environmental factors. A number of relationship factors may contribute to problems with ED. These include decreased trust and respect, decreased physical attraction to partner, communication difficulties, and power conflicts, among others (Carey et al., 1993). In addition, men who experienced sexual abuse as children have a three-fold risk of developing problems with erectile dysfunction, compared with men without a history of being abused (Laumann et al., 1999).

Specialty Mental Health

Specialty mental health interventions for ED often include the following components: providing information and education, training in communication and conflict resolution, improving sexual technique, implementing cognitive interventions, as well as using structured behavioral techniques (e.g., sensate focus). In a summary of interventions that meet evidenced-based practice standards, Gambescia and Weeks (2006) found empirical support for individual therapy involving psychoeducation, cognitive interventions to change maladaptive sexual thoughts, behavioral methods to reduce anxiety, and behavioral homework (e.g., guided self-stimulation). Empirical support was also found for couples counseling, including psychoeducation; interventions to reduce fear, anxiety, and pessimism; communication strategies; and sensate focus exercises. For detailed descriptions of the approaches, see Masters, Johnson, and Kolodny (1995); the biopsychosocial approaches of Carey et al. (1993) and Millner and Ullery (2002); and the cognitive–interpersonal model from Rosen et al. (1994).

Behavioral Health in Primary Care

Our review of the literature revealed no published studies of behavioral treatment of ED in primary care settings by behavioral health professionals.

197

The following section, therefore, is based on our clinical experiences in adapting specialty mental health treatments for ED to approaches that are consistent with a primary care behavioral health consultation model.

Primary Care Adaptation

To adapt approaches from specialty mental health, we often focus on education, supplemented by handouts to assist patients. The 5A's model provides a useful structure for guiding BHC discussions about erectile dysfunction.

Assess.   A functional assessment for ED should include questions regarding factors that may be relevant to the etiology and/or treatment of ED, as well as to the assessment of the effect of ED on functioning, symptoms, and quality of life. Peterson and Fuerst (2007) delineated several screening questions for psychological factors in ED. Two primary questions include the following:

- Do you have naturally occurring erections in the morning, and can you get an erection by yourself (i.e., via masturbation)?
- Have you ever been sexually molested or sexually assaulted, either as a child or as an adult?

Additional ED-symptom specific questions from Lue et al. (2004) and Gambescia and Weeks (2006) include the following:

- Was the onset of your problem gradual or sudden?
- Is your erectile dysfunction partner or situation specific?
- When was your last normal erection?
- On a scale of 0 to 5, rate your rigidity during sex (where 0 is *not rigid at all* and 5 is *completely rigid*).
- When you have erections with sexual stimulation, how often were your erections hard enough for penetration?
- During sexual intercourse, how difficult was it to maintain your erection to completion of intercourse?
- Do you have to concentrate to maintain an erection?

Other areas of inquiry relevant to ED include presence of other psychological symptoms or disorders (e.g., depression, anxiety), relevant medical problems (e.g., cardiovascular disease, diabetes) or medications that might affect ED, behavioral habits that could worsen ED (e.g., tobacco, alcohol, drug use), relationship problems (i.e., prior to and subsequent to the development of ED), and anxiety or guilt related to sexuality. Finally, assessing the patient's interest in or history of medical treatments for ED provides useful information for treatment planning. Whenever possible, we recommend reviewing the patient's medical record for medical diagnoses and medications that may affect ED because this typically yields more detailed information than patient self-report of medical history.

Advise.   After conducting the assessment, we advise the patient on intervention approaches. At this point, we typically introduce two concepts. First, we discuss that it is often not helpful in treatment to draw a sharp line between organic and psychogenic ED, and that even ED that is primarily organic in origin has a psychological effect that may perpetuate and worsen the problem. This can decrease concerns about being seen by a behavioral health provider for what the patient may see as a purely physical problem. Second, we share our belief that, in most cases, it is helpful to involve the patient's partner in future appointments. Finally, if patients have a history of being sexually abused, or if there is significant dysfunction in the partner relationship, we consider recommending a referral for specialty mental health individual or marital treatment.

Agree.   With the proliferation of medical treatments for ED, including medications such as Viagra, patients may be hesitant to engage in behavioral health treatments for ED, preferring a medical management approach to the problem. Sharing with the patient a biopsychosocial conceptualization of the problem, highlighting not only the relevant biological factors influencing ED but also the ways thoughts, emotions, and behaviors may cause or worsen his experience may help decrease patients' reluctance to try behavioral health approaches, either alone or in conjunction with medical management.

Assist.   The following section describes the interventions we commonly use in primary care for ED, including education, support of medical interventions for ED, sensate focus, communication training, cognitive restructuring and anxiety management, and changing lifestyle habits. As mentioned earlier, we generally prefer to work jointly with the couple rather than with the individual alone.

Education. Many couples experiencing erectile problems may benefit from education regarding general sexuality and ED in particular. Discussing and providing written materials (i.e., handouts or books) on ED definition, risk factors, and treatments; the sexual response cycle; the role of sexual stimulation; male and female sexual anatomy; as well as specific behavioral strategies for ED is a foundational intervention. Figures 13.1 and 13.2 contain sample psychoeducational handouts for general information about the nature and treatment of ED. Figure 13.3 lists books we frequently recommend to patients experiencing a variety of sexual problems. Within this list, the books by Milstein and Slowinski (1999) and Metz and McCarthy (2004) focus on ED and incorporate information and strategies for men and their partners. Zilbergeld's (1992) book contains readings relevant for ED, and Gottman and Silver's (1999) work focuses on more general communication strategies and pitfalls that may be relevant for patients with ED.

Support of medical intervention. With the increased availability of medical treatment options for ED, BHCs can help patients succeed with treatments that are not as easy as an oral medication, such as penile injections, a urethral suppository, or a vacuum device. You may work with couples on ways to integrate these interventions into their sexual behavior in ways that feel comfortable to both partners. Assisting couples in openly discussing their concerns or embarrassment about the treatments may be a first-line intervention. For other couples, discussing ways to have the partner involved with the intervention (e.g., having the partner give the injection or help with the vacuum device) as part of foreplay can enhance sensuality and arousal.

Use of an oral medication such as Viagra may have unforeseen negative consequences on the relationship and sexual functioning of some couples. For example, some partners may have adapted to a low frequency or absence of intercourse and may resent or feel uncomfortable with the increased sexual requests from the patient taking Viagra. You can assume a helpful role in facilitating appropriate communication and problem solving between partners with these concerns.

Sensate focus. Sensate focus was developed by Masters and Johnson (1970). Implementing sensate focus interventions with patients in primary care first relies on psychoeducation. Initially, you should ensure that the couple understands the rationale for the proscription on sexual intercourse (i.e., creating a relaxing environment free from demands and expectations for an erection and intercourse), the purpose of the exercise (i.e., to give and receive sensual pleasure in a non-demanding, non-sexual context; to focus on sensations rather than performance), and its progressive nature (i.e., over time, gradually moving from sensual touch to sexual touch of the breasts and genitals, to an eventual transition to intercourse). In addition to a discussion of these topics during the appointment, you may want to provide written materials that describe the approach in more detail. Figure 13.4 describes an initial behavioral exercise that we have found useful as a starting point with couples who can then further develop and tailor their specific activities. We also encourage additional reading to further guide this sensate focus approach (e.g., Milstein & Slowinski, 1999). Gambescia and Weeks (2007) provide concise descriptions of physical homework assignments related to sensual and sexual touch for patients with sexual problems that BHCs might find useful.

Communication training. Some couples may benefit from improving their ability to communicate in an appropriate manner, either on general topics or on those specific to sexuality. Chapter 3 reviews specifics on developing assertive communication skills. Examples tailored for couples who have difficulty talking about sexual topics appropriately might include statements such as:

- I feel unloved when you rush right into sex without cuddling first. I'd like it if you would spend a few minutes snuggling and holding me before we take off our clothes.

Questions and Answers About Erectile Dysfunction

What is Erectile Dysfunction?

Erectile dysfunction (ED) is the repeated inability to get or keep an erection firm enough for sexual intercourse. ED can be a total inability to achieve an erection, an inconsistent ability to do so, or a tendency to sustain only brief erections.

How Common is ED?

Estimates range from 15 million to 30 million, depending on the definition used. Incidence increases with age: About 5% of 40-year-old men and between 15% and 25% of 65-year-old men experience ED. But it is not an inevitable part of aging.

What Are the Risk Factors for ED?

In older men, ED usually has a physical cause, such as disease, injury, or side effects of drugs. Any disorder that causes injury to the nerves or impairs blood flow in the penis has the potential to cause ED.

What Causes ED?

Damage to nerves, arteries, smooth muscles, and fibrous tissues, often as a result of disease, is the most common cause of ED. Diseases such as diabetes, kidney disease, chronic alcoholism, multiple sclerosis, atherosclerosis, vascular disease, and neurologic disease account for about 70% of ED cases. Between 35% and 50% of men with diabetes experience ED.

Lifestyle choices that contribute to heart disease and vascular problems also raise the risk of ED. Smoking, being overweight, and avoiding exercise are possible causes of ED. In addition, surgery, especially radical prostate surgery for cancer, can injure nerves and arteries near the penis, causing ED. In addition, many common medicines such as blood pressure drugs, antihistamines, antidepressants, tranquilizers, appetite suppressants, and cimetidine (an ulcer drug) can produce ED as a side effect.

Experts believe that psychological factors such as stress, anxiety, guilt, depression, low self-esteem, and fear of sexual failure cause 10% to 20% of ED cases. Men with physical reasons for ED frequently experience the same sort of psychological reactions (e.g., stress, anxiety, guilt, depression).

Other possible causes are smoking, which affects blood flow in veins and arteries, and hormonal abnormalities, such as not enough testosterone.

How is ED Treated?

Most physicians suggest that treatments proceed from least to most invasive. For some men, making a few healthy lifestyle changes may solve the problem. Quitting smoking, losing excess weight, and increasing physical activity may help some men regain sexual function.

Cutting back on any prescribed or over-the-counter medications with harmful side effects is considered next. If you think a particular drug is causing problems with erection, tell your doctor and ask whether you can try a different class of medicine.

Psychotherapy and behavior modifications in selected patients are considered next if indicated, followed by oral or locally injected drugs, vacuum devices, and surgically implanted devices. In rare cases, surgery involving veins or arteries may be considered.

FIGURE 13.2. Questions and answers about erectile dysfunction handout. From *Erectile Dysfunction* (National Institutes of Health Publication No. 06-3923, pp. 1–5), by the National Kidney and Urologic Diseases Information Clearinghouse, 2005, Bethesda, MD: National Institutes of Health. Copyright 2005 by the National Institutes of Health. In the public domain.

- I feel aroused when you gently stroke me right here.
- When you are completely silent during sex, I feel isolated. I'd prefer if you would be a bit more vocal, such as sighing and telling me what feels good.
- When I lose my erection, I feel anxious and embarrassed when you try to directly stimulate my penis right away. I'd like it if you would kiss me and stroke my thighs instead.
- I feel irritated when you approach me for sex so late at night. I'm tired and worry about getting up for work the next morning. I'd really like it if we could agree on some other times of the day for sex, before 11 p.m.

Recommended Readings for Improving Intimacy and Sex

Barbach, L. (2000). *For yourself: The fulfillment of female sexuality.* New York: Bantam Doubleday.
Comfort, A. (1994). *The new joy of sex.* New York: Crown House Publishing.
Friday, N. (1998). *Men in love.* New York: Dell.
Friday, N. (1998). *My secret garden: Women's sexual fantasies.* New York: Pocket Books.
Gottman, J., & Silver, N. (1999). *The seven principles for making marriage work: A practical guide from the country's foremost relationship expert.* New York: Three Rivers.
Heiman, J., & LoPiccolo, J. (1988). *Becoming orgasmic: A sexual and personal growth program for women.* New York: Simon & Schuster.
Metz, M. E., & McCarthy, B. W. (2003). *Coping with premature ejaculation: Overcome PE, please your partner, and have great sex.* Oakland, CA: New Harbinger.
Metz, M. E., & McCarthy, B. W. (2004). *Coping with erectile dysfunction: How to regain confidence and enjoy great sex.* Oakland, CA: New Harbinger.
Milstein, R., & Slowinski, J. (1999). *The sexual male: Problems and solutions.* New York: Norton.
Zilbergeld, B. (1992). *The new male sexuality.* New York: Bantam Books.

FIGURE 13.3. Recommended readings for improving intimacy and sex handout.

In addition, we frequently recommend Gottman and Silver's (1999) book for couples who show general dysfunctional communication patterns. If couples have more severe marital problems or communication problems that do not improve with brief intervention, referral for couples therapy and/or sex therapy may be warranted.

Cognitive restructuring and anxiety management. When the evaluation suggests that performance anxiety may be causing or worsening ED, we initiate interventions to change anxious thought patterns. Identifying and modifying inaccurate beliefs about male sexual functioning may help decrease unrealistic expectations and performance anxiety. Thought stopping and thought substitution can be used when patients begin having thoughts that are counterproductive (e.g., "I must be 100% hard to satisfy my partner," "If I lose my erection again, I'll disappoint my partner," "If I can't get an erection soon, my partner will leave me."). Encouraging the patient to focus on sensations or sexual behaviors, rather than alarming thoughts, may also prove beneficial. Finally, we also include training in general relaxation methods (see chap. 3, this volume) to help decrease anxiety and tension and promote relaxation before sexual activity. Carey et al. (1993) provided further discussion of cognitive restructuring applications for ED.

Changing lifestyle habits. Use of tobacco and alcohol can cause or worsen problems with erectile dysfunction. We discuss the role that substance use may have in worsening ED when this appears to be a factor and assist individuals in quitting tobacco (see chap. 6, this volume) and avoiding use of alcohol prior to sexual activity.

Arrange. Recurrence of problems with ED posttreatment is common; increased attention in the literature has been given to relapse prevention for ED (McCarthy, 2001). Therefore, after the patient has seen improvements in ED, we recommend arranging one to two relapse prevention appointments over the course of the ensuing 6 to 12 months. For patients who have not experienced significant improvements, we facilitate a referral to a specialty mental health provider for treatment, ideally one with expertise in treating sexual dysfunction.

PREMATURE EJACULATION

Premature ejaculation is a disorder characterized by ejaculation that persistently occurs earlier than desired (i.e., either before, during, or shortly after penetration), with minimal sexual stimulation; it causes distress or interpersonal difficulty and is not exclusively caused by the use of a substance. Consideration should be given to the novelty of the situation or partner, age, and frequency of sexual activity (American Psychiatric Association, 2000, p. 552). The prevalence rate of premature ejaculation

Sexual Problems and Self-Help Interventions

Sexual problems occur for many people and result from both medical and nonmedical reasons. Sexual problems can include things such as reduced desire to have sex, difficulty feeling aroused, not being able to have or keep an erection (for men) or become lubricated (for women), difficulty staying aroused, and/or difficulty having an orgasm.

Medications Can Cause Sexual Side Effects

Medications can affect desire, arousal, and orgasm. The following are some medications that can affect sexual functioning:

- Antidepressants, mood stabilizers, tranquilizers, and other drugs given for anxiety
- Oral contraceptives and hormonal therapies
- Chemotherapy medications
- Alcohol, narcotics, and other controlled substances
- Some medications for treatment of allergies, hypertension, and glaucoma
- Anticonvulsant medications

Medical Problems and Surgeries That Can Cause or Worsen Sexual Problems

- Diabetes
- Emphysema
- Recent surgery (e.g., mastectomy, hysterectomy, or removal of ovaries for females; prostatectomy, orchiectomy for men)
- Cardiovascular disease
- Sleep loss (i.e., insomnia)
- Thyroid conditions
- Chronic pain
- Cancer

Relationship Difficulties

- Dissatisfaction, resentment, or struggles for power or control within the relationship
- Poor communication
- Having different value systems
- Lack of intimacy, emotional expression, or physical affection
- Discrepancies in sexual preferences

Personal and Psychological Factors

- Fatigue
- Depression
- Anxiety and stress
- Age. As we get older, our sexual response slows down and we need more stimulation and time
- Performance anxiety (i.e. fears about sexual response or loss of control)
- Negative beliefs about sex or certain sexual practices
- Low self-esteem and poor body image
- Narrow or unrealistic standards for sexual interactions

Do-It-Yourself Activities That Can Help Sexual Problems
Alone:

- Self-exploration and stimulation. This can help you increase awareness of your own body and make it easier to communicate likes and dislikes to your partner.
- Changing negative thoughts and assumptions about sex with more positive and realistic thoughts about what feels good and right for you.
- Challenging negative thoughts about your partner by focusing on what is attractive and positive about him or her.
- Challenging negative thoughts about yourself by focusing on what is attractive and positive about you.
- Physical exercise increases blood flow, reduces tension, enhances body image, and can improve other conditions that hinder sexual functioning.

FIGURE 13.4.   Sexual problems and self-help interventions handout. (*Continued*)

With Your Partner:

- Rebuild or establish emotional intimacy
  - Schedule time together when you simply talk to each other. Use the time to share feelings and get reacquainted with what is attractive and unique about your partner.
  - Share leisure activities.
  - Add small expressions of affection back into your daily routine if this is lacking (e.g., an affectionate note, phone call, or e-mail; hugs or hand-holding)
- Increase communication
  - Discuss sexual interests, desires, needs, and difficulties when you are NOT engaged in sexual activity.
  - Talk about what is going well and what you would like to be different in the relationship overall, then work together to come up with doable solutions.
- Add something new to sexual encounters (e.g., place, position, clothing, technique, erotica).
- Allow more time for foreplay and provide more partner-guided stimulation.
- During sexual encounters, focus on sensations rather than thoughts, performance, expectations, and appearances.

<u>Behavioral Exercise</u>

This exercise is designed to help you and your partner learn more about what types of stimulation you like. It also encourages physical intimacy and provides a way for you give as well as receive pleasure. It is not a prelude to sex and does not include intercourse or orgasm, so there are no sexual performance demands.

- Pick a time and place for you and your partner to be together. Allow at least 1 hour. The place should be private, comfortable, and free of distractions.
- Both partners should, at most, wear comfortable, light underclothes, although you may find being nude more comfortable.
- Without touching genitals, take turns giving and receiving stimulation (e.g., massaging, fondling, caressing). Take about half an hour per partner.
- Each partner should focus on the sensations of touching and being touched.
- The receiving partner should direct the giving partner by providing feedback about what is pleasurable or not or what could be done differently. The giving partner should adjust their stimulation accordingly. Use various strokes (e.g., long, short, soft, hard). Try using the palms, fingertips, and so forth.
- Partners should do only what is comfortable for them, and let the other person know when something feels pleasurable or becomes uncomfortable.
- Remember, this exercise is designed to increase intimacy and decrease performance expectation, pressure, and anxiety, so NO SEX!

FIGURE 13.4. *(Continued)* Sexual problems and self-help interventions handout.

in the U.S. population is 21% (Laumann et al., 1999), making it the most frequent male sexual disorder.

Key Biopsychosocial Factors in Premature Ejaculation

Understanding the biopsychosocial factors associated with premature ejaculation improves the BHC's ability to assess and treat this disorder. The following review highlights these important factors.

Physical factors. Some medical conditions may cause problems with PE (e.g., multiple sclerosis, epilepsy, prostatitis, pelvic or neurologic injury). Side effects of certain medications (e.g., desipramine, cold medications with ephedrine or pseudoephedrine) or withdrawal symptoms from medications (e.g., trifluoperazine, opiates) may also contribute to PE (Metz & McCarthy, 2003).

In the absence of these conditions or medications, a number of other biological variables have been proposed as etiological factors for PE, including hypersensitivity of the penis, genetic factors, hypersensitivity of serotonin receptors, and endocrinopathy, among others. Currently, however, there is limited empirical data to support many of these hypotheses (McMahon et al., 2004).

Pharmacological approaches may be helpful in decreasing problems with PE. There is some evidence that daily or as needed treatment (e.g., 4–6 hours before sexual activity) with selective serotonin reuptake inhibitors may be effective in reducing PE (e.g., McMahon & Touma, 1999; Waldinger, Zwinderman, & Olivier, 2001). In addition, treatment with topical anesthetics has proven useful for some individuals with PE (Atikeler, Gecit, & Senol, 2002). It should be noted that use of antidepressants or topical anesthetics for treatment of PE is off-label; there are no medications approved by the Food and Drug Administration for treatment of PE (Perelman, 2006). McMahon et al. (2004) recommended that medication treatment be considered as a first line approach for individuals with lifelong PE, whereas those with acquired or situational PE first receive behavioral or psychological intervention.

Emotional and cognitive factors. Individuals experiencing difficulty managing stress and other emotions are more likely to have problems with PE (Laumann et al., 1999). Similarly, correlations exist between PE, emotional problems (e.g., depression, low self-confidence, anxiety), and relationship problems (Symonds et al., 2003); however, the causal direction of these relationships remains unclear. Some (e.g., Masters & Johnson, 1970) have hypothesized that cognitive factors, including lack of attention to physiological cues and levels of sexual tension before orgasm, contribute to PE. More recent research suggests that during sex, men with PE have more preoccupations regarding controlling ejaculation and higher levels of anxiety than men without PE (Hartmann, Schedlowski, & Kruger, 2005).

Behavioral factors. Deficits in psychosexual skills may contribute to PE. Some standard behavioral treatments for ED, such as the stop–start technique (Semans, 1956) and the squeeze technique (Masters & Johnson, 1970) are based on the assumption that individuals with PE do not adequately recognize signs of, or exert control over, ejaculation. Other researchers (e.g., Ruff & St. Lawrence, 1985) have theorized that conditioning from earlier sexual experiences may contribute to PE (e.g., early sexual experiences that emphasized rapid ejaculation to avoid detection, masturbation).

Environmental factors. Male victims of child sexual abuse have twice the risk of developing problems with PE compared with men without an abuse history (Laumann et al., 1999). Problems in current relationships are also correlated with PE (Symonds et al., 2003), although it is unclear to what extent these problems cause or result from the problems with PE.

Specialty Mental Health Treatment

Rosen and Leiblum (1995) reviewed the literature on traditional behavioral treatments for PE (e.g., stop–start technique, squeeze technique) and noted that although initial reports of success were high (e.g., 90%), later studies showed lower rates of improvement and significant relapse. Expert consensus guidelines (McMahon et al., 2004) recommend the following treatment components: stop–start technique, squeeze technique, sensate focus, and relationship counseling. Behavioral treatments are recommended for men with acquired (i.e., rather than lifelong) PE or as adjuncts to medication treatment for men with lifelong PE.

Behavioral Health in Primary Care

Interventions for PE through primary care behavioral health services have not yet been empirically studied. The following discussion represents our adaptation of specialty mental health treatment for PE into our primary care behavioral health practices.

Primary Care Adaptation

Adapting the evidence-based techniques for premature ejaculation to a primary care setting requires the BHC to have skill in educating the patient. We supplement this education with a useful structure for organizing contacts with these patients.

Assess. Assessment of relevant biopsychosocial factors for PE in primary care often begins with questions to determine whether problems with PE are lifelong or acquired. This distinction may be helpful in selecting appropriate interventions because consensus guidelines recommend medication use for lifelong PE. Assessment could begin as follows:

Dr. Jones referred you to me because of some concerns about sexual functioning. Is that your understanding of why you are meeting with me today? [Patient responds affirmatively.] Dr. Jones said that you spoke with him specifically about trouble with premature ejaculation—ejaculating earlier than you would like—when you're having intercourse with your partner. Is this right? How long has this been a problem for you? [Patient responds that PE only has been a problem for about 6 months.] What changes can you think of that happened in your life, or in your relationship, around the time the problem started? Did you have any changes in your health or medications around that time?

Other relevant questions include the following:

- How much control do you feel you have when you ejaculate?
- Does premature ejaculation occur in all situations (e.g., with different partners and with masturbation)?
- Do you usually ejaculate before entering your partner, as you enter, or after?
- How much time passes between when you enter your partner and when you ejaculate? [Modify question as needed on the basis of the response to prior question.]
- What thoughts go through your mind when you are having sex? What do you focus on?
- Have you had difficulty with getting erections, or getting as hard as you would like, during sex?
- What strategies have you tried to help yourself "last longer"?
- How would you describe your relationship with your partner?
- How has premature ejaculation affected your sex life?
- How has premature ejaculation affected your relationship?
- What health problems do you have? What medications do you take?

- How has your mood been lately? Have you felt down or depressed much of the time? Anxious or stressed?

The Premature Ejaculation Severity Index (PESI; Metz & McCarthy, 2003) is an additional assessment tool appropriate for the primary care setting. The PESI is a brief, 10-item self-report inventory measuring severity of problems with PE and can quickly be completed by patients before the behavioral health appointment.

Polonsky (2000) differentiated between four clinical presentations of PE: *simple,* in which the patient presents alone with a desire to achieve better control over ejaculation, and does not have significant relationship problems; *simple plus relational,* in which the patient and the partner seek assistance in developing better control over ejaculation, and in improving relationship skills; *complicated,* in which the patient has more serious psychological problems that affect relationships and PE; and *complicated and relational,* in which the patient has both significant psychological and relationship problems. Attending to these clinical presentations during the assessment may help differentiate between patients who may respond well to interventions in the primary care environment (i.e., simple or simple plus relational) versus the more complicated presentations that may require referral to specialty mental health treatment.

Advise. If a medical evaluation has not been conducted, particularly if the onset of PE is recent, we advise the referring provider to rule out any medical problems or medications that may be contributing to problems with controlling ejaculation. If organic factors do not appear primary, we may advise that the patient and his partner attend several BHC appointments to learn specific behavioral and communication skills to help improve control over ejaculation. We strongly encourage partners to attend the appointments. Although the patient himself can complete some aspects of the intervention, others require cooperation from the sexual partner (e.g., transitioning from use of the squeeze technique during masturbation to using the method during intercourse).

Agree.   Reaching agreement on the goals of the intervention may be hampered by unrealistic expectations. It is common for patients with PE to believe that they should be able to have complete control over the timing of their ejaculation or that they should always be able to postpone it indefinitely, even during long periods of intense stimulation. Identifying these rigid beliefs and working to develop more reasonable goals and measures of success may help prevent early discouragement and subsequent abandonment of efforts to change.

Assist.   Consistent with expert consensus guidelines (McMahon et al., 2004), the intervention components we use with PE patients as a BHC includes education, sensate focus, stop–start and squeeze techniques, and relationship interventions.

Education.   We typically begin work with a patient and partner, if available, by providing psychoeducation regarding sexual functioning, behavior, and attitudes. Normalizing problems with PE (i.e., by emphasizing that they are not alone, that PE is the most common sexual problem men experience) can help reduce embarrassment and reluctance to talk about their experiences. We routinely discuss the nature and physiology of the sexual response cycle. We highlight the differences between the two stages of ejaculation, emission (i.e., when seminal fluid enters the urethra) and expulsion (i.e., when seminal fluid is expelled from the penis), emphasizing the fact that once emission occurs, expulsion is inevitable (Perelman, 2006). We also spend time discussing whether the patient can recognize premonitory sensations (i.e., sensations that immediately precede emission), because the ability to identify precursors to emission is key in using the stop–start technique described later. Finally, we highlight the role thoughts play in the sexual response cycle, with mental focus influencing arousal. Metz and McCarthy's (2003) self-help book for PE can provide patients with greater depth of information, as well as a series of home-based strategies for PE.

Sensate focus.   Although not all PE treatment approaches include a sensate focus treatment component, expert consensus guidelines (McMahon et al., 2004) include sensate focus as a recommended element of PE treatment. Some couples may find

that sensate focus exercises designed to decrease emphasis on performance may help reduce anxiety, which may contribute to PE. See the discussion of sensate focus earlier in this chapter, as well as in Figure 13.4, for additional information.

Stop–start and squeeze techniques.   The goal of the stop–start and squeeze techniques, described initially by Semans (1956) and Masters and Johnson (1970), respectively, is to learn to recognize signs of impending emission and then do something different to learn to decrease the physical and/or mental stimulation leading to ejaculation and hence improve control over its timing.

We rely on an approach described by Polonsky (2000). Figure 13.5 is the handout we use with patients. In implementing this approach, we initially advise the patient to masturbate without lubrication. When he notices sensations indicating he is close to emission, he should stop masturbating and if helpful, firmly squeeze his penis at the juncture between the head and the shaft or at the base. After waiting for the sensations to lessen (about a minute), he should begin masturbating again. This cycle is repeated several times. With practice, the patient will learn more about his own sensations as well as how to control them through changes in stimulation. The patient may then progress to exercises involving continuous stimulation (i.e., rather than stopping or squeezing) but at varied or lower levels (e.g., slowing down the masturbation rhythm) to keep arousal levels high but still controlled. After he has achieved greater control over ejaculation with the prior exercises, he may add a lubricant while masturbating, which typically increases pleasurable sensations. We advise the patient to practice these exercises at least three times per week.

The final phase involves intercourse between the patient and his partner. If the partner has not yet attended an appointment with the patient, we encourage the patient to allow the partner come in for joint consultation at this point in the intervention. We stress the need for open communication about PE and the behavioral techniques being used. The couple is advised to initially continue to use the stop–start or squeeze techniques during intercourse. When he feels sensations indicating emission is close, he either stops thrusting or

---

Gaining Control Over Premature Ejaculation

The first step in working toward gaining control over premature ejaculation involves masturbating without lubrication. When you notice sensations that you are close to ejaculation, STOP! Wait a full minute for the sensations to decrease. Then resume masturbation, repeating the cycle several times. You may find that using your thumb and forefinger to firmly squeeze your penis may help delay ejaculation. You can experiment with squeezing at the base of your penis, or where the shaft joins the head of your penis. After you have repeated this exercise several times, allow yourself to ejaculate, focusing on the sensations. Practice this exercise several times per week.

After you have begun developing greater control over delaying ejaculation with the first technique, you can progress to the second step. This involves altering the amount or type of stimulation during masturbation, rather than stopping stimulation altogether, to delay ejaculation. As before, begin by masturbating without lubrication. When you notice sensations indicating that you are close to ejaculating, experiment with changing the type of stimulation. For example, you might slow down the strokes or make them lighter. The goal is to learn how to keep your arousal level high but still controlled. Repeat the cycle several times, and practice the entire exercise at least three times per week.

The next step is simply to add lubrication during masturbation. Lubrication typically increases sensations of pleasure. Work on mastering the above techniques while masturbating with lubrication.

The final step involves progressing to intercourse with your partner. Continue to use the same basic principles you have already developed. Notice the sensations in your body that indicate you are close to ejaculating. When these sensations occur, stop moving or thrusting. Wait about a minute for your stimulation level to decrease. You may find it helpful to also squeeze the base of your penis during this time. When you resume movement, begin slowly. Repeat the process several times prior to allowing yourself to ejaculate. Finally, ask what you can do for your partner.

Remember that continued practice will help develop the skills for controlling ejaculation. However, as with most skills, perfection is not a realistic goal. There will still be times when you ejaculate earlier than you would like. This is normal and should not be cause for alarm. Remember the improvements you have made, and return to practicing some of the exercises described earlier.

FIGURE 13.5. Gaining control over premature ejaculation handout. Data from pages 305–332 of Polansky (2000).

squeezes the base of his penis until sensations decrease. When movement is resumed, it should be slow. This cycle is repeated several times before the patient then allows himself to ejaculate. The couple should then discuss what the partner would like in terms of sexual stimulation before ending the encounter.

Relationship interventions. Communication skills between partners, particularly regarding sexuality, may need to be improved. The assertive communication strategies discussed earlier in the chapter and included in chapter 3 may be useful for couples with PE. One theme unique to PE that may need to be addressed involves the partner's perception of the cause of the PE. It is common to find that the partner harbors the belief that the PE is somehow due to the patient's selfishness and lack of concern for the partner's pleasure. This may

lead to resentment and further relationship problems. In this situation, we work with couples to openly communicate about their beliefs about the cause of PE and the effect PE has on the partner. We also may provide recommendations for the couple to enhance the partner's pleasure during sexual interactions.

Arrange. As mentioned previously, not all patients benefit from brief, psychoeducationally and behaviorally based interventions in the primary care setting. Patients whose PE involves more complex etiology (e.g., significant psychological or relationship problems) may require more intensive specialty mental health services (e.g., sex therapy, cognitive–behavioral therapy, relationship counseling). You will want to develop an awareness of local resources for these services and recommend referral if it becomes apparent that a higher level of care is necessary for improvement of PE.

FEMALE ORGASMIC DISORDER

Female orgasmic disorder is defined as persistent delay or absence of orgasm, despite a normal excitement phase, that causes distress or interpersonal problems. Clinicians must consider the woman's sexual experience level, degree of sexual stimulation, and age in making the diagnosis. Furthermore, the disorder cannot be directly caused by medical conditions, medications, or another mental disorder. Most cases of female OD are lifelong rather than acquired, but some women may develop orgasmic problems later in life as a result of trauma (e.g., rape), relationship problems, sexual communication problems, or medical conditions. (APA, 2000, pp. 547–548). Prevalence estimates of female OD in community samples range from 7% to 26% (Laumann et al., 1999; Simons & Carey, 2001), making it the most common sexual disorder in women.

Key Biopsychosocial Factors in Female Orgasmic Disorder

As with ED and PE, understanding the biopsychosocial factors that contribute to female orgasmic disorder help the BHC operate more easily in the primary care environment. This knowledge can help improve patient education and communication with primary care providers (PCPs).

Physical factors.   Medical problems (e.g., diabetic neuropathy, vascular disease) and medications (e.g., antidepressants, benzodiazepines, antihypertensives, opioids, neuroleptics) can impair ability to achieve orgasm (APA, 2000; Lewis et al., 2004; Regev, Zeiss, & Zeiss, 2006). There currently are no medications with proven efficacy for female OD (Regev et al., 2006; Segraves, 2003).

Emotional and cognitive factors.   Women who experience problems with managing emotions and stress are at heightened risk for all sexual dysfunctions, including OD (Laumann et al., 1999). Women with psychiatric disorders, including depression and anxiety, are more likely to experience problems with OD (Lewis et al., 2004; Regev et al., 2006). Low lev-

els of sexual assertiveness and belief in myths about orgasm and sexuality may also contribute to problems with orgasm in women (Hurlbert, 1991; Regev et al., 2006).

Behavioral factors.   Lack of appropriate sexual stimulation from a partner, limited experience with masturbation, and limited skill with specific sexual techniques that may enhance arousal and orgasm have been thought to be primary causes of primary female OD (Regev et al., 2006; Wakefield, 1987). Indeed, researchers have found that women who feel comfortable with masturbation tend to have fewer problems with OD (Kelly, Strassberg, & Kircher, 1990).

Environmental factors.   Women who have experienced sexual abuse or trauma may be more likely to experience problems with orgasm (APA, 2000, p. 548; Regev et al., 2006). Current problems with intimate relationships, including conflict or communication problems surrounding sexuality or low levels of comfort with the sexual partner, also may contribute to orgasmic difficulty (Regev et al., 2006).

Specialty Mental Health

Summaries of the treatment outcome literature for female OD indicate that lifelong OD can successfully be treated with guided masturbation training or cognitive behavioral sex therapy. These treatments typically show high success rates for women with lifelong OD, with 80% to 90% achieving orgasm through masturbation. Success rates are lower (20%–60%), however, for achieving orgasm with partner stimulation (Regev et al., 2006; Rosen & Leiblum, 1995). Although acquired OD is more difficult to treat, some success has been found with guided masturbation training (LoPiccolo & Stock, 1986). If acquired OD is related to problems that are more complex, such as history of sexual trauma or significant relationship difficulties, interventions may need to focus on these areas (Regev et al., 2006; Rosen & Leiblum, 1995).

Behavioral Health in Primary Care

No studies examining the effect of brief behavioral health consultation in primary care settings on female OD could be identified. However, literature suggests that minimal contact approaches based in bibliotherapy can be as effective for female OD as more intensive specialty treatments (van Lankveld, 1998). Integrating guided self-help or bibliotherapy into primary care-based interventions may prove effective.

Primary Care Adaptation

Structuring the assessment and intervention using the 5A's format can promote efficiency in information collection and effectiveness in intervention for this potentially sensitive subject. We detail how to use the 5A's for successful BHC–patient interaction.

Assess.   Functional assessment of female OD should include assessment of the ways in which physical, emotional, cognitive, behavioral, and environmental factors may contribute to the onset or maintenance of the anorgasmia. Figure 13.6 summarizes recommended assessment questions for female OD (Heiman, 2000; Regev et al., 2006). Inquiring about medications (e.g., antidepressants, antihypertensives, benzodiazepines, neuroleptics, opioids), use of substances (e.g., alcohol), and medical problems (e.g., back problems, nerve damage, multiple sclerosis, diabetic neuropathy, history of abdominal

surgery, hysterectomy, vascular disease) can help determine whether physical factors may be contributing to problems achieving orgasm. Particularly close attention to the possible role of physical factors should be given when a patient's OD is acquired rather than lifelong. Similarly, close assessment of environmental factors (e.g., current relationship problems, recent sexual trauma) is warranted when a woman who previously was able to achieve orgasm presents with new orgasmic difficulties.

Advise.   The advice given to patients regarding treatment options varies on the basis of information gathered in the assessment, particularly the evaluation of which biopsychosocial factors are most relevant in the onset and maintenance of the orgasmic difficulties. If it appears that health problems or medications may be involved but this has not yet medically evaluated, we advise patients and the PCP to assess whether physical factors are playing a significant role in the orgasmic dysfunction before working with these patients further. If the etiology seems largely related to significant relationship problems, we typically advise that the patient participate in

---

Sample Assessment Questions for Female Orgasmic Disorder

When did your problems with achieving orgasm develop?

Were there changes in your health, relationships, or other areas when the problem began?

Have you ever experienced an orgasm?

During what types of sexual activity have you had orgasms (e.g., masturbation, intercourse)?

Do you always have trouble achieving orgasm or just in specific situations?

Do you experience any pain with intercourse?

Have you experienced any kind of sexual trauma, either as a child or adult? [If yes, screen further for posttraumatic stress disorder.]

How often do you do the following?

- Feel sexual desire? Find you are interested in sex? Engage in sexual activity, including masturbation?
- Become aroused (e.g., lubrication, swelling) with a partner? Through masturbation?
- Experience orgasm with a partner? Through masturbation?
- Feel satisfied by your sexual experience?
- What medications or substances do you use? [Screen for antidepressants, alcohol, illicit drugs.]
- What medical conditions do you have? (e.g., back problems, nerve damage, multiple sclerosis, diabetic neuropathy, history of abdominal surgery, hysterectomy)
- Are you aware of any fears or thoughts that might be getting in the way of having orgasms?
- Are you having problems in your relationship (e.g., communication problems, conflicts)?
- Do you feel down or sad much of the time? Have you lost interest in activities you enjoyed?
- How often do you feel anxious or stressed?
- What do you think is causing your difficulties with achieving orgasm?

FIGURE 13.6.   Sample assessment questions for female orgasmic disorder.

interventions that initially focus on improving the couple's relationship, either BHC-provided services or through a specialty mental health referral if the severity of the relationship distress is high. If significant psychological problems such as posttraumatic stress disorder (PTSD) or depression appear largely responsible for the OD, as may be the case with acquired OD, we often advise the patient to receive treatment for these problems before explicitly focusing on treatment of OD. Depending on the nature of the problem, we again would either recommend follow-up with BHC services (e.g., in the case of mild to moderate depression) or advise that the PCP consider a referral for specialty mental health treatment (e.g., in the case of PTSD or severe depression). Patients presenting with lifelong OD that appears related to lack of sexual knowledge, skills, or experience seem to be the best candidates for brief psychoeducational and behavioral interventions that can be accomplished in primary care. We typically advise these patients to continue services through the BHC.

Agree. The core intervention for female OD, as discussed previously, involves masturbation training. The degree to which patients feel comfortable with an approach founded on masturbation varies greatly. Personal, cultural, and religious beliefs may influence whether a patient is open to this form of intervention. Therefore, as you are attempting to reach agreement with patients on the goals of intervention and the specific strategies used to reach these goals, it is critical to assess a patient's views on masturbation and her willingness to engage in this type of intervention. Providing a detailed rationale for how masturbation training may help with the problem can be helpful in many instances. Treatment approaches need to be modified for women who strongly oppose masturbation. For example, if a woman is unwilling to masturbate, you might work with the couple to increase skills and comfort with sexual experimentation and communication (e.g., open discussion about what types of sexual touch are most stimulating), to minimize thoughts that interfere with sexual assertiveness or that increase anxiety, or to increase use of sexual fantasy.

Assist. The interventions we use most frequently with female patients with OD include psychoeduca-

tion, sensate focus, masturbation training, and sexual communication.

Psychoeducation. We provide psychoeducation aimed at increasing knowledge about physiology, the sexual response cycle, types of stimulation that often produce pleasure, and the role of cognition in enhancing arousal and orgasm. Exploring myths that patients may hold about orgasm can provide an opportunity to develop helpful beliefs about sexuality. Figure 13.7 is a handout that we use to facilitate discussion with patients about beliefs they may hold that might perpetuate their problems with OD. Having anatomical models or diagrams available in the clinic can aid in educating patients about relevant anatomy and ensuring that patients and partners are communicating accurately about anatomy. We also routinely recommend that patients engage in additional psychoeducational reading about female OD, which we can then incorporate in a guided self-help format. The list of readings in Figure 13.3 contains material specifically written for improving female sexuality and orgasmic disorder.

Sensate focus. Although sensate focus exercises have not been shown to substantially decrease female OD, they may be helpful with particular subsets of women with OD, particularly those who experience sexual anxiety or who feel uncomfortable communicating with their partner about needs for specific types of sexual stimulation (Gambescia & Weeks, 2007; Meston, Hull, Levin, & Sipski, 2004). If these factors appear to play a role in the maintenance of OD, we incorporate sensate focus as an intervention. See the discussion of sensate focus earlier in this chapter, as well as Figure 13.4, for additional information.

Masturbation training. A core intervention, guided masturbation training gives patients the opportunity to learn about their own sexual preferences and responses and to discover what types of stimulation may lead to orgasm. We typically begin with a discussion of the patient's prior history of how, or if, she has masturbated in the past. We encourage patients to consider various approaches to masturbation, including using different pressures, rhythms, and speeds with manual stimulation; using a vibrator; or experimenting with rhythmically tightening and relaxing the pelvic floor muscles (i.e., as in Kegel exercises) and the leg

Developing Helpful Beliefs for Enhancing Arousal and Orgasm	
Unhelpful belief	**Helpful belief**
It is my partner's job to give me an orgasm.	I can take control of my own sexuality and pleasure.
The only acceptable method of having an orgasm is through intercourse.	Intercourse is just one way to have an orgasm. An orgasm through rubbing, oral sex, or using a vibrator has the same physiological response and can give me pleasure.
An orgasm is the most important aspect of sexuality.	An orgasm is one aspect of my sexuality. I can enjoy desire and emotional satisfaction without an orgasm.
I should be able to have an orgasm every time I have sex.	It is not realistic to expect an orgasm every time. The majority of women do not have an orgasm each time they have sex. Sexuality is complex and variable. I can enjoy the sexual experience even without an orgasm.
If I tell my partner what I want, I'll be seen as "pushy" or "slutty."	My partner wants to give me pleasure. By talking about our desires, we can both increase our arousal and pleasure.

FIGURE 13.7.   Developing helpful beliefs for enhancing arousal and orgasm handout.

muscles. We often encourage the patient to incorporate sexual fantasy during masturbation, particularly if anxiety or self-consciousness is present. Self-help books for female OD, such as those from Barbach (2000) and Heiman and LoPiccolo (1988), can provide patients with more detailed exercises and can be integrated into BHC interventions in a guided self-help approach.

Sexual communication. As women transition from masturbation to sexual activity with a partner, communication about sexual preferences is essential. Some women may benefit from interventions to increase their ability to discuss sexual matters and preferences openly. Assertive communication training (see discussion earlier in this chapter and in chap. 3) can be incorporated to increase patient comfort in telling their partners the types of sexual stimulation they like and do not like or the types of sexual behavior they might like to try.

Arrange.   As discussed previously, we are more likely to initially coordinate a referral for specialty mental health treatment of female OD when the patient presents with acquired (i.e., vs. lifelong) problems achieving orgasm. Women with lifelong OD who do not benefit from the primary care

behavioral health intervention described earlier are considered for referral to specialty care.

SUMMARY

Sexual dysfunctions affect the functioning and quality of life of substantial numbers of individuals. With the greater availability of medical treatments for some of the sexual dysfunctions (e.g., medication for erectile dysfunction), primary care medical providers are seeing larger numbers of individuals presenting with sexual dysfunction concerns. However, medical providers may not feel adequately prepared to offer treatment that incorporates more than medication or surgery. BHCs can offer a unique service by conducting a biopsychosocial evaluation and tailoring recommendations for intervention to target underlying cognitive, emotional, behavioral, or environmental factors that may be causing or maintaining sexual dysfunction. As outlined in this chapter, evidence-based specialty mental health interventions can be tailored to be consistent with a brief, structured primary care behavioral health model. Outcome research is needed to empirically demonstrate that primary care behavioral health interventions truly lead to improvement in these sexual dysfunctions.

CHAPTER 14

SPECIAL CONSIDERATIONS FOR OLDER ADULTS

American adults age 65 years and older (i.e., older adults) are expected to account for 20% of the U.S. population by 2030 (Centers for Disease Control and Prevention [CDC] and The Merck Company Foundation, 2007). Of all medical visits made by older adults between 2003 and 2004, 42.7% were to a primary care provider (PCP; i.e., family or internal medicine; National Center for Health Statistics, 2007b). Although some may assume that older adults are seen in internal medicine clinics, family medicine physicians provide care from "cradle to grave," and as many as 25% of patients seen in family medicine clinics are over 65 years old. Often, older age is associated with illness and poor functioning; however, almost three quarters of older adults describe their health as "good" or "excellent/very good" (National Center for Health Statistics, 2007a). Medical care for older adults can be quite complex. On average, older adults are diagnosed with at least two chronic medical conditions (CDC, 2003) and are taking 4.5 medications. When working in primary care settings, it is essential to have the breadth of knowledge and resources available to provide appropriate recommendations for helping to successfully manage the health care of older adults.

SPECIALTY MENTAL HEALTH

Although most psychologists report that they see older adults in their practice, relatively few have received formalized training to work with this population (Qualls, Segal, Norman, Niederehe, & Gallagher-Thompson, 2002). The American Psychological Association (APA, 2003) published

20 guidelines providing practitioners with a frame of reference and basic information about aging and special concerns related to working with older adults. These guidelines address areas including attitudes and knowledge about older adults, knowledge about adult development, aging, and older adults; clinical issues (e.g., cognitive changes, problems in daily living, psychopathology); assessment; interventions and consultations; and continuing education (APA, 2003). Although most psychologists work in specialty mental health settings, these guidelines are useful for those working in primary care.

BEHAVIORAL HEALTH CARE IN PRIMARY CARE

In this chapter, we highlight some of the presenting problems seen more frequently in primary care settings, such as problems with cognitive functioning and incontinence. These concerns are not unique to older adults but tend to be more common among this cohort. Integrating behavioral health providers into primary care increases the likelihood that older adults will engage in behavioral health services (Bartels et al., 2004). Primary care clinicians indicated that the integration of behavioral health professionals into the primary care setting enhances the behavioral health care of older adults (Gallo et al., 2004). We briefly discuss special considerations for caregiver stress, depression and anxiety, sexual functioning, and social role changes and bereavement. Finally, we discuss practical adaptations for the care of older adults in primary care.

COGNITIVE FUNCTIONING

Concern about dementia among older adults is common in primary care; however, 26% to 76% of cases in primary care in which dementia is, or may be, present are not diagnosed (Holsinger, Deveau, Boustani, & Williams, 2007). Although Alzheimer's disease is most commonly cited as the reason for dementia, other medical conditions, including cerebrovascular diseases (e.g., strokes) and Parkinson's disease, can be associated with impaired cognitive functioning. Aside from dementia, cognitive abilities, including processing speed, reasoning, and memory decline as people age (Salthouse, 2004).

Assess

One challenge associated with memory complaints is distinguishing whether problems with memory are associated with dementia, depression, delirium, or reflect normal aging. A variety of standardized measures can help providers assess the extent of cognitive impairment; however, many of these measures would take too long to administer in the context of a primary care visit. Your main task in assessing memory problems is not necessarily to determine what the problem is and how to treat it but instead to help determine whether there is a significant cognitive impairment that needs further assessment in a specialty clinic by a neuropsychologist, neurologist, or geriatrician.

Two measures that are often recommended to screen for cognitive deficits include the The Mini-Mental State Examination (MMSE; Folstein, Folstein, & McHugh, 1975) and the Clock Drawing Test. The MMSE is one of the most widely used measures for screening for cognitive functioning in older adults; the test consists of 30 questions assessing orientation, registration, attention and calculation, recall, and language. The advantages of this measure are its brevity (i.e., it takes approximately 5–10 minutes to administer) and the extensive research examining its use. However, the MMSE is not sensitive to mild cognitive impairment, changes that occur with severe Alzheimer's disease, or damage to the right hemisphere of the brain, which is involved in executive functioning (Tombaugh & McIntyre, 1992). In addition, age, level of education, ethnicity, and sociocultural background have been shown to affect the score of the MMSE (Tombaugh & McIntyre, 1992), although adjusted norms for age and educational level are available (Crum, Anthony, Bassett, & Folstein, 1993). Using corrected MMSE cutoff scores, Tangalos et al. (1996) demonstrated 82% sensitivity and 98% specificity for detecting dementia in an older adult primary care sample. The MMSE can be ordered from Psychological Assessment Resources, Inc. through their Web site (http://www.minimental.com/).

The Clock Drawing Test is a measure of executive functioning (e.g., how well an individual can plan behaviors). According to Shulman (2000), the most common method of conducting the Clock Drawing Test includes the following steps:

1. Hand the patient a predrawn 4-inch diameter circle.
2. State, "This circle represents a clock face. Please put in the numbers so that it looks like a clock and then set the time to 10 minutes past 11."

There are a wide variety of ways to score the Clock Drawing Test. On average, the scoring methods demonstrate good sensitivity (85%) and specificity (85%) for dementia (Shulman, 2000). One of the quickest scoring methods is to divide the clock into four quadrants by drawing a line between the 12 and the 6 and a line perpendicular to the original line to divide the circle into four equal quadrants. Errors in the first through third quadrant are assigned a 1, and an error in the fourth quadrant is assigned a 4. Scores 4 and higher are considered clinically significant and indicate that more extensive testing should be performed. Essentially, a clock drawing with any significant abnormalities is a cue that more testing is needed.

Harvan and Cotter (2005) recommended the combined use of the MMSE and the Clock Drawing Test, which has demonstrated the best sensitivity (100%) and specificity (91%) to screen for dementia in primary care settings (Yamamoto et al., 2004). According to the review by Cullen, O'Neill, Evans, Coen, and Lawlor (2007), additional measures that may be useful for screening for dementia in primary care settings include the Modified Mini-Mental State Examination (3MS), Cognitive Abilities Screening Instrument (CASI), Short and Sweet Screening

Instrument (SASSI), Short Test of Mental Status, and Addenbrooke's Cognitive Examination-Revised (ACE-R). The 3MS, CASI, SASSI, and ACE-R are all modifications of the MMSE (Cullen et al., 2007).

When we are screening for cognitive problems we ask the patient about the changes that they have noticed. However, asking patients to remember what they are forgetting may not be the most effective method to screen for cognitive decline. Asking family members about a patient's memory problems is more likely to elicit accurate information about decline than a patient's self-report (Carr, Gray, Baty, & Morris, 2000; Holsinger et al., 2007). In addition, behavioral and emotional problems (e.g., depressive symptoms, social withdrawal, paranoia, sleep disturbance) may be present before changes in memory are evident (Jost & Grossberg, 1996). To screen for memory problems, we would ideally talk with family members and ask the following:

- What have you noticed your dad forgetting? Does he forget your name? The names of people he knows well? What are some examples?
- Does he get lost easily, including in places that he has been to before?
- Does he have difficulty operating common appliances? Has he left the stove on? Is this a change for him?
- Does his mood change frequently? Is this unusual for him?
- Have you noticed changes in his behavior or thinking, such as not spending time with others, hopelessness, or paranoia? Have you noticed changes in his sleeping patterns?

It is also valuable to ask about Activities of Daily Living (ADLs; Katz, Ford, Moskowitz, Jackson, & Jaffe, 1963), those activities that are essential for self-management (e.g., bathing, walking, climbing stairs), and Instrumental Activities of Daily Living (IADLs; Lawton & Brody, 1969), which are higher level skills, such as shopping, managing money, and using public transportation. Some questions you could ask about ADLs include the following:

- Can he bathe himself?
- Does he brush his teeth?
- Can he dress himself?

- Can he use the bathroom on his own?
- Does he have any difficulties feeding himself?
- Does he walk on his own without assistance?
- Can he climb stairs on his own?

Some questions you could ask about IADLs include the following:

- Does he do his own cooking? Shopping?
- Does he keep his living area or home clean?
- How does he get around when he wants to go somewhere?
- Has he had difficulties managing his money? Does he pay bills on time?
- Does he take his medication on his own?

With these questions, you are looking for changes in functioning. Dementia is usually associated with gradual changes, unless it is due to a sudden event such as a stroke. Loss of ADLs implies that a significant dementia may be present. Skill deficits may become suddenly apparent when a caregiver becomes incapacitated or dies. For example, an older man who relied on his wife to cook and clean may not be able to prepare his own meals and maintain his living space.

Impairments in cognitive and behavioral functioning can affect an individual's ability to make decisions that are necessary to sustain an independent lifestyle (e.g., managing health and finances). Determining someone's capacity to make decisions requires balancing clinical, legal, and ethical concerns, because the consequences of finding someone incapacitated may result in the appointment of a surrogate decision maker (Moye, Armesto, & Karel, 2005). Although in the past a distinction was made between competence (i.e., a legal determination) and capacity (i.e., an informal evaluation), the legal system has increasingly adopted the term *capacity* (Moye et al., 2005). Formal capacity evaluations are unlikely to be performed in the primary care setting, but behavioral health consultants (BHCs) should be aware of the factors that are important in the determination of capacity, because many informal decisions about capacity are made in this setting. The definitions of *incapacity* vary between states, but generally include an assessment of one or more the following: (a) a disabling condition, including mental illness; (b) impaired cognitive or decision-making abilities; (c) an impaired ability to manage property or person; (d) an inability to maintain essential health requirements (e.g., medical care, nutrition); and (e) an impairment causing an endangerment to the person or to others (Moye et al. 2005; Sabatino & Basinger, 2000). Additional information about formal capacity evaluations can be found in the volume by the American Bar Association and American Psychological Association (2006), which is available online at http://www.abanet.org/aging/docs/judges_book_5-24.pdf.

Informal (i.e., nonlegal) decisions about capacity are more common in primary care, wherein decisions are made through evaluations of functioning and discussions with the patient and family member(s). Ultimately, clinical judgment remains the "gold standard" for determining capacity because measures for assessing capacity are not well studied (Moye, Gurrera, Karel, Edelstein, & O'Connell, 2006).

Advise

The possibility of significant cognitive impairment can be overwhelming for patients and their families. Again, in primary care settings, we are not making the diagnosis of a dementia but alerting patients and their family members to the possibility of a dementia process. We advise patients, their family members, and the PCP when there appears to be a sufficient reason to pursue a more detailed evaluation of the patient's cognitive functioning. For those individuals who do not screen positive for significant memory decline, we may recommend to the PCP and the patient that he or she return in 6 months for a reevaluation. In addition, regardless of whether we believe that an individual may meet criteria for a dementia diagnosis, we discuss techniques that could be used to manage memory concerns. For example, we might say, "There are multiple things you can do that may improve your ability to remember, including using reminder devices, memory exercises, physical exercise, and relaxation. Would you be interested in spending sometime learning how to use these techniques?"

We also advise patients about available resources. An important resource for older adults and their families is the local Area Agency on Aging (http://www.n4a.org/), which consolidates community resources for older adults. Depending on the level of functioning, we may also encourage patients and caregivers to contact community organizations that serve older adults, such as the Alzheimer's Association (http://www.alz.org), the state's department of human services, or local senior centers. If we know that a patient may have difficulty managing his or her meals, then we may encourage the use of a group such as Meals on Wheels (http://www.mowaa.org/). If the patient belongs to a religious organization, we encourage the patient and the family to explore what services that group might offer.

Agree

When we believe individuals need more testing, we discuss with the patients and their family members the purpose of the testing and help schedule appointments with appropriate clinics (e.g., neuropsychology). In these cases, as well as in cases in which the memory loss does not appear to be related to dementia, we offer to discuss methods that could be used to improve remembering.

Assist

Despite the lack of evidence supporting the "use it or lose it" assumptions about memory, experts continue to recommend mentally stimulating activity, in part because there is no evidence that such a practice is harmful (Salthouse, 2006). However, some more recent evidence suggests that cognitive training may decrease functional decline (Willis et al., 2006). We encourage patients to engage in cognitive training exercises, but avoid making unsubstantiated claims about the impact of these exercises. We may recommend memory cues and devices, engaging in cognitively stimulating activities, physical exercise, and using relaxation techniques, particularly when one is having difficulty remembering, may be helpful for improving remembering skills.

Memory cues and devices. Developing systems to help patients remember everyday tasks or objects may help reduce some of the stress associated with memory difficulties. These memory cues and devices might include identifying common areas where things are placed, using reminder notes or a calendar to plan tasks and appointments, or learning skills to remember information more efficiently. So you might say the following:

> It can be helpful to incorporate the use of reminders and devices to help you remember. Establish a place to put important objects, such as a hook by the door for keys, a bin on your dresser for your wallet and cell phone. You can use daily to-do lists to help you remember what you need to do each day. Memory strategies, such as remembering things together in groups, can help you remember. For example, rather than trying to remember the individual numbers in a phone number, try putting the numbers together. So instead of 5-5-5-7-3-0-9, remember the number as five hundred and fifty-five and seven thousand, three hundred, and nine.

Cognitive exercises.   Engaging in tasks and games that are stimulating and require sustained concentration and planning may help to "exercise" the patient's memory. For example, you could say the following:

> Exercising your memory by engaging in activities that require careful thinking may also help your memory. Some examples of these activities are learning a new skill, learning to play an instrument, or playing games or completing puzzles that require complex thinking, such as chess, crossword puzzles, or sudoku. Some older adults enjoy writing or orally sharing their life stories as a way to exercise their memory. Is there anything that you used to do or would like to do to "exercise" your memory?

Physical activity.   We often talk with PCPs about a patient's physical limitations and make appropriate recommendations about increasing physical activity. It may be necessary to have a physical therapist develop an appropriate program for physical activity; however, if the PCP recommends increased

physical activity, we help the patient get started by saying the following:

> Physical activity may improve your ability to think and remember. Would it be reasonable for you to start a walking program? Because you haven't been walking for physical activity, perhaps we could start out by just walking for 10 minutes a day. What days and times could you plan to do that walk?

Relaxation.   When someone has difficulty remembering something, it is common for that person to become increasingly frustrated or distressed. Teaching a relaxation technique, such as relaxed breathing, which patients could use when they become distressed about remembering, may help reduce unnecessary sympathetic arousal and distress. The techniques we discussed in chapter 3 may be useful to consider when introducing relaxation strategies. You could say the following:

> When you are having difficulty remembering something, it is important to try to remain calm. If you get upset, your stress response makes it even harder for you to remember. Taking a couple of deep breaths can help to reduce the stress response that sometimes interferes with remembering.

Arrange

If you are seeing many older adults, it is helpful to have relationships with neuropsychologists or other medical professionals who can assist with more extensive testing for dementia when necessary. In addition, relationships with social workers and hospice staff can help the PCP manage the care of older adults more efficiently. Because of the progressive nature of many dementias (e.g., Alzheimer's disease), it can be helpful to the PCP for you to schedule follow-up appointments with the patient and family member to help monitor changes in functioning. Setting follow-up appointments (e.g., 6 months–1 year) for individuals with memory complaints who do not screen positive for memory problems can also be helpful to monitor for any significant changes. In addition, knowing local resources for older adults can help patients and their families get more immediate support for difficulties that they may be encountering.

INCONTINENCE

Among community dwelling older adults in the United States, 38% of women and 17% of men reported being incontinent (Anger, Saigal, & Litwin, 2006; Anger, Saigal, Stothers, et al., 2006). Although urinary incontinence gradually increases until midlife, the prevalence rises more rapidly after age 70 (Hannestad, Rortveit, Sandvik, & Hunaskaar, 2000). Incontinence can have a profound impact on an individual, as it can affect employment, leisure activities, avoidance of sexual activities, and is a primary reason older adults move into a residential or nursing care facility (National Institute for Health and Clinical Excellence [NICE], 2006).

If incontinence results from physical exertion (e.g., sneezing, climbing stairs, running), it is called *stress incontinence,* whereas if the incontinence occurs when the individual needs to void, it is called *urge incontinence.* The combination of stress and urge incontinence is termed *mixed incontinence.* Two other forms of incontinence are *overflow* and *functional incontinence.* Frequent urination, increased urgency, or constant dripping of urine is a symptom of overflow incontinence, which occurs because the bladder is overdistended. Functional incontinence refers to individuals who can normally control their urine; however, because of some impairment (e.g. mobility limitations, dementia) the patient is not able to get to the bathroom in time to urinate.

Behavioral interventions for urinary incontinence have often been used in primary care clinics as well as in other medical settings (e.g., urology, obstetrics and gynecology clinics). A systematic review of the literature revealed that pelvic floor muscle training (PFMT), also known as Kegel exercises, significantly reduces incontinence for women (Hay-Smith & Dumoulin, 2006; NICE, 2006), and there is some evidence that PFMT is effective for men as well (Macdonald, Fink, Huckabay, Monga, & Wilt, 2007). PFMT using at least eight contractions three times per day is recommended as a first-line treatment for a period of at least 3 months for women with stress or mixed urinary incontinence (NICE, 2006). In addition, adjunctive biofeedback, which is more common in a specialty mental health clinic, has been shown to be a useful treatment for urinary incontinence (Glazer & Laine, 2006).

Assess

A BHC will not make the diagnosis of incontinence, but he or she may spend time assessing its effect on functioning. As with any functional assessment, it is important to gain an understanding of the frequency, duration, intensity, what is associated with it or triggers it, and the consequences of the symptoms. The following are some helpful questions:

- How long has incontinence been a problem? How much urine do you lose?
- How many times a day do you lose urine? Do you lose urine when you're physically active?
- What situations seem to make the incontinence worse? Better?
- When do you have an urge to urinate? Do you avoid situations or activities because you are concerned that you may lose control? If so, what situations or activities?

Increased caffeine use (e.g., greater than 100 mg per day), being obese, and excessive fluid intake may also increase the risk of urinary incontinence (NICE, 2006), so these factors should also be assessed as potential contributing factors. In addition, if the PCP has not medically evaluated the incontinence, it is important to work with that individual to rule out medical conditions or medications that may be contributing to the incontinence (Weiss, 1998).

Advise

We discuss behavioral methods of managing incontinence, which may supplement or substitute for pharmacological interventions, such as oxybutynin, that may be used to treat incontinence, as follows:

> One method for improving your ability to control your urine flow is to strengthen the muscles that you use to control your urine. Strengthening these muscles is just like strengthening other

muscles in your body; by repeatedly contracting these muscles they will increase in strength over time, and your ability to control your urine will likely improve.

We inform patients that these exercises are considered the first-line of intervention for incontinence and can be an effective intervention that will allow them to engage in activities that they may be avoiding.

Agree

The behavioral interventions for incontinence require regular practice to be effective. Before we teach the behavioral interventions, we determine patients' motivation to change, as we discussed in chapter 3, by assessing the importance of the change, their confidence in change, and their willingness to practice these skills. We emphasize that the muscle training may not have an immediate effect on their ability to control their urine, but with time and practice those skills will gradually improve. Once we have some acceptance from the patient, we move to the assist phase.

Assist

When we teach PFMT, we spend time educating patients about urinary incontinence and how PFMT can help improve control of their incontinence as follows:

> Sometimes we develop incontinence because the muscles that we use to control our urine get weaker as we age. Just like other muscles in our body, if we exercise those muscles we can make the muscles stronger. If the muscles are stronger, we can control our urine flow more easily. Therefore, we're going to discuss an exercise routine to help you strengthen those muscles. As you are sitting here, see whether you can squeeze the muscles that you use to control your urine flow. The squeezing should not cause you any pain and you shouldn't need to move your body, just gently squeeze those muscles. Are you able to do that? To practice, squeeze the muscles that you use to stop the flow of urine and hold that squeeze for 10 seconds, then let the muscles relax for 10 seconds. Repeat the squeezing and relaxing eight times at least three times a day.

If patients have difficulty identifying which muscles to contract, encourage them to practice stopping their urine in mid-flow or for women to place a finger into the vagina and practice squeezing their finger. Individuals should practice this technique for at least 3 months before determining whether the technique is effective (NICE, 2006).

In addition to PFMT, bladder training should also be considered as a first-line treatment for women with urge or mixed urinary incontinence (NICE, 2006). Bladder training requires the patient to wait for increasingly longer periods between voiding. The amount of time is shaped by starting out with the current amount of time between voiding and increasing the amount of time by a length that is accepted by the patient.

If the patient is drinking caffeine or appears to be consuming an excessive amount of liquids, we will discuss ways to reduce consumption, such as gradually tapering by one daily glass or cup per week. If the person is obese, we may offer to use the interventions we discuss in chapter 6 for targeting weight.

Arrange

We like to have patients return in 2 to 3 weeks to assess whether they are continuing to practice the skills; they come back again after 3 months of practice to determine the effectiveness of the intervention. Should the PFMT and bladder training not work, it is recommended that oxybutynin, an antimuscarinic medication, be added as a treatment (NICE, 2006); however, this medication is not recommended for patients with dementia. If available, biofeedback may be useful to add as an adjunctive treatment. Complementary interventions, such as acupuncture, hypnosis, and herbal medications, have not been found to have significant therapeutic benefits (NICE, 2006). If the more conservative treatments for urinary incontinence fail, then it is common for physicians to consider surgical interventions.

CAREGIVER STRESS

When working with older adults in primary care, it is important to assess whether that person is a caregiver or whether anyone else (e.g., significant others, family members, friends) is helping to care for the patient. Caring for another adult can be a chronic stressor for a caregiver, which may contribute to increased risk of physical health problems in the caregiver him- or herself (Vitaliano, Zhang, & Scalan, 2003). If a caregiver's physical or behavioral health is significantly impaired, the person who is being cared for may be at risk as well. In specialty mental health settings, psychoeducational interventions, psychotherapy, and multicomponent therapy (e.g., individual and family therapy) were found to be useful for reducing caregiver distress (Gallagher-Thompson & Coon, 2007). Measures are available to help screen for caregiver stress, such as the Modified Caregiver Strain Index (Thorton & Travis, 2003). Parks and Novelli (2000) provided several practical recommendations to assist caregivers, including educating the caregiver about the family member's disease and the signs of progression, encouraging respite care, discussing methods for managing behavioral problems, and developing ways to manage stress, which could involve using the techniques we discussed in chapter 3. Evidence shows that providing stress management techniques, in addition to education about managing the patient in need, result in better caregiver functioning compared with that of those who receive only education (Burns, Nichols, Martindale-Adams, Graney, & Lummus, 2003). It can also be important for the BHC to give the caregiver "permission" to take care of him- or herself and/or to get outside assistance for a few hours per week. For example, you might say the following:

> It sounds like almost all of your time is devoted to taking care of your spouse. I wonder what toll that takes on you. It can be helpful to take some time for yourself to do something you might enjoy or just to take a break. By taking those little breaks, caregivers can find more energy to take care of their loved ones. Is that something you could consider doing?

It is common for caregivers to believe that they would be doing something wrong by taking time for themselves. Telling them that it is important to take care of themselves as well can help them to be more willing to engage other activities. The National Family Caregivers Association (http://www.thefamilycaregiver.org) provides many excellent resources for caregivers.

DEPRESSION AND ANXIETY

As many as 37% of older adults seen in primary care settings demonstrate significant depressive symptoms (U.S. Department of Health and Human Services, 1999). Integrating behavioral health providers into the primary care setting to enhance the assessment and treatment of older adults demonstrating depressive symptoms has been "strongly recommended" (Steinman et al., 2007). The Geriatric Depression Scale (GDS; Yesavage et al., 1983) was developed specifically for use with older adults. The original scale may be too lengthy for regular use in primary care settings; however, the GDS-5 and the GDS-15 (see Figure 14.1) are valid, shorter versions that take less than 5 minutes to administer (Karlin & Fuller, 2007). Other measures of depressive symptoms such as the Patient Health Questionnaire-9 (Kroenke, Spitzer, & Williams, 2001) and the Beck Depression Inventory-II (Beck, Steer, & Brown, 1996) may not be appropriate for patients with limited physical functioning. When assessing depressive symptoms, it is particularly important to ask about suicidal thoughts. As many as 75% of older adults who completed suicide had been seen in a primary care clinic within a month before their suicide (Conweil, 2001; Karlin & Fuller, 2007). Cognitive and behaviorally based treatments, such as the ones that we discussed in chapter 5, have been shown to be effective with older adults in the primary care setting (Skultety & Zeiss, 2006; Steinman et al., 2007).

Assessment and treatment of anxiety in older adults has not been widely studied, and most studies are not conducted in primary care settings (Wetherell, Sorrell, Thorp, & Patterson, 2005). Although community estimates indicate that at least 3.5% to 10.2% of older adults experience significant anxiety symptoms, only 1.3% are diagnosed with an anxiety disorder in primary care, suggesting that anx-

---

GDS 5 / 15 Geriatric Scale

Section I

1. Are you basically satisfied with your life?	YES	**NO**
2. Do you often get bored?	**YES**	NO
3. Do you often feel helpless?	**YES**	NO
4. Do you prefer to stay home rather than going out and doing new things?	**YES**	NO
5. Do you feel pretty worthless the way you are now?	**YES**	NO

Calculate score in the box below. Answers in **bold** are worth 1.

Score from first five questions = [   ]

If a score of 2 or more above, please continue with remaining 10 questions; otherwise depression may not be a problem.

Section II

6. Have you dropped many of your activities and interests?	**YES**	NO
7. Do you feel that your life is empty?	**YES**	NO
8. Are you in good spirits most of the time?	YES	**NO**
9. Are you afraid that something bad is going to happen to you?	**YES**	NO
10. Do you feel happy most of the time?	YES	**NO**
11. Do you feel you have more problems with memory than most?	**YES**	NO
12. Do you think it is wonderful to be alive now?	YES	**NO**
13. Do you feel full of energy?	YES	**NO**
14. Do you feel your situation is hopeless?	**YES**	NO
15. Do you think that most people are better off than you are?	**YES**	NO

Calculate below the totals from both section one and section two. Answers in **bold** are worth 1.

Score from all 15 questions = [   ]

For clinical purposes, a score greater than 5 points is suggestive of depression and should warrant a follow-up interview. Scores greater than 10 are almost always depression.

FIGURE 14.1. GDS 5/15 Geriatric Scale. From "Development and Validation of a Geriatric Depression Screening Scale: A Preliminary Report," by J. A. Yesavage et al., 1983, *Journal of Psychiatric Research, 17*, p. 41. Copyright 1983 by Elsevier. Adapted with permission. Scoring method from "Comparing Various Short-Form Geriatric Depression Scales Leads to the GDS-5/15," by S. K. Weeks, P. E. McGann, T. K. Michaels, and B. W. Penninx, 2003, *Journal of Nursing Scholarship, 35*, p. 133. Copyright 2003 by Blackwell. Adapted with permission.

iety symptoms may not be appropriately identified in primary care settings (Stanley, Roberts, Bourland, & Novy, 2001). In contrast to the assessment of depression in older adults, there are no measures specifically designed to screen for anxiety disorders in older adults. The Generalized Anxiety Disorder-7 (Spitzer, Kroenke, Williams, & Löwe, 2006) and the Beck Anxiety Index for primary care (Beck & Steer, 1993) have been examined in a broad age range of patients, but it is unclear how useful these measures are for older adults (Karlin & Fuller, 2007).

When screening for anxiety among older adults, it is important to assess the patient's fear of falling. Among older adults who have not fallen, 20% to 30% report a fear of falling, and 48% to 56% of those who have fallen report the same fear. This can be assessed by asking questions such as the following:

Have you fallen or had near misses or unsteadiness when you were afraid that you might fall? Do you worry about falling or losing your balance when you walk inside? What about outside? Do you avoid or limit activities because of your concerns about falling?

To help reduce the risk of falling and the fear of falling, BHCs should encourage the development of an appropriate exercise regime, including Tai Chi. Medical evaluations and interventions regarding orthostatic blood pressure changes, vision impairments, activities of daily living, medications, cognitive functioning, and environmental hazards should also be encouraged. Assessment and interventions across these areas have been shown to reduce the risk of falling (Chang et al., 2004; Zijlstra et al., 2007).

Overall, we have found techniques such as those presented in chapter 5 to be clinically useful for targeting anxiety symptoms among older adults, although there is an obvious need for more empirical studies in this area.

SEXUALITY

The majority of older women and men up to age 85 are engaged in regular sexual activity, particularly if they consider their health to be at least "good" (Lindau et al., 2007). There are discussions in chapters 13 and 15 of many of the sexual problems most commonly reported by older adults, including, for men, erectile dysfunction and premature ejaculation and, for women, orgasmic disorder, lubrication difficulties, and pain (Lindau et al., 2007). Often, older adults do not discuss their sexual functioning problems with their medical providers (Lindau et al., 2007). Therefore, it is important for the BHC to integrate questions about sexual functioning and health into their assessments and be prepared to provide recommendations for targeting these problem areas. Nusbaum and Hamilton (2006) provided some practical advice for assessing sexual history in primary care patients. It is perhaps most important to ask about sexual health in a matter-of-fact and sensitive manner, such as in the following example:

> Sexual functioning is often an important part of an individual's life that isn't discussed in medical appointments. Would it be OK for me to ask a few questions about your functioning in

this area? [If yes, then ask the following.] Do you have any concerns about your sexual functioning, including concerns about a lack of interest in sex or problems during sex, such as pain, difficulty with lubrication, or having an orgasm [women] / maintaining an erection or premature ejaculation [men]?

If the patient answers affirmatively, then, asking the questions presented in chapter 13 may provide important information the BHC can use to design interventions that would be appropriate. As part of the primary care team, BHCs must be comfortable with discussing all aspects of functioning, no matter what the person's age.

SOCIAL ROLE AND SOCIAL SUPPORT CHANGES

Older adults often cope with significant changes in their social roles (e.g., retirement) and social support structure. As we age, our social support networks often get smaller but the relative importance of the individuals within that support network significantly increases (Lang & Carstensen, 1994). Therefore, the loss of individuals within a close network of support may be particularly difficult for the older adult. In primary care, behavioral health professionals can help physicians screen for whether a particular symptom presentation is more consistent with depression or bereavement.

Following a significant loss, approximately 50% of individuals demonstrate a *common grief response,* which is associated with higher levels of grief and depressive symptoms shortly after the loss, which diminish over several months (Ott, Lueger, Kelber, & Prigerson, 2007). Studies suggest that another 34% to 46% of individuals demonstrate *resilient grief,* which is associated with low levels of grief and depression (Bonanno et al., 2002; Ott et al., 2007). A smaller percentage of adults demonstrate *chronic grief,* which is associated with higher levels of grief, depression, and a failure to maintain health behaviors. Some individuals demonstrate symptoms of *complicated grief,* which is defined as separation distress (e.g., crying, preoccupation with thoughts of the deceased individual, yearning, searching) and traumatic distress (e.g., feeling disbelief, being stunned by the loss) lasting at least 6 months (Prigerson et al., 1995).

When seeing someone who is bereaved, the first step is to evaluate whether the patient's grief response is a common grief response, chronic grief response, or depression. One of the most important indicators of healthy functioning is whether the patient is beginning to engage or reengage with activities, friends, and family members after the loss. If patients report staying at home and avoiding activities, we recommend that you establish a behavioral activation plan to help the patient reengage with activities and other people. We use a handout, such as the one in Figure 14.2 to educate patients and describe possible methods of coping with their distress. In addition, you may use the strategies we presented in chapter 3 and 5 to help patients decrease the depressive and anxiety symptoms they may demonstrate. Consider following-up with these patients in two to four weeks so you can reassess their functioning.

PRACTICAL CONSIDERATIONS

Irrespective of disease processes, as people age, physical functioning, including vision, hearing, and mobility, decreases. If you commonly have older adults as patients, there are some practical considerations for working as a BHC, such as the following:

- Write down all recommendations for the patient with the specific plan for how to implement those recommendations.

- Handouts should use font sizes of 14 to 16 points to increase readability and should not be printed on high-gloss paper that may increase glare. Consider having magnifying glasses available for use when you are reviewing handouts with patients.

- Remember that the current cohort of older adults has a lower literacy rate than other cohorts of adults. Determine whether the patient has difficulty reading when interpreting testing or using handouts to guide interventions.

- Consider keeping a pocket amplifier available to assist those older adults who may have difficulty

hearing or who have forgotten to bring their hearing aids.

- Maximize lighting in the room and ensure that there is good light on your face. Look toward patients when talking as older adults may use the movement of lips to supplement their hearing.

- Have room in your office space for a wheelchair, or a plan for how you would accommodate someone who relies on a wheelchair for mobility.

- Have enough seating available for the patient and caregivers.

- Consider slowing your rate of speech and avoiding multiple, complex questions.

- Goals for change and interventions should be concise and specific. Consider asking the patient to repeat back to you the plan for change.

- Consider the impact of medication side effects on functioning. Although this is true for any patient, older adults are more likely to be taking multiple medications. The complex interactions of medications may affect functioning. It may be helpful to evaluate when patients take their medications and what impact those medications have on the patient's functioning.

- Among older adults, physical activity is an important recommendation for a variety of health reasons, including disease management, memory improvement, and emotional regulation. However, the types of physical activities that are recommended should be considered in close coordination with the medical provider. Particular consideration should be given to avoiding falls and managing fear of falling.

SUMMARY

Older adults are a diverse population who are often living active lifestyles. As the baby boom generation continues to age, more individuals will become part of this group and thus the group may significantly change. If you work with older adults, it is important that you become familiar with some of the common problems that older adults experience. The information in this chapter can be used as a foundation on which to build your assessment and intervention skills.

Bereavement, Grief, and Mourning

Bereavement is the state of having lost a significant other to death. *Grief* is the personal response to the loss. *Mourning* is the public expression of that loss.

What Is "Normal" Grief?

Grief reactions vary depending on who we are, who we lost, our relationship with that person, the circumstances around their passing, and how much their loss affects our day-to-day functioning. Different people may express grief differently; you may even have different grief responses between one loss and another. Reactions to grief and loss include not just emotional symptoms but also behavioral and physical symptoms. These reactions often change over time. All are normal for a short period. The following are some of the symptoms you may experience:

- **Emotional.** Shock, denial, numbness, sadness, anxiety, guilt, fear, anger, irritability.
- **Behavioral.** Crying unexpectedly, sleep changes, not eating, withdrawing from others, restlessness, trouble making decisions.
- **Physical.** Concentration problems, exhaustion or fatigue, decreased energy, memory problems, upset stomach, pain, and headaches. Symptoms that are not normal and may signal the need to talk to a professional include, use of drugs or alcohol, violence, and thoughts of killing oneself.

Duration

The duration of grief varies from person to person. Research shows that the average recovery time is 18 to 24 months. Grief reactions can be stronger around significant dates, like the anniversary of the person's death, birthdays, and holidays.

Giving Yourself Time to Grieve

It is normal and important to express your grief and to work through the concerns that arise for you at this time. Avoiding your feelings may not be helpful and may delay or prolong your grief. The following are some suggestions that may help you:

- **Find supportive people to reach out to during your grief.** This is the time when the support of others may be the most helpful. Don't be afraid to tell them how they can best help, even if it means just listening. It is often very helpful to talk about your loss with people who will allow you to express your emotions.
- **Take care of your health.** Often after a loss, we stop doing the things we need to for health care, such as exercising, eating correctly, or taking prescribed medications. If you are on a health care regimen, it is important to continue to follow that plan.
- **Postpone major life changes.** Give yourself time to adjust to your loss before making plans to change jobs, move or sell your home, remarry, and so forth. Grief can sometimes cloud your judgment and ability to make decisions.
- **Consider keeping a journal.** It is often helpful, as a way to work through your feelings, to write or tell the story of your loss and what it means to you.
- **Participate in activities.** Staying active through exercise, enjoyable activities, outings with supportive others, or starting new hobbies can help you get through tough times while providing opportunities for constructive development and use of energy.
- **Find a way to memorialize your loved one.** Planting a tree or garden in the name of your loved one, dedicating a work to their memory, contributing to a charity in their name, and other such activities can be helpful.
- **Consider joining a grief-support group or contacting a grief counselor for additional support and help.** Remember that depressive symptoms (e.g., feeling sad) are a fundamental part of normal bereavement. Staying active and finding support from others can help you to work through the grief process.

FIGURE 14.2. Bereavement, grief, and mourning handout.

CHAPTER 15

WOMEN'S HEALTH

Women have unique health care needs and concerns. In addition to being knowledgeable about common physiological problems among women, such as gynecological and premenstrual disorders, individuals providing health care to women must be prepared to address issues such as infertility, family planning and pregnancy, termination of pregnancy or pregnancy loss, partner relationship discord, and domestic violence. Although these latter issues do not exclusively affect women, they are prevalent among women and health care providers must understand the unique ways in which they affect women and be skilled in addressing their effects and implications. Women's health clinics have become an increasing popular model for addressing the specific needs of women, including delivering gynecological care as well as general primary care.

Behavioral health providers working in women's health clinics can use the integrated, consultative model we have advocated throughout this book and can apply the clinical guidance as one would in a general primary care practice. This chapter, however, provides special guidance for behavioral health consultants (BHCs) working in women's health clinics on three clinical areas that are specifically relevant in that environment: antepartum and postpartum depression, chronic pelvic pain, and menopause.

ANTEPARTUM AND POSTPARTUM DEPRESSION

Medical care for antepartum (i.e., pregnant) and postpartum women can be provided in a specialty obstetrics and gynecology (OB/GYN) clinic, a women's health clinic, or a family medicine clinic. When this service is offered in a specialty clinic (i.e., OB/GYN), that clinic, typically becomes the woman's primary care clinic during pregnancy and postpartum care. At some point following the completion of the pregnancy, care is transitioned back to a general medical practice. This transition can create problems for continuity of care as well as for screening and intervention for postpregnancy complications such as post-partum depression. When working in an OB/GYN clinic, it is important to consider these factors and develop a plan that optimizes the transition of care back to the primary care provider (PCP). Likewise, if you are working in a primary care or women's health clinic, you should carefully consider when and how postpartum depression (PPD) screening should take place and the most effective modes of intervention within your primary care setting.

Screening for PPD is essential because of the high prevalence of this condition. A meta-analytic review estimated PPD to have a prevalence rate of 13% (O'Hara & Swain, 1996). A more recent prospective cohort study of 14,000 women identified 13.5% of the women during pregnancy and 9.1% of the postpartum women scoring 13 points or greater on the Edinburgh Postnatal Depression Scale (EPDS), which indicates a probable depressive disorder (Evans, Heron, Francomb, Oke, & Golding, 2001). A diagnosis of postpartum depression is a diagnostic specifier for a major depressive disorder occurring within 4 weeks after delivery, as detailed in the *Diagnostic and Statistical Manual of Mental Disorders, Fourth Edition, Text Revision* (American Psychiatric Association, 2000, pp. 422–423). Risk factors and etiology are not different from nonpostpartum periods (Riecher-Rössler & Hofecker Fallapour, 2003). The types of treatments for and the outcomes of PPD are similar to those of other depressive disorders (Elkin et al., 1989). Thus, the treatment of depression in women who are pregnant or in the postpartum period is likely to be similar to the treatment of depression in women at other times during their life (Bledsoe & Grote, 2006), except that medication concerns may be greater because of pregnancy and breastfeeding. Nonetheless, PPD is a public health priority (U.S. Department of Health and Human Services [USDHHS], 2000) as it not only has an impact on the woman and her functioning but also can negatively affect her infant and spouse (Clark, Tluczek, & Wenzel, 2003).

Primary Care Adaptation

Consistent screening is an important part of identifying women who might benefit from BHC services. The following highlights important screening and assessment strategies in primary care.

Assess. The U.S. Preventive Services Task Force ([USPSTF], 2002a) recommends screening for depression in primary care settings when a system is in place to confirm an accurate diagnosis and provide effective treatment and follow-up. There is good evidence that screening increases the accurate identification of individuals with depressed mood in primary care; treatment of those identified decreases clinical morbidity (USPSTF, 2002b). Despite this and despite the recommendation for improved recognition of PPD (Logsdon, Wisner, Billings, & Shanahan, 2006), medical providers often fail to screen for and/or recognize depression during or after pregnancy (Beck & Gable, 2000), with up to 50% of the incidences of PPD going undetected (USDHHS, 2000). BHCs in primary care or women's health clinics have a significant opportunity to educate and support an active screening program. In our experience, PCPs are much more likely to implement a standard screening practice if they know they have support to effectively further assess and treat patients who screen positive for the problem.

Edinburgh postnatal depression scale. There are a number of screening instruments that can be used during pregnancy and postpartum (see Boyd, Le,

& Somberg, 2005 and Gaynes et al., 2005, for reviews). The best measure to use will depend on the setting and resources available; however, we recommend using the EPDS as a primary screening tool (Figure 15.1; Cox, Holden, & Sagovsky, 1987). This instrument measures cognitive and emotional symptoms of depression and excludes somatic symptoms, except for sleep problems, that are more likely to occur during these times, which would increase the number of false positives (Boyd et al., 2005). It is the most widely researched and used screening measure for pregnant and postpartum women, demonstrating moderate to good reliability with women from different countries and languages (Boyd et al., 2005; Gaynes et al., 2005). One study (Murray & Cox, 1990) has examined screening accuracy during pregnancy, showing a sensitivity of 100% and a specificity of 87%. As a postpartum measure, it has shown 68% to 86% sensitivity and 78% to 96% specificity (Cox et al., 1987; Murray & Carothers, 1990). The positive predictive value for depression at a score of 13 or more ranges from 70% to 90% (Buist et al., 2002). It can be easily administered by a variety of primary care personnel and typically takes less than 5 minutes to complete. In one large study (Buist et al., 2006), 90% of the women found it easy to complete.

Times for screening. The current literature is unclear as to what are the best antepartum and postpartum times to screen for depressive symptoms. Optimum screening would take place every visit during pregnancy and every visit for a year postpartum. However, money, time demands, and personnel make this difficult in many clinics. The Australian Postnatal Depression Project (Buist et al., 2002) is examining optimal screening times during pregnancy for 97,000 women at 12, 28, and 36 weeks of pregnancy, and Gaynes et al. (2005) suggested future studies should examine the utility of screening at 6 weeks, 3, 6, and 12 months postpartum. We have successfully implemented screening for all newly pregnant women and all transfer obstetrical patients, during all visits between 28 to 32 weeks of pregnancy and again at 6 weeks postpartum.

Once a positive screen exists, conducting a further assessment and differential diagnosis is likely a

---

Edinburgh Postnatal Depression Scale (EPDS)

Date/Time:_____ Baby's Date of Birth:_____

As you have recently had a baby, we would like to know how you are feeling. (As you will soon have a baby, we would like to know how you are feeling.) Please UNDERLINE the answer which comes closest to how you have felt IN THE PAST 7 DAYS, not just how you feel today.
Here is an example, already completed.
I have felt happy: Yes, all the time; <u>Yes, most of the time</u>; No, not very often; No, not at all
   This would mean: "I have felt happy most of the time" during the past week.
Please complete the other questions in the same way. **In the past 7 days,**

1. I have been able to laugh and see the funny side of things
   - 0 As much as I always could
   - 1 Not quite so much now
   - 2 Definitely not so much now
   - 3 Not at all

2. I have looked forward with enjoyment to things
   - 0 As much as I ever did
   - 1 Rather less than I used to
   - 2 Definitely less than I used to
   - 3 Hardly at all

3. I have blamed myself unnecessarily when things went wrong
   - 3 Yes, most of the time
   - 2 Yes, some of the time
   - 1 Not very often
   - 0 No, never

4. I have been anxious or worried for no good reason
   - 0 No, not at all
   - 1 Hardly ever
   - 2 Yes, sometimes
   - 3 Yes, very often

5. I have felt scared or panicky for no very good reason
   - 3 Yes, quite a lot
   - 2 Yes, sometimes
   - 1 No, not much
   - 0 No, not at all

6. Things have been getting on top of me
   - 3 Yes, most of the time I haven't been able to cope at all
   - 2 Yes, sometimes I haven't been coping as well as usual
   - 1 No, most of the time I have coped quite well
   - 0 No, have been coping as well as ever

7. I have been so unhappy that I have had difficulty sleeping
   - 3 Yes, most of the time
   - 2 Yes, sometimes
   - 1 Not very often
   - 0 No, not at all

8. I have felt sad or miserable
   - 3 Yes, most of the time
   - 2 Yes, quite often
   - 1 Not very often
   - 0 No, not at all

9. I have been so unhappy that I have been crying
   - 3 Yes, most of the time
   - 2 Yes, quite often
   - 1 Only occasionally
   - 0 No, never

10. The thought of harming myself has occurred to me
   - 3 Yes, quite often
   - 2 Sometimes
   - 1 Hardly ever
   - 0 Never

FIGURE 15.1. Edinburgh Postnatal Depression Scale (EPDS). From "Detection of Postnatal Depression: Development of the 10-item Edinburgh Postnatal Depression Scale," by J. L. Cox, J. M. Holden, and R. Sagovsky, 1987, *British Journal of Psychiatry, 150,* p. 786. Copyright 1987 by the Royal College of Psychiatrists. Reprinted with permission.

role the BHC will fulfill. See chapter 5 for suggestions on depression assessment.

Advise. Results from research on effective treatments for pregnant and postpartum women are consistent with those for others who are depressed. Treatments include medication, cognitive and behavioral therapies, and group treatment, education, and support (Bledsoe & Grote, 2006; Shaw, Levitt, Wong, & Kaczorowski, 2006). See chapter 5 of this volume for suggestions for treatment of depression within a primary care setting. Roughly two-thirds of depressed individuals in primary care prefer a nonpharmacological treatment for their symptoms (van Schaik et al., 2004); it is likely that a higher percentage of pregnant and breastfeeding women will not consider medication treatment as a first option because of concerns about how it might affect the fetus or child. Medications can be effective, however, and should be included as an option, weighing the pros and cons of risk to mother and fetus or child. Although empirical data are limited, there is general support and extensive use of selective serotonin reuptake inhibitors (SSRIs) as a first-line medication treatment for PPD (Abreu & Stuart, 2005). Data show Zoloft (i.e., sertraline) and Paxil (i.e., paroxetine) as the least detectable in breast milk (Weissman et al., 2005). Abreu and Stuart (2005) present a detailed literature review of SSRI treatment of PPD. We suggest you inform yourself on the latest research on antidepressant medications, to assist mothers and/or medical staff in making informed decisions based on the most up-to-date data from well-controlled studies.

Another option to consider for this population is class or group treatments within the primary care setting. This might include new parent education support classes or psychoeducational depression treatment classes. We suggest group treatments that specifically target pregnant or postpartum women, allowing the patients to get valuable information from each other on how they are managing common challenges, which goes beyond what they might get through individual treatment, for example a baby stroller walking group. In these walking groups, mothers walk together with their infants in a stroller. Preliminary evidence suggests that a stroller walking group can be an effective adjunctive treatment for depression (see Daley, Macarthur, & Winter, 2007, for a review). Walking for as little as 40 minutes two times a week with a group of mothers and their infants in strollers and one time a week alone at a moderate intensity (i.e., 60%–75% of maximum heart rate) has been shown to significantly lower EPDS scale scores in 12 weeks when compared with a social support control group.

Agree. In our experience, most women are willing to agree to try the changes you suggest because they are motivated to improve their functioning so they can take better care of their child. If the patient agrees to make multiple changes, it may be beneficial to start on one change to avoid having her feel overwhelmed and to create the best chances for successful change. Initiating the easiest change (e.g., increasing frequency of exercise by walking with the baby in the stroller three times a week for 10 minutes) might be the best place to start.

Assist. There are several standard depression interventions you might start:

- behavioral activation (i.e., increasing exercise or other fun, valuable, enjoyable activities);
- cognitive disputation (i.e., developing more accurate ways to view the situation); and
- problem-solving.

See chapter 5 for more specific guidance on behavioral activation and cognitive disputation. Additional information on goal setting, cognitive disputation, and problem-solving can be found in chapter 3.

Group intervention may also be useful. Structured psychoeducational depression classes for women with PPD may offer multiple benefits. Classes allow intervention to occur for a large number of patients (e.g., 10) in a relatively short period. Patients can make the same changes as in an individual consultation appointment and might learn additional effective coping strategies from other class participants. Interacting in a group setting may also increase motivation to continue with a treatment strategy that has yet to produce results, because other patients may be having similar difficulties and are continuing the treatment.

Stroller walking groups could be scheduled after a psychoeducational class or a person from the clinic could meet with the group and lead the patients through muscle stretches before and after walking. Where and how this group meets will depend on the weather, location, and resources available at each clinic.

Arrange. At a minimum, we recommend at least one follow-up consultation after the initial appointment to help determine whether the patient was able to follow the plan. If she did not follow through, problem solve barriers, reinitiate or change the plan and suggest an additional follow-up visit with you. If symptoms are improving, then a follow-up might be arranged with you or the PCP in 2 weeks to reassess symptoms and functioning. Follow-up appointments can vary between individuals because of their life circumstances and the severity of their depressive symptoms. In our experience, it is usual for patients to return after the initial consultation appointment and report that they have successfully implemented the plan and are functioning more effectively; depressed mood has usually decreased and other symptoms, such as energy level, are improving. Some individuals may return for two or three appointments and report that they have not changed their thinking or behaviors and that their symptoms remain unchanged. Consider recommending these patients for specialty mental health treatment, if obvious barriers cannot be overcome.

CHRONIC PELVIC PAIN

Chronic pelvic pain (CPP) is defined by the American College of Obstetricians and Gynecologists (ACOG) as noncyclical pain of at least 6 months duration that appears in the pelvis, anterior abdominal wall, lower back, or buttocks, and is serious enough to cause disability or lead to medical care (ACOG, 2004). An estimated 9.2 million women in the United States suffer with CPP at an annual outpatient medical cost of $881.5 million dollars (Mathias, Kuppermann, Liberman, Lipschutz, & Steege, 1996). CPP symptoms and pathology can include endometriosis, pelvic floor muscle tension,

dyspareunia, dysmenorrheal, ovulation pain, chronic pelvic inflammatory disease, pelvic congestion syndrome, fibroids, interstitial cystitis, myofascial pain with trigger points, and pelvic pain of unknown etiology or pathology. Often, women initially present to their PCP (e.g., gynecologist, family medicine physician), with 39% of the women in gynecological and family medicine settings reporting symptoms consistent with CPP (Jamieson & Steege, 1996).

Childhood sexual abuse is reported by 20% to 30% of women with CPP, with the percentage as high as 64% among those whose pain is of an unknown etiology (McDonald & Elliott, 2001). Women with CPP are also more likely to report a history of childhood physical abuse which is directly associated with somatization, anxiety, and depression in women with CPP (Walling et al., 1994). Women with CPP who report an abuse history compared to women with CPP who do not report an abuse history acknowledge having (a) more psychological distress, (b) less life control, (c) greater perceived punishing responses from individuals in their environment, and (d) greater focus on body and physical sensations (Toomey, Hernandez, Gittelman, & Hulka, 1994). Stressful life events in concert with psychological factors may lead pain receptors to be more sensitive. This, in conjunction with increased stress hormones (e.g., cortisol), neuroendocrine changes, and dysregulation of the hypothalamic–pituitary–adrenal axis, may play a role in the development and persistence of CPP (McDonald & Elliot, 2001; Wesselmann, 2001).

CPP is one of the most difficult challenges in medicine from a diagnostic and management perspective because it may involve complicated interactions between vascular, visceral, neuropathic, and muscular systems (McDonald & Elliot, 2001; Wesselmann, 2001). The relationship between pain and tissue damage or pathology in the female pelvic region is not well understood; in fact, one-third to over one-half of all individuals with CPP have no identifiable reason for their pain (Mathias et al., 1996; Rapkin, 1990; Wesselmann, 2001). Women often endure many exams and procedures and see multiple specialists with no definitive diagnosis or treatment. This can leave both the provider and patient frustrated with unrelieved suffering during this time. Furthermore, when a referral is made to a behavioral health pain specialist, it is frequently made as a last resort and the individual may feel abandoned by the medical system or believe that others think the pain is purely psychological. It has been suggested that once a diagnosis of CPP is made, surgical procedures that offer no pain relief or an exacerbation of the condition should be minimized. Instead, treatment should be multidisciplinary, and focused on symptomatic pain management, (McDonald & Elliott, 2001; Wesselmann, 2001). Working in primary care gives behavioral health providers a ripe opportunity to create processes for care within the clinic whereby every woman who has a CPP diagnosis, regardless of whether there is evidence of pathology, receives a focused biopsychosocial assessment and treatment as part of comprehensive pain management.

Specialty Mental Health

Mental health treatments are generally not designed exclusively for CPP. The studies examining mental health treatments for CPP have been done outside of the primary care setting and include management strategies effective for other chronic pain conditions. A variety of interventions may lead to decreased frequency and/or intensity of pain and improved functioning. Strategies with some empirical support include stress management self-control activities such as relaxation and hypnosis, cognitive–behavioral therapy for depression and anxiety control, psychodynamic therapy, sex therapy and education, pacing, progressive relaxation training, imagery, deep breathing, self-disclosure through writing, and cognitive therapy for beliefs, thoughts, feelings, and stress (Albert, 1999; McDonald & Elliott, 2001; Norman, Lumley, Dooley, & Diamond, 2004; Wesselmann, 2001).

Primary Care Adaptation

Assessing and treating women with CPP will require asking questions about areas that can be uncomfortable or elicit strong emotional responses. The 5A's approach is likely to help the BHC assess and interview efficiently and effectively while helping to minimize patient discomfort.

Assess.   Assessing CPP is similar to the assessment of other chronic pain conditions. Main areas of assessment might include (a) variability in pain and factors associated with increased or decreased pain, (b) effect of pain on daily activities, (c) adaptive coping responses to pain, and (d) social and environmental influences on pain perception. Guidance on specific questions for a pain assessment is found in chapter 11. In addition to these foundational assessment areas, there are several additional important areas to assess.

Sexual and physical abuse. Because psychological trauma stemming from childhood and/or adult sexual or physical abuse is often associated with CPP, it is important to use screening questions to assess this history and its current effect. The provider should carefully balance eliciting detail with minimizing distress during this focused assessment to avoid retraumatizing the patient. Furthermore, we suggest that questions about sexual and physical abuse be asked toward the end of the functional assessment to avoid having the patient believe that the BHC thinks her pain is psychological in nature. Focused questions for sexual and physical abuse in primary care might include the following:

- Have you experienced any physical or sexual abuse or traumas as a child or adult? [If yes, then ask the following:]
- Was it physical, sexual, or both? Was it as a child, adult, or both?
- Have those incidents been affecting you in any way over the last 6 months? [If yes, then ask the following:]
- How have those incidents affected you?

The symptoms and impairments a patient may be experiencing as a result of abuse might include anxiety, depression, posttraumatic stress disorder (PTSD), partner intimacy problems, and/or intense anxiety or fear during gynecological exams. All of these conditions have the propensity to make CPP worse and significantly interfere with effective CPP management. If physical or sexual abuse is endorsed, you may want to consider a brief screen using the Primary Care PTSD Screen (PC-PTSD; Prins et al., 2004) found in chapter 5 of this volume.

Sexual dysfunction. As might be expected, given the anatomical location of pain in individuals with CPP, patients often have sexual dysfunction, including female orgasmic disorder, dyspareunia, postcoital pain, dissatisfaction with sexual frequency, and decrease in sexual desire. In addition to lubrication problems, increased pain during thrusting and in different sexual positions can be common and seems to be more prevalent among patients with CPP than in comparison with gynecologic control samples (see McDonald & Elliott, 2001, for a review). In addition to pain exacerbation, sexual dysfunction may inhibit intimate relationships in a manner that starts or increases a stress response, anxious and/or depressed mood, anger, and resentment, and as such, can interfere with effective pain management. The assessment and management of sexual dysfunction is important with any pain condition, however, it may be especially relevant for CPP. The following questions will allow you to make a reasonable assessment of sexual dysfunction, the data from which can be used to make recommendations for treatment as indicated (see chap. 13, this volume, for additional questions).

- On a scale of 0 to 10, with 0 being not satisfied at all with your current sexual activities and 10 being the most satisfied you can imagine being with your sexual activities, how satisfied are you with your current sexual activities? [If the answer is below 7, consider asking the following questions.]
- Do you have pain before, during, or after sex or intercourse? [If yes, ask the following questions.]
  - When does the pain occur?
  - Where is the pain located? [Ask about frequency, duration, and intensity.]
  - Is the pain worse with your partner's thrusting?
  - Is the pain worse in different positions?
- Is lubrication a problem?
- Do you have orgasms? [If yes, ask the following questions.]
  - Do you have pain during orgasm?
  - Does your partner know you are in pain? [If yes, ask the following.] How does your partner respond to your pain?
- Do you have distressing or stressful thoughts during sex?

Summary. If a patient is focused exclusively on physiological or disease-based explanations for CPP, she may not be as interested in pursuing nonmedical, nonsurgical pain management strategies. Therefore, it is important to strike a balance in communicating your understanding of her symptoms and functional impairments and summarizing psychosocial and behavioral factors that may be contributing to the CPP. Suggest that ongoing medical evaluations, if still needed, should be pursued and, at the same time, you may be able to get her started on managing her current pain differently, in a way that decreases pain and suffering. Highlight how thoughts, emotions, and physical symptoms are interconnected. The summary might sound like the following:

> For the last 6 months, you have had recurring pelvic pain. You've had multiple tests that have not shown a specific diagnosable condition that your doctor can treat. That doesn't mean your pain is in your head. There are a host of reasons, including tests not being sensitive enough to identify the problem, past injuries, activities, and genetic vulnerabilities that could be interacting to produce your pain. Even if there was a definitive diagnosis, it doesn't necessarily mean there would be a medical or surgical treatment that could eliminate your pain. Being frustrated or stressed seems to increase your pain. On good days, you go full-force, then end up paying the price over the next 2 days with increased pain and decreased activity. You are more irritable than you would like to be, you've decreased sexual activity in response to the pain, and you feel like you are not being the kind of partner you would like to be. The thought of continuing like this leads you to feel more desperate and depressed. You're not sleeping well and you are feeling hopeless regarding your future.

Advise. The results of your assessment will guide what you advise for treatment or self-management.

Common areas for intervention might include negative emotions (e.g., anxiety, depressed mood), negative thinking, improving communication, increasing activities, pacing, and physiological arousal management. A primary goal of pain management is to reduce exacerbation of pain and improve functioning with pain. It is important to explain what the management strategies you are advising are designed to accomplish, so the patient does not get the false hope that her pain is going to be eliminated. See chapter 11 for additional recommendations on the advise process for pain management, including an example of how to describe the gate-control theory of pain (Melzack & Wall, 1965) and how different interventions may help to improve pain management.

If sexual or physical abuse is affecting current functioning to the extent that the patient may be experiencing PTSD, we suggest you recommend and assist the patient in getting specialty mental health treatment outside of the clinic for these problems. A 30-minute appointment is generally inappropriate for addressing issues of sexual or physical abuse because there may be insufficient time to deal with the extreme distress that may be elicited. The advice you give might be as follows:

> One of the things I recommend is that we set you up with an appointment with a provider outside of primary care who can spend more time with you to further assess and treat the difficulties you are experiencing with your past physical and sexual abuse. We can do a lot together in the 30-minute consult appointments to help you manage your pain and I'm going to lay out what some of those things are in a minute. However, 30-minute appointments typically are not long enough to treat difficulties with past physical or sexual abuse. At the same time, effective treatment for past abuse is an important part of maximizing your pain management plan. Ongoing communication between myself, your PCP, and the provider outside this clinic may be important to maximize your

treatment response. With your permission, we would communicate with each other as part of a team effort to assist you in managing your symptoms and improving your functioning.

If sexual dysfunction is a concern, then also advise on how treatment of sexual dysfunction may be helpful. Advice might focus on improving lubrication, decreasing muscle tension or bracing, altering the focus of sexual activity to nonintercourse interactions, changing intercourse positions and movement, and improving communication. Goals of these changes would be to decrease pain and to improve the frequency and enjoyment of sexual activity. See chapter 13 for additional recommendations on the advise process for female orgasmic disorder.

Agree, assist, and arrange. Chapter 11 elaborates on strategies to use in the agree, assist, and arrange phases for chronic pain management, and in chapter 13 we discuss strategies to use in the agree, assist, and arrange phases for female orgasmic disorder. For sexual or physical abuse and/or PTSD, you may want to have a list of mental health professionals within your system or local community that you know and work with on a regular basis who have expertise in evidence-based treatment for these problems. You might offer this list to the patient or help their PCP to initiate a consult.

MENOPAUSE

Natural *menopause* is the term used to mark the permanent cessation of menstruation for 12 months (Nelson et al., 2005). *Perimenopause* is the transition time from regular cycling to complete cessation, which can last 4 to 5 years or longer (Mayo Clinic, 2005). During this time the duration, frequency, and amount of bleeding is less predictable. *Postmenopause* is the time after the 12 months without menstruation. Throughout this chapter, we use the term menopause to refer to perimenopause and postmenopause in addition to the 12-month span when menstruation has first stopped.

As a result of fluctuating hormone levels during menopause, a variety of problematic symptoms can occur, the most common being vasomotor symptoms such as hot flashes or flushes and night sweats, which are reported by an average of 50% of women across studies (Nelson et al., 2005). Vasomotor symptoms are also the most common menopausal sequelae for which women seek medical assistance (Barlow, Grosset, Hart, & Hart, 1989). Vaginal dryness is reported by up to one third of women and sleep disturbances range from 40% to 60% because of vasomotor symptoms (Nelson et al., 2005). Most studies show no relationship between mood and/or behavioral health conditions and stage of menopause when compared with women not in menopause (Nelson et al., 2005). However, a large cohort study of 16,065 women by Bromberger et al. (2001) did show a significantly higher rate of distress among early perimenopausal women.

It is hypothesized that vasomotor symptoms are related to hormonal changes affecting the hypothalamus, which is responsible for temperature regulation in the body. The exact mechanism of action is unclear; however, fluctuating estrogen levels may cause the hypothalamus to perceive the body to be hot and therefore respond by trying to dissipate heat, which produces the hot flash (Breastcancer.org, 2006; Freedman, 2001). Increased frequency of vasomotor symptoms has been associated with increased stress (Gannon, Hansel, & Goodwin, 1987; Swartzman, Edelberg, & Kemmann, 1990), alcohol use, hot beverages or food, caffeine, smoking (Gannon et al., 1987; Mayo Clinic, 2005), and higher environmental temperatures (Freedman, 2001). Hormone replacement therapy (HRT) can effectively reduce vasomotor symptoms and vaginal dryness, but for a variety of health and personal reasons (e.g., personal history of breast cancer or migraine headaches), women may choose not to engage in HRT and thus alternative symptom-management strategies are needed.

Specialty Mental Health

There are a handful of studies examining specific interventions to reduce menopause symptoms. These studies were primarily targeted to reduce hot flashes and included relaxed breathing (Freedman & Woodward, 1992), progressive muscle relaxation (Germaine & Freedman, 1984), relaxation response

training in "mental focusing" using diaphragmatic breathing (Irvin, Domar, Clark, Zuttermeister, & Friedman, 1996), and applied relaxation, including progressive relaxation, release-only relaxation, cue-controlled relaxation, differential relaxation, and rapid relaxation (Wijma, Melin, Nedstrand, & Hammar, 1997). Other studies used multicomponent treatment, including relaxed breathing, medication, and counseling or group support (Ganz et al., 2000). Hunter and Liao (1996) used a cognitive–behavioral therapy intervention that included relaxed breathing, muscle relaxation, education about hot flashes and menopause, and how to cope with hot flashes in social situations using relaxed breathing and self-talk. Finally, Stevenson and Delprato (1983) used relaxation training, systematic desensitization, thought stopping, imagery, marital contingency contracting, and biofeedback. The intervention in each study showed a reduction in frequency and/or intensity of hot flashes. We were unable to find any study that specifically examined symptom management with behavioral health interventions within primary care.

Primary Care Adaptation

Adapting specialty mental health treatments for menopause can be done smoothly using the 5A's approach. Education of symptom monitoring and behavior change are likely to be primary BHC intervention strategies.

Assess. The primary care functional assessment that we presented in chapter 2 is an appropriate generic assessment for women with menopause symptom complaints. Focusing on assessment and treatment of vasomotor symptoms related to stress, sleep problems related to night sweats, and sexual difficulties related to vaginal dryness are appropriate primary areas of focus. Recommendations by Dobmeyer (2004) in conjunction with our own clinical experience regarding questions to ask in these areas are listed in Figure 15.2.

The following is an example of how a summary might sound at the end of the assessment phase:

> You've had symptoms for the last
> 6 months that include hot flashes one
> to three times a day each lasting for

Additional Functional Assessment Questions for Hot Flashes

Women experiencing menopause may have a variety of problem symptoms. Some of the most common are hot flashes, sleep problems, and vaginal dryness. Do you have any of these or other bothersome symptoms?

Hot Flashes
Inquire about stressful environments and other triggers as follows:

"Over the last month, did you find you were stressed, worried, anxious, frustrated or agitated?" [If yes, then ask the following questions.]
"What times and in what situations do you feel this way?"
"What are the physical symptoms you notice?"
"What thoughts do you have in these situations?"
"How do others respond to you?"
"What do you do to manage these symptoms?"
"Is there anything that makes the symptoms better or worse?"
"Were there other times in your life when you felt this way?"
If not specifically identified, assess caffeine & alcohol use, hot drinks, and hot environments as triggers.

Sleep Problems or Night Sweats
Use the standard sleep behavior assessment from chapter 5. Ask the following questions:

- "When do night sweats wake you?"
- "Once awake, what do you do to manage?"
- "What thoughts typically go through your mind when you can't sleep?"
- "Is there anything that makes your night sweats better or worse?"
- "Does room temperature seem to have an impact on the number of night sweats?"

Sexual Difficulties Related to Decreased Lubrication
"Do you have problems with vaginal lubrication (i.e., being too dry during sex)?" [If yes, then inquire specifically about the problem/s and ask the following question.]
"Have you done anything to help improve vaginal lubrication?"

Expectations and Interpretations
"On a 0 to 10 scale, with 0 being the *worst coping ever* and 10 being the *best coping ever,* how would you rate your ability to cope with your symptoms?"
"Sometimes women feel embarrassed about their symptoms. Do you feel that way?"
"Do you worry about not being in control of your symptoms?"
"What do you know about menopause?"

FIGURE 15.2.   Additional functional assessment questions for hot flashes.

about 5 minutes in which you are sweating and have a flushed face. Sometimes these seem to happen for no reason at all; at other times, they seem to happen when you're feeling stressed. You have night sweats that wake you two to three times a night; you have trouble falling back to sleep and lie awake in bed for about 45 minutes worrying about falling back to sleep and how that will affect your ability to perform at work the next day. You don't feel rested in the morn-ing and you have increased your coffee intake from 16 ounces a day to 48 ounces a day so that you can concentrate better at work. You've noticed that you don't have as much lubrication during inter-course, but that isn't a problem as you and your husband use lubricants. Over the last 3 months, your symptoms have gotten worse; it seems to be related to increased job stress given the extra responsibility in your new position. You feel embarrassed at work because people see your face flush and they ask what is going on. You don't like people at work to know your personal health business and you are becoming increasingly worried about when hot flashes will occur in the future. Do I have it right, or is there something I've missed?

Advise. On the basis of the unique symptoms, behavioral, and functional impairments of the patient provide advice on treatment options that might best address problems, explaining what the intervention is and how it might help. Common areas of advice might include the following.

General education about menopause. You might say, "Most people don't know a lot about menopause, so it might be helpful to go over what is typical, what to expect, and other specific information on the topic." The following Web sites contain free educational material that can be downloaded for an interactive discussion, as needed:

- http://www.mayoclinic.com/health/menopause/DS00119,
- http://www.medicinenet.com/menopause/article.htm, and
- http://www.nlm.nih.gov/medlineplus/menopause.html.

Monitoring symptoms. You might say, "You have some idea of what triggers the hot flashes, but at other times they seem come out of the blue. It might be helpful to track your symptoms to see whether we can identify other triggers that you could avoid or modify." (See Figure 15.3 for self-monitoring sheet.)

Hot Flash Symptom Diary

Please use this form to record all hot flashes. The "severity scale" ranges from 0 (*no symptoms*) to 10 (the *most extreme* hot flash symptoms you can imagine). "Situation or triggers" could include stressors, activities, thoughts, alcohol, or other factors you believe may trigger or worsen your hot flashes. "Action taken" refers to what you did when the hot flash occurred (e.g., left the room, removed clothing, took some deep breaths, told yourself calming thoughts).

Date	Time	Severity 0–10	Length	Situation/triggers	Action taken

FIGURE 15.3. Hot flash symptom diary.

Questioning thoughts. You might say the following:

At work and in bed at night, your mind gets you stressed or anxious. We know that the more stressed or anxious you get, the more difficult it is to fall back to sleep, and that increased stress response is associated with increased number and intensity of hot flashes. We can't stop your mind from initially telling you things that are stressful, but we can help you get better at noticing those thoughts, not reacting to them, and generating more helpful reassuring thoughts that can decrease your stress response and help you fall back to sleep more easily and perhaps decrease the number of hot flashes at work. [See Figure 15.4, for reassuring thinking sheet.]

Relaxation. You might say the following:

By helping you to decrease your body's physiological stress response, we can likely help you improve your sleep and decrease your hot flashes. One of the ways we can do that is to teach you how to do relaxed breathing so you can turn the volume down on your stress response. We can also make a plan for physical relaxation to be a habit throughout the day. [See chap. 3 for relaxation training guidance.]

Altering sleep behaviors. See chap. 5 for a discussion on improving sleep.

Altering environment and avoiding triggers. You might say the following:

By avoiding or decreasing things such as caffeine and alcohol that seem to trigger your hot flashes, you can probably decrease the number of hot flashes you have each day. Also, by making your room cooler at night, we can probably decrease or eliminate night sweats.

Agree. After describing the options, ask what the patient would like to do. If there are several areas she would like to target, ask what is the most important and/or easiest for the patient to initiate and start there.

Assist. There are varieties of treatment options appropriate to target symptoms and improve functioning. What you do should be tailored to the individual. Common areas of intervention are as follows:

- Education. Review fact-related information about menopause.
- Have the patient monitor symptoms for further assessment of problem areas and as a way to assess symptom change (see chap. 3, this volume, for additional details on self monitoring).
- Teach strategies for questioning and challenging stressful or anxiety-provoking thoughts (see chap. 3, this volume, for additional details).
- Teach deep breathing and cue-controlled relaxation (see chap. 3, this volume, for additional details).
- If deep breathing and cue-controlled relaxation do not produce maximal effect, use passive or progressive muscle relaxation as an additional relaxation strategy (see chap. 3, this volume, for additional details).
- Establish a sleep behavior change plan (see chap. 5, this volume, for additional details).
- Have the patient alter her substance use (e.g., caffeine, alcohol, tobacco use) associated with symptoms.
- Have the patient lower the temperature in her bedroom to 64 degrees to decrease night sweats. Freedman and Roehrs (2006) showed a significant reduction in the number of night sweats at this temperature.

Arrange. We suggest you start whatever intervention you can on the first appointment. If you are unable to start anything, the patient should return to establish the planned changes and learn new skills, and implement the plan. You might suggest having one or more return appointments to ensure the plan is working, to solve problems, or to add additional skills, as needed.

SUMMARY

Undetected or ineffectively treated depression during and after pregnancy, CPP, and menopausal symptoms, such as hot flashes, can lead to unnecessary suffering. In addition to the patient's personal

Managing Menopausal Hot Flashes With Reassuring Thinking

Stressful, alarming thoughts may increase the severity of menopausal hot flashes. Alarming thoughts about the hot flashes may also lead to more difficulty coping effectively with the symptoms. One tool to help better manage menopausal symptoms is to change or disrupt a pattern of alarming thoughts by replacing them with more reassuring or supportive statements.

Identify Your Negative Self-Talk.
The first step in changing alarming thinking is to identify your negative, alarming self-talk related to menopausal symptoms. Here are some examples of common thoughts women may have about these symptoms. Place a check mark next to any thoughts that seem relevant to you.

☐ Oh no—here it comes.
☐ Everyone is noticing how much I'm sweating right now.
☐ I can't deal with this right now.
☐ People will think I'm strange/anxious/old/etc.
☐ Something is physically wrong with me.
☐ I can't stand this.
☐ This sweating is so embarrassing.

What other alarming or negative self-talk do you notice when you experience hot flashes? Please list them below:

_____

_____

Develop Reassuring Coping Statements.
The second step in changing alarming thinking is to accept what is happening by saying reassuring, calming statements to yourself. This may help to keep your initial symptoms from escalating to higher levels and can give you a greater sense of control over the situation.

Some people find it helpful to write several coping statements on a 3×5 index card. When hot flash symptoms begin, pull this card out, and repeat the coping statements to yourself to help manage the symptoms and your reaction in a healthier manner.

Here are some examples of positive coping statements that people have found helpful when they first feel the symptoms of a hot flash coming on. Put a check in the boxes of coping statements you believe could be most helpful for you.

☐ I don't like feeling this way, but I can accept it.
☐ I can feel like this and still be okay.
☐ I can handle these symptoms or sensations.
☐ These symptoms are natural; I'm perfectly healthy.
☐ I'm going to go on with what I'm doing and wait for my symptoms to decrease.
☐ I'll just let my body do its thing. This will pass.
☐ I can use my coping strategies (e.g., relaxation) and allow this to pass.
☐ Fighting and resisting isn't going to help, so I'll just let it flow.
☐ My symptoms are not very noticeable; they feel stronger than they look to others.
☐ So what.

What additional coping statements do you believe would be helpful for you to combat your own alarming self-talk? Please list them below.

_____

_____

FIGURE 15.4.   Managing menopausal hot flashes with reassuring thinking handout.

functional impairments stemming for these conditions, other important individuals in women's lives can be affected as well. Effective behavioral health treatment for women with these problems is certainly possible and, likely, preferable in the primary care setting using a behavioral health consultation model.

An active screening program for depression during and after pregnancy is vital. If you do not know it is there, you cannot treat it. Behavioral health assessment and intervention early in the course of CPP is consistent with a multidisciplinary model believed to offer the best management approach and has the possibility of reducing suffering and disability, regardless of whether an organic explanation for the pain is identified. We strongly recommend you discuss with your medical team the possibility of developing a standard process of care within the clinic to include giving most women with CPP an initial behavioral health assessment to determine whether effective behavioral health interventions for managing symptoms is indicated. Finally, women going through menopause can vary greatly in the physiological changes they experience. HRT works well for many women in managing these symptoms. For other women who cannot, or choose not to, engage in HRT consider implementing a standard process of care whereby these women get an initial assessment to determine what, if any, management strategies might help.

CHAPTER 16

HEALTH ANXIETY (HYPOCHONDRIASIS)

According to the *Diagnostic and Statistical Manual of Mental Disorders, Fourth Edition, Text Revision* (American Psychiatric Association, 2000), the primary feature of health anxiety, or hypochondriasis, is the preoccupation with the false belief or idea that one has, or is in, significant danger of catching or developing a serious illness (p. 507). This preoccupation produces significant impairment or distress in occupational, social, family, or other important areas of functioning. It persists over time, despite appropriate medical evaluation and reassurance that there is no evidence of disease and that the patient is in good health. Health anxiety has been characterized as a problem consisting of thinking errors regarding the appraisal or meaning of various body sensations (Salkovskis, Warwick, & Deale, 2003) that are amplified and/or maintained by the behavioral responses to those appraisals (see Abramowitz & Braddock, 2006; Salkovskis & Warwick, 2001; Taylor & Asmundson, 2004 for reviews of the cognitive–behavioral model of health anxiety). Prevalence of health anxiety in outpatient medical clinics has been estimated to range from 4% to 6% (Barsky, Wyshak, Klerman, & Latham, 1990) with a clinical presentation that may include various combinations of the following (Taylor & Asmundson, 2004).

Fears of

- Being exposed to a disease pathogen or catching a disease in the future.
- Having a disease now that has been missed by exam or test.

Physical symptoms that are

- Not dangerous or life-threatening (e.g., skin discoloration, sores, swelling).
- Stress or anxiety related (e.g., tight chest, upset stomach, tingling hands).
- Diffuse and vague (e.g., muscle weakness all over, feeling "spaced out").

Behaviors, such as

- Multiple medical appointments for the same medical test previously performed.
- Multiple medical appointments for medical provider reassurance they are not ill.
- Multiple requests for reassurance they are not ill from important people in their lives.
- Medical information gathering (e.g., Internet, books).
- Repeated body checking (e.g., blood pressure, temperature, breast exam).
- Avoiding or escaping situations in which they believe they might catch a disease.
- Scanning the body for symptom change.

Thoughts, such as

- "What if my doctor is wrong and/or the test is wrong and I have a disease?"
- Of disease, death, suffering, or detailed images of disease and death.
- Perseveration and/or conviction they have a disease that has not been identified.

Patients with health anxiety use the health care system in ineffective and inefficient ways, such as to make appointments for symptoms that have already been evaluated, to go to emergency rooms for evaluation of benign or normal body changes, and/or to leave multiple phone messages for their providers on a given day in a panicked manner. These behaviors result in medical appointments that are more frequent and at higher costs (Barsky, Ettner, Horsky, & Bates, 2001). Primary care providers (PCPs) and their patients can become frustrated with this ongoing interaction (Barsky, Wyshak, Latham, & Klerman, 1991; Lin et al., 1991). Patients can feel they are not being taken seriously, and PCPs can feel frustrated and ineffective.

SPECIALTY MENTAL HEALTH

Over the past 2 decades, new behavioral, cognitive–behavioral, and pharmacotherapy interventions have been developed and shown to be successful in the management and/or treatment of health anxiety (see Abramowitz & Braddock, 2006; Taylor & Asmundson, 2004; Taylor, Asmundson, & Coons, 2005, for reviews). Empirically supported treatment packages have included various combinations of time management training; stimulus control for worry reduction; assertive communication training; relaxation training; systematic exposure; cognitive restructuring; thought, emotion, and body sensation monitoring; education about causes of body sensations and the role of attention; and warmth and empathy (see Taylor & Asmundson, 2004, for details). A meta-analysis by Taylor and Asmundson showed all psychosocial and drug treatments have better effect than no treatment. Cognitive–behavioral treatments appear to work best for severe health anxiety, whereas psychoeducation may be adequate for mild health anxiety (Taylor & Asmundson, 2004). Other data suggest that clomipramine (i.e., Anafranil; 25–225 mg/day), imipramine (i.e., 125–150 mg/day), fluoxetine (i.e., Prozac; 20–80 mg/day), fluvoxamine (i.e., Luvox; 300 mg/day), paroxetine (i.e., Paxil; up to 60 mg/day), or nefazodone (i.e., Serzone; 200–500 mg/day) can reduce physical symptoms, worry, fears, behavioral avoidance, and reassurance seeking (Fallon, 2001; Fallon et al., 1996; Taylor & Asmundson, 1994; Wesner & Noys, 1991). Fluoxetine may be the drug of choice, but

further long-term evaluation is still needed (Taylor & Asmundson, 1994).

BEHAVIORAL HEALTH IN PRIMARY CARE

To date, no study has examined the delivery of cognitive and/or behavioral treatment for health anxiety exclusively within a primary care setting. Data on patients unwilling to accept a mental health treatment referral are not available. However, some data (Craig, Boardman, Mills, Daly-Jones, & Drake, 1993) as well as clinical experience (Barsky et al., 2001) suggest that patients with health anxiety are commonly not willing to accept a referral for mental health treatment. Other clinical impressions (Taylor et al., 2005; Tyrer, Seivewright, & Behr, 1999) suggest that patients with health anxiety may be more willing to accept mental health treatment when it is provided in a medical setting. The challenge for behavioral health providers is to adapt these evidence-based treatments so that they are likely to succeed when delivered in a time-limited primary care appointment.

PRIMARY CARE ADAPTATION

Adapting evidence-based care to the primary care setting is crucial if behavioral health consultants (BHCs) are going to assist PCPs with the management of health anxiety. The 5A's model is detailed here to assist the BHC with this challenging endeavor.

Assess

We believe the following factors are important to attend to when conducting an initial assessment.

- An appropriate medical evaluation has been completed.
- There is a genuine interest in the patient's problem, taking symptoms and impairments seriously.
- There has been a differential diagnosis.
- There has been a detailed functional assessment of physical symptoms, triggers, safety behaviors, fears and maladaptive beliefs, occupational and social functioning, and stressors.

Medical evaluation. It is imperative before assessing for health anxiety that an appropriate medical examination and testing has ruled out the likelihood of disease, injury, or substance (e.g., medication) as the cause of the patient's symptoms. Roughly 2% of those individuals seen for health anxiety outside of primary care have a general medical condition that is responsible for their symptoms (Warwick, Clark, Cobb, & Salkovskis, 1996).

Taking the patient's problem seriously. By the time you see patients who meet criteria for health anxiety, they have often received multiple messages that their symptoms are not physical but psychological. Because this is not a satisfactory explanation for these patients, they reject it and continue to look for someone who they believe will take their problems seriously (Salkovskis et al., 2003; Taylor & Asmundson, 2004). To effectively engage the patient from the start and to increase the chances that you can collect the information you need in 30 minutes, we suggest that you are clear with the patient that you believe his or her symptoms are real and that you want to understand the symptoms, functional impairment(s), and concerns. One way to achieve this might be to say something such as the following before starting your functional assessment:

> It is really important that I understand your symptoms, concerns, how you're functioning, and how your quality of life is impaired. I'm going to ask you a variety of questions during the next 15 minutes and I'll want to hear any additional information that I haven't asked about that you think is important for me to know before I summarize my understanding of your current difficulties. If we need to spend more than 15 minutes to get additional information, we can. Before I make any suggestions for treatment, I'm going to summarize my understanding of your current condition and concerns to make sure I've gotten it right; if I haven't gotten it right, I want you to let me know what parts I've missed.

It may also be useful to summarize what you have heard as you are collecting information so the patient knows you are engaged and listening (Salkovskis et al., 2003). Summarize in a manner that conveys understanding without leaving an opening after the summary that he or she may fill by expanding on what he or she has already said. Make the summary statement and use the momentum of the statement to launch into another question. For example, you could say the following:

> If I've understood you correctly so far, you notice pain in the lower right part of your stomach that seems to never go away. Some days it is more painful than usual. Because your brother died of pancreatic cancer, you are certain that this must be pancreatic cancer or some type of gastrointestinal cancer that just hasn't been detected by the tests yet, because they may not be sensitive enough to pick it up.

Transition to another question without a pause after the summary:

> Often, people who have symptoms such as yours have to change how they function in various areas of their life, such as in social relationships, work performance, exercise, and/or valuable and enjoyable activities. In response to your symptoms and concerns, have any areas of your life changed? If so, how?

Differential diagnosis. Patients with health anxiety share a number of overlapping symptoms with those who have somatization disorder and other anxiety disorders such as generalized anxiety disorder, specific phobia, panic disorder, and obsessive–compulsive disorder (Noyes, 2001). Conducting an assessment that identifies health anxiety while ruling out other anxiety disorders and collecting clinically relevant information can be difficult given the limited amount of time allotted for primary care appointments. Stewart and Watt (2001) and Taylor and Asmundson (2004) have published excellent reviews of structured clinical interviews and standardized questionnaires used for differential diagnosis of health anxiety. The use of and/or adaptation of the Health Anxiety Inventory Short Version (HAIS; Salkovskis, Rimes, Warwick, & Clark, 2002) can be valuable for making differentiations during your health anxiety assessment. The HAIS is an 18-item measure specifically designed for use as a screening measure in medical settings. Analyses showed the combined score to have a high specificity in identifying health-anxious patients in comparison with other anxious groups of individuals and with individuals with physical illness. Those scoring 31.1 or higher on this measure have a greater likelihood of being health-anxious. We have included the HAIS in Figure 16.1. If you decide to use the HAIS, consider titling it the "Illness Questionnaire" to avoid eliciting a negative response from the patient.

Functional assessment.   Collecting information in the following areas is important to understand the cognitive and behavioral factors maintaining or exacerbating the patient's problems; you might target these factors for treatment. In addition to the standard functional assessment questions in chapter 2, see Figure 16.2 for a list of additional health anxiety questions.

Triggers.   Ask about specific situations or times when patients notice or become more concerned about their health problems. This information can help you better target cognitive and/or behavioral treatments and identify new thoughts and behavioral responses that can decrease fear, anxiety, and physical symptoms instead of maintaining and increasing them. After identifying specific triggers, ask questions about thoughts, beliefs, fears, and behaviors in response to the trigger.

Physical symptoms.   Assess how the patient responds physiologically to triggers. For each physical response the patient reports, ask about thoughts, beliefs, fears, and behaviors that follow the onset of the physical symptoms.

Safety behaviors and safety signals.   Safety behaviors are performed in excess by the patient to decrease his or her perceived risk of danger. These behaviors might include measuring blood pressure or temperature; avoiding people, places, or objects; or

seeking reassurance from their medical provider, friends, or online support group.

Safety signals are typically objects or information a patient associates with not having a bad outcome (Taylor & Asmundson, 2004). Another way of thinking about a safety signal is as a "safety blanket" the patient believes he or she needs to be safe. Examples include having a cell phone with them, knowing where the closest emergency room is located, or always having medication with them. Patients come to believe safety signals are crucial for being healthy or protected; however, they serve as continual cues for thinking about disease and poor health and may increase their sense of vulnerability and helplessness (Taylor & Asmundson, 2004). Safety signals perpetuate anxiety; it can be useful to target them for treatment. It may be helpful to preface your questions about safety behaviors and signals by telling the patient about common behaviors health-anxious patients engage in, as a way to normalize these behaviors. This can lead the patient to feel more at ease and be more honest when responding.

Fears and maladaptive beliefs.   Maladaptive beliefs and fears may be direct targets for intervention because they may be prompting maladaptive behaviors and/or body reactions that perpetuate the problem. As recommended by Taylor and Asmundson (2004), you should systematically question the patient about recent events when he or she becomes anxious about his or her health so that you elicit what the patient believes is so awful or bad. This can be done using a downward-arrow technique (Beutler, Harwood, & Caldwell, 2001). This technique initially elicits a thought related to increased anxiety. The provider then continues to ask questions in the form of "If that were true, then what?" to help identify the patient's beliefs related to increased anxiety. This may help to elicit valuable information quickly.

Occupational and social functioning and stressors. In patients presenting with health anxiety symptoms, functional impairments and stressors are assessed in a manner similar to other behavioral health problems. The goal is to assess and highlight how his or her anxiety symptoms and behaviors are negatively affecting important areas of the patient's life. In our experience, answering these questions can help motivate patients to change because they are

Health Anxiety Inventory—Short Version

Illness Questionnaire

Each question in this section consists of a group of four statements. Please read each group of statements carefully and then select the one which best describes your feelings, over the past six months. Identify the statement by circling the letter next to it. For example if you think that statement (a) is correct, circle statement (a); it may be that more than one statement applies, in which case, please circle any that are applicable.

1. (a) I do not worry about my health.
   (b) I occasionally worry about my health.
   (c) I spend much of my time worrying about my health.
   (d) I spend most of my time worrying about my health.
2. (a) I notice aches/pains less than most other people (of my age).
   (b) I notice aches/pains as much as most other people (of my age).
   (c) I notice aches/pains more than most other people (of my age).
   (d) I am aware of aches/pains in my body all the time.
3. (a) As a rule I am not aware of bodily sensations or changes.
   (b) Sometimes I am aware of bodily sensations or changes.
   (c) I am often aware of bodily sensations or changes.
   (d) I am constantly aware of bodily sensations or changes.
4. (a) Resisting thoughts of illness is never a problem.
   (b) Most of the time I can resist thoughts of illness.
   (c) I try to resist thoughts of illness but am often unable to do so.
   (d) Thoughts of illness are so strong that I no longer even try to resist them.
5. (a) As a rule I am not afraid that I have a serious illness.
   (b) I am sometimes afraid that I have a serious illness.
   (c) I am often afraid that I have a serious illness.
   (d) I am always afraid that I have a serious illness.
6. (a) I do not have images (mental pictures) of myself being ill.
   (b) I occasionally have images of myself being ill.
   (c) I frequently have images of myself being ill.
   (d) I constantly have images of myself being ill.
7. (a) I do not have any difficulty taking my mind off thoughts about my health.
   (b) I sometimes have difficulty taking my mind off thoughts about my health.
   (c) I often have difficulty in taking my mind off thoughts about my health.
   (d) Nothing can take my mind off thoughts about my health.
8. (a) I am lastingly relieved if my doctor tells me there is nothing wrong.
   (b) I am initially relieved but the worries sometimes return later.
   (c) I am initially relieved but the worries always return later.
   (d) I am not relieved if my doctor tells me there is nothing wrong.
9. (a) If I hear about an illness I never think I have it myself.
   (b) If I hear about an illness I sometimes think I have it myself.
   (c) If I hear about an illness I often think I have it myself.
   (d) If I hear about an illness I always think I have it myself.
10. (a) If I have a bodily sensation or change I rarely wonder what it means.
    (b) If I have a bodily sensation or change I often wonder what it means.
    (c) If I have a bodily sensation or change I always wonder what it means.
    (d) If I have a bodily sensation or change I must know what it means.

FIGURE 16.1.   Health Anxiety Inventory—Short Version. Score this measure 0–3 for each question: A = 0, B = 1, C = 2, D = 3. A score of above 31 indicates a greater likelihood of being health anxious. The words "ringing" and "ring" in the original instructions were replaced using the words "circling" and "circle." The word "definite" in the instructions for numbers 15–18 was replaced with the word "sure." From "The Health Anxiety Inventory: Development and Validation of Scales for the Measurement of Health Anxiety and Hypochondriasis," by P. M. Salkovskis, K. A. Rimes, H. M. C. Warwick, and D. M. Clark, 2002, *Psychological Medicine, 32*, pp. 851–853. Copyright 2002 by Cambridge University Press. Reprinted with permission. (*Continued*)

11. (a) I usually feel at very low risk for developing a serious illness.
    (b) I usually feel at fairly low risk for developing a serious illness.
    (c) I usually feel at moderate risk for developing a serious illness.
    (d) I usually feel at high risk for developing a serious illness.
12. (a) I never think I have a serious illness.
    (b) I sometimes think I have a serious illness.
    (c) I often think I have a serious illness.
    (d) I usually think that I am seriously ill.
13. (a) If I notice an unexplained bodily sensation I don't find it difficult to think about other things.
    (b) If I notice an unexplained bodily sensation I sometimes find it difficult to think about other things.
    (c) If I notice an unexplained bodily sensation I often find it difficult to think about other things.
    (d) If I notice an unexplained bodily sensation I always find it difficult to think about other things.
14. (a) My family/friends would say I do not worry enough about my health.
    (b) My family/friends would say I have a normal attitude to my health.
    (c) My family/friends would say I worry too much about my health.
    (d) My family/friends would say I am a hypochondriac.

For the following questions, please think about what it might be like if you had a serious illness of a type which particularly concerns you (such as heart disease, cancer, multiple sclerosis and so on). Obviously you cannot know for sure what it would be like; please give your best estimate of what you think might happen, basing your estimate on what you know about yourself and serious illness in general.

15. (a) If I had a serious illness I would still be able to enjoy things in my life quite a lot.
    (b) If I had a serious illness I would still be able to enjoy things in my life a little.
    (c) If I had a serious illness I would be almost completely unable to enjoy things in my life.
    (d) If I had a serious illness I would be completely unable to enjoy life at all.
16. (a) If I developed a serious illness there is a good chance that modern medicine would be able to cure me.
    (b) If I developed a serious illness there is a moderate chance that modern medicine would be able to cure me.
    (c) If I developed a serious illness there is a very small chance that modern medicine would be able to cure me.
    (d) If I developed a serious illness there is no chance that modern medicine would be able to cure me.
17. (a) A serious illness would ruin some aspects of my life.
    (b) A serious illness would ruin many aspects of my life.
    (c) A serious illness would ruin almost every aspect of my life.
    (d) A serious illness would ruin every aspect of my life.
18. (a) If I had a serious illness I would not feel that I had lost my dignity.
    (b) If I had a serious illness I would feel that I had lost a little of my dignity.
    (c) If I had a serious illness I would feel that I had lost quite a lot of my dignity.
    (d) If I had a serious illness I would feel that I had totally lost my dignity.

FIGURE 16.1. *(Continued)* Health Anxiety Inventory—Short Version. Score this measure 0–3 for each question: A = 0, B = 1, C =2, D = 3. A score of above 31 indicates a greater likelihood of being health anxious. The words "ringing" and "ring" in the original instructions were replaced using the words "circling" and "circle." The word "definite" in the instructions for numbers 15–18 was replaced with the word "sure." From "The Health Anxiety Inventory: Development and Validation of Scales for the Measurement of Health Anxiety and Hypochondriasis," by P. M. Salkovskis, K. A. Rimes, H. M. C. Warwick, and D. M. Clark, 2002, *Psychological Medicine, 32,* pp. 851–853. Copyright 2002 by Cambridge University Press. Reprinted with permission.

reminded that they are not living their life in a way that is consistent with their desires, values, and goals.

Summary.   Because of the nature of health anxiety, the summary and acceptance phase can be compli-cated. Because health-anxious patients strongly believe they have a disease or illness, they may be reluctant to give up this view. Summarizing your understanding of their problem in a way that reflects what they have said while empathically highlighting

---

Additional Functional Assessment Questions for Health Anxiety

---

Triggers
- During the last month, have there been places, people, experiences, or things you heard or read about that seemed to start increased anxiety, worry, or fear about your health?
- Have these triggers in the last month been similar to what you've experienced in the last year or have there been different triggers?
- What are the thoughts you have in these situations?
- When you're in these situations are there things you do or don't do that help decrease your concern?
- Are there things you do or don't do that increase your concern?

Physical Symptoms
- When people get more concerned about their health or symptoms, they often notice additional physical changes they didn't notice before, or the physical symptoms they were concerned about seem to get worse. Does that happen for you?
- If so, what are the physical symptoms or changes?

Safety Behaviors and Safety Signals
- When feeling more worried about your health, what do you do to decrease worry?
- It is usual for people who are concerned about their health to get opinions from other individuals or professional sources. Do you do this?
- Sometimes, people avoid certain people, places, or things to feel less vulnerable to disease or illness. Do you avoid people, places, or things to feel less vulnerable or safer?
- When people have objects, such as medication, or information, such as where a hospital or clinic is located, or when they have others with them, such as a friend, their worry about their health can be less. Do you do things such as this or similar things?
- Sometimes, people will check themselves physically, take their temperature, take their blood pressure, check heart rate, or check various body products when concerned about their health. Do you do anything like this?

Fears and Maladaptive Beliefs
- What was running through your mind at the point that your worry about your health was most upsetting or frightening to you?
- So, if that did happen, then what? What are you concerned would happen then?
- Alternatively, you could ask the following:
  - Let's assume what you were thinking actually happened. How would your life change?
  - And if that did happen or your life did change, then what?
  - And if that happened, what would that lead to?

FIGURE 16.2. Additional functional assessment questions specific for health anxiety.

that what they have been doing has not improved their condition, can lead patients to consider an alternative explanation for their symptoms. If possible, highlight how thoughts, emotions, and physical symptoms are interconnected. The summary might sound as follows:

For the last 2 years you have had recurring pain or bloating and discomfort in your stomach. Because your brother died of pancreatic cancer, you're certain that this must be pancreatic cancer or some type of stomach cancer. You've had multiple tests that have not shown any signs or symptoms of cancer, which reassure you for a few days. You even notice that at times after tests, the stomach pain or bloating may go away or is significantly less. You avoid watching television because anything that is medically related triggers increased worry that you have cancer that has not been discovered. As a result, you don't watch TV at night with your spouse and children the way you once did. You have trouble concentrating at work, so you're less productive. You have more arguments with your spouse and don't spend as much time with your children because you don't feel well. [If the patient agrees with your summary, move to offering an alternative explanation for the patient to consider.]

On the basis of the information I've gathered, in combination with the examinations and tests your PCP has conducted, I'm convinced your symptoms are real and distressing *AND at* the same time, I do not believe you have pancreatic cancer. I believe you have excessive concern and worry when you have normal or uncomfortable body changes that are not harmful. When this happens, you may notice even more symptoms. You've stopped living your life the way that you would really prefer to and spend a significant amount of time focused on these symptoms.

When I work with people who have similar problems and concerns, they tell me they have doubts about the role their thoughts, emotions, or behaviors are playing in their current difficulty. I'd like to discuss in more detail the different factors that I think may be important in your case and make sure I answer any questions you have before we discuss your goals for treatment and possible treatment options based on those goals.

As you discuss the role of emotional, cognitive, and behavioral factors, stop periodically and ask patients to tell you their understanding of what you have been discussing. If they have misunderstood you, correct the misperceptions and assess understanding before moving on. At this point, you should tell patients that you think they have health anxiety and use the "Health Anxiety" handout in Figure 16.3 to explain further what health anxiety is and the types of things people can do to manage it.

Health Anxiety

What is health anxiety? Health anxiety is the ongoing, persistent fear or belief that one has, is going to have, or is at high risk of developing a serious medical illness or disease. This fear continues even when medical examinations or tests show no signs of serious disease or illness.

What about all my symptoms? Your symptoms are real. People with health anxiety can experience symptoms caused by normal, yet uncomfortable, biological processes, for example pain, bloating, and gas. Symptoms could also be from other medical conditions that are not life threatening, such as irritable bowel syndrome. Increased concerned about symptoms, anxiety, or worry can turn on the body's stress response, which can produce symptoms like tight chest, upset stomach, dizziness, flushed face, racing heart, difficulty breathing, and fatigue. Healthy patients who are anxious about their health pay more attention to these body changes and become more concerned or worried about harmless body sensations.

What if something really is wrong with me and I'm not just excessively anxious or worried? Your provider has found no evidence of serious disease or illness. There is no test or exam that is ever going to be 100% accurate or assure you that you will never develop an illness. However, collecting additional information about your symptoms through your own experiments that examine how your symptoms are or are not related to ways of thinking and engaging or not engaging in certain behaviors can be valuable in providing evidence that your symptoms are not related to a serious disease.

My main concern is fear of getting sick. How can you help? Fear of developing an illness can also be addressed by developing a systematic way of confronting what you fear most. The behavioral health consultant can further detail these strategies.

FIGURE 16.3. **Health anxiety handout.**

After explaining health anxiety, you might tell the patient that you have some specific ideas for what he or she might change or do to minimize symptoms, increase functioning, and decrease suffering. However, before you lay out your recommendations, you should tell him or her that you would like to specifically hear what he or she wants to change. If the patient has a goal that is not attainable (e.g., complete elimination of physical symptoms or worry), it is important discuss this and negotiate a more realistic goal. The following is an example of what you might say before describing options for treatment:

> On the basis of what we've discussed, I would like to lay out some options for you to consider. I'd like to try to examine in a more scientific way how thoughts, emotions, and behaviors affect your symptoms, your functioning, and your suffering and how changing those factors might be helpful. Are you interested in hearing what you might be able to do?

Advise

Your next step is to advise patients on treatment options that would best address their problems, explaining what the intervention is and how it might help. See Figure 16.4 for a handout you can use to discuss the advantages and disadvantages of medication, and cognitive and behavioral interventions. Highlight advantages and disadvantages of medication versus cognitive and behavioral treatment approaches and explain what each option is designed to do.

Agree

Elicit from the patient what he or she is willing to attempt, and ask what the patient would like to try first and what seems most achievable. Early success may increase the patient's confidence and enhance his or her motivation to engage in interventions that are more difficult. If the patient seems ambivalent about making changes, you may want to engage in a style of interacting based on motivational interviewing strategies to delineate their ambivalence and to help promote the discrepancy between their current thoughts, behaviors, and values, and their motivation and belief in their change. See chapter 3 for general motivational interviewing strategies and documents you might use to increase motivation to change. Also, see Taylor and Asmundson (2004) for guidance that is more detailed. Do not move on to a treatment intervention until the patient has agreed that he or she is willing to try some intervention. If at this point the patient is not willing to engage in treatment, we recommend you simply let the patient know that you are available in the future if he or she changes his or her mind. This may also be the point at which you work with the PCP to develop a pattern of regularly scheduled appointments for the patient as a way to effectively manage the patient's desire for frequent health care visits.

Assist

There are a variety of treatment options for health anxiety that we believe are adaptable and effective for use in primary care, including education and stress management, cognitive disputation, worry control, interoceptive exposure, situational exposure, and behavioral experiments. These cognitive and behavioral strategies are well defined and have been used for a variety of stress and/or anxiety-related difficulties. This chapter does not allow for explicit detail on these strategies, so the following focuses on goals and how the strategies can be altered for efficient and effective use in a 30-minute appointment.

Education and stress management. Depending on the patient's symptoms and functional impairment, you might use education and stress management as an introduction to treatment, as a main treatment, or as a introduction to other treatments. This approach might be particularly useful for those who also present with depressed mood, other anxiety disorders, or other problems affected by autonomic arousal, such as irritable bowel syndrome, insomnia, headache, or muscle soreness (e.g., neck, shoulders, low back) which can be initiated or made worse by increased autonomic arousal (Taylor & Asmundson, 2004). It is important to reduce the likelihood that stress management

---

Treatment for Health Anxiety

Medication

Research suggests it is effective. Treatment is 6 to 12 months.

Advantages. (a) Easy to get, (b) easy to take.

Disadvantages. (a)Normal side effects—dry mouth, constipation, drowsiness, trouble falling asleep, blurred vision, headache, nausea, loss of appetite; (b) symptoms may return when medication is stopped.

You are having real body sensations that you are responding to in unhelpful ways. Your responses can even increase your body sensations and worry about those sensations. Medications can help decrease your sensitivity to these body sensations, making it easier to change unhelpful behaviors and helping to decrease worry about symptoms.

Thinking and Behavioral Treatments

Research shows them to be effective. Treatment varies from 3 to 12 months.

Advantages. (a) No side effects, (b) long-term effectiveness once treatment is complete.

Disadvantages. (a) Requires more time and effort, (b) might involve increased anxiety for short periods of time.

- *Stress management strategies.* Some people become worried about their health in response to the harmless, yet uncomfortable stress response symptoms they experience. Stress management strategies help you learn about your unique stress response, its harmless effects, and what you can do to reduce these unpleasant harmless reactions.
- *Thinking modification strategies.* Changing your thinking can help reduce misinterpretations of body symptoms, not necessarily eliminate them. It can be the misinterpretation of harmless body symptoms that leads you to engage or not engage in activities, which increases your suffering and affects how you function in different areas of your life. Thinking modification helps you examine anxious and worrisome thinking and how you can question that thinking to look at multiple explanations for what you perceive. The goal is to help you learn how your thoughts affect you physically, emotionally, and behaviorally and how you can develop ways of thinking that are more accurate so that you can spend your time engaging in the other valued activities in your life.
- *Exposure to feared objects, people, or environments.* The general goals of this treatment are to (a) decrease general fear, (b) decrease avoidance, and (c) decrease safety behaviors. This treatment could include the following methods:
- Interoceptive exposure. You engage in activities that turn on or increase feared physical symptoms. This treatment is designed to help you learn that your feared prediction about what might happen is not true and to desensitize you to these sensations.
- Situational exposure. This treatment is used to desensitize you to people, places, objects you avoid due to fear of catching a disease by having you purposely be in those situations. The goal is to test your belief and decrease anxiety in relation to the avoided people, places, or objects.
- Behavioral experiments. This can be used in a variety of ways, but may be best used as a way to test the effect of safety behaviors (i.e., actions you take to feel safe). Are they more helpful or harmful? This might be done by having you do something such as increasing the safety behavior to see how that affects your fear or physical symptoms. More should be better, right?

FIGURE 16.4.   Treatment for health anxiety handout.

becomes a safety behavior to avoid frightening symptoms that patients believe will cause great harm (Taylor & Asmundson, 2004). Appropriate use might be to decrease gastric discomfort that is occurring and interfering with a patient's enjoyment of an activity. An inappropriate use, for example, would be to avoid discussing gastric discomfort because the patient thinks that the discomfort signals the pres-

ence of pancreatic cancer. Some patients become worried about their health in response to nonpathological, yet uncomfortable, stress response symptoms they experience. The focus of these interventions is to help the patient learn about the stress response, understand that it is normal, and teach what can be done to reduce these unpleasant but harmless reactions.

Goals of education and stress management. The goals of stress management are to (a) learn that sensations are a result of increased autonomic arousal, not disease and (b)learn to decrease unpleasant physical sensations through relaxation and questioning thoughts.

Tailoring education and stress management to the primary care setting. Carefully constructing your education on stress management interventions are important in successfully working with patients who have health anxiety. The following details how a BHC can do this.

1. At the end of the initial appointment, or before seeing the patient for a follow-up, give the patient the handouts titled "Stress Response and How It Can Affect You" (see Figure 16.5) and "Your Physical Reactions to Stress" (see Figure 16.6). Ask patients to review these handouts, complete Your Physical Reactions to Stress, and bring it to the return appointment.

2. Tell them that in this consultation appointment you want to make sure they understand the stress response (i.e., what turns it up, what turns it down, their unique responses) and have them begin to learn and practice some specific strategies they can use to minimize it.

3. Spend the first 10 minutes of the next appointment reviewing the two handouts. Highlight the multiple stress responses people can have and how some of the patient's stress responses are common, normal responses. Spend the next 20 minutes explaining how changing the way he or she breathes can help decrease his or her stress response. Take the patient through a deep breathing exercise, explain cue-controlled relaxation, and set a plan for cue-controlled relaxation and deep breathing practice (see chap. 3, this volume).

4. Have the patient come for a 30-minute return visit to assess their use of relaxed and cue-controlled breathing. Resolve difficulties, and then spend 10 minutes taking the patients through four-group progressive muscle relaxation (PMR) or imagery if the patient has a chronic pain condition. See chapter 3 for PMR and imagery delivery suggestions. To help patients begin to recognize and question thoughts that may be increasing their stress response, take 10 minutes to review the handout titled "How to Question Stressful, Anxious, or Depressed Thinking" in chapter 3. Have patients continue to use the "Your Physical Reactions to Stress" monitoring form (Figure 16.6), and have them bring the form to return appointments.

5. Have the patient return for another 30-minute appointment to assess the use of relaxation and thought-questioning strategies. If duration and intensity of symptoms are not decreasing and/or concern over symptoms is not decreasing, have the patient continue for another week or 2, and if there is still no shift, incorporate additional cognitive modification or exposure.

Consistent with the primary care mode of operation, we suggest a stepped-care approach. Our clinical experience suggests that education and stress management fit well within brief primary care appointments, makes sense to patients, and are relatively easy for people to successfully complete. In addition, if this does not produce the desired results, you can use it as a foundation that will help facilitate the more intensive interventions that we discuss next.

Cognitive intervention. Cognitive interventions should be designed to help patients identify evidence in support of and against their beliefs about their health (Abramowitz & Braddock, 2004) and may include cognitive disputation, worry control, and exposure, as described in chapters 3 and 5. Taylor and Asmundson (2004) suggest that beliefs about the following might be targeted:

- Risk of disease.
- Current health.
- Effect of reassurance seeking.
- Effect of body checking.
- Effect of avoidance.

Cognitive Disputation.

1. At the end of the initial or follow-up appointment, give the patient the handout titled "How to Question Stressful, Angry, Anxious, or Depressed Thinking" (Figure 3.3). The patient should

---

Stress Response and How It Can Affect You

The *stress response,* or "fight or flight" response is the emergency reaction system of the body. It is there to keep you safe in emergencies. The stress response includes physical and thought responses to your perception of various situations. When the stress response is turned on, your body may release substances like adrenaline and cortisol. Your organs are programmed to respond in certain ways to situations that are viewed as challenging or threatening.

The stress response can work against you. You can turn it on when you don't really need it and, as a result, perceive something as an emergency when it's really not. It can turn on when you are just thinking about past or future events. Harmless, chronic conditions can be intensified by the stress response activating too often, with too much intensity, or for too long. Stress responses can be different for different individuals. Below is a list of some common stress related responses people have. (Circle the responses you have had in the last 2 weeks.)

Physical Responses

Muscle aches	Insomnia	↑ Heart rate	Headache
Weight gain	Nausea	Constipation	Dry mouth
Muscle twitching	Weight loss	Low energy	Weakness
Tight chest	Diarrhea	Dizziness	Trembling
Stomach cramps	Chills	Hot flashes	Sweating
Pounding heart	Choking feeling	Chest pain	Leg cramps
Numb hands/feet	Dry throat	Appetite change	Face flushing
↑ Blood pressure	Light-headedness	Feeling faint	Trouble swallowing
Rash	↑ Urination	Neck pain	Tingling hands/feet

Emotional and Thought Responses

Restlessness	Agitation	Insecurity	Worthlessness
Anxiety	Stress	Depression	Hopelessness
Guilt	Defensiveness	Anger	Racing thoughts
Nightmares	Intense thinking	Sensitivity	Expecting the worst
Numbness	Lack of motivation	Mood swings	Forgetfulness
↓ Concentration	Rigidity	Preoccupation	Intolerance

Behavioral Responses

Avoidance	Withdrawal	Neglect	↑ Alcohol use
Smoking	↑ Eating	Arguing	Poor appearance
↑ Spending	Poor hygiene	↓ Eating	Seeking reassurance
Nail biting	Skin picking	↑ Talking	↑ Body checking
Sexual problems	Foot tapping	Fidgeting	Rapid walking
↓ Exercise	Teeth clenching	Multitasking	Aggressive speaking
↓ Fun activities	↑ Sleeping	↓ Relaxing activities	Seeking information

The parasympathetic nervous system in your body is designed to turn on your body's *relaxation response.* Your behaviors and thinking can keep your body's natural relaxation response from operating at its best.

Getting your body to relax on a daily basis for at least brief periods can help decrease unpleasant stress responses. Learning to relax your body, through specific breathing and relaxation exercises as well as by minimizing stressful thinking, can help your body's natural relaxation system be more effective.

FIGURE 16.5. Stress response and how it can affect you handout.

review the exercises in this handout and bring them to the next appointment. At the follow-up, spend 15 minutes reviewing the "Thinking Mistakes that Increase Stress, Anger, Depression, Anxiety, and Worry" section of the handout.

Tell the patient that people with similar concerns about their health often have developed thinking mistakes that contribute to anxiety. Go over the common thinking mistake categories and, once you have reviewed it, have the

---

Your Physical Reactions to Stress

Complete this form between now and your next appointment for all the stressful experiences you have and for the physical reactions, symptoms, or sensations you notice before, during, or after the stressful event.

An example

Date/time	Stressful situation or event	Physical reaction, symptoms, sensations	Highest intensity 0–10	Minutes before intensity below 2
3/3/07 @ 8:00	Overslept 45 minutes	Tight chest, trembling	7 or 8	60 to 120

Your monitoring form

Date/time	Stressful situation or event	Physical reaction, symptoms, sensations	Highest intensity 0–10	Minutes before intensity below 2

FIGURE 16.6.   Your physical reactions to stress handout.

patient briefly tell you whether he or she sees his or her own thinking falling into some of these categories. Most people recognize that they engage in thinking patterns falling into one or more of these areas.

2. Spend the remaining 15 minutes reviewing "Disputing or Challenging Thoughts and Beliefs" section of the handout. Explain that this is one way of looking at how thoughts can produce bodily sensations, emotions, and behaviors. The handout can be a tool to examine how the patient's thoughts in response to different situations are affecting him or her and can help him or her discover other ways of thinking that might produce different results.

3. At the next follow-up, spend 25 minutes reviewing the "Disputing or Challenging Thoughts and Beliefs" section of the handout.

4. Spend the last 5 minutes devising a plan to continue using the "Disputing or Challenging Thoughts and Beliefs" section of the handout and/or, as time allows, to introduce worry control, to be reviewed in more detail in the follow-up appointment.

Worry control. Worry control treatment might be delivered as a stand-alone intervention or paired with cognitive disputation. The goal of worry control is to decrease overall daily worry by creating a specific place and time for the patient to engage in worry. See chapter 5 as well as intervention handouts for additional detail on this strategy.

Exposure. Taylor and Asmundson (2004) described several types of exposure exercises that might be useful to treat health anxiety. In our opinion, those that lend themselves best to primary care are interoceptive and situational exposure and behavioral experiments. The goals of exposure are to decrease general fear, avoidance, and safety behaviors. See chapter 5 of this volume for information and patient handouts on interoceptive and situational exposure.

Behavioral experiments can be used in a variety of ways, but may be best used as a way to test the effect of safety behaviors, particularly body checking behavior. Such experiments can assist the patient in determining whether safety behaviors are more helpful or harmful. Behavioral experiments should be presented as a way to gather information and can be presented to the patient like this:

1. Take 10 minutes to list potential advantages and disadvantages of safety behavior.
2. Set a plan to increase the safety behavior over the following week and assess what changes occur as a result of increasing this behavior.

As an example, for the patient who is anxious that he or she might have stomach cancer you might discuss how repeatedly pushing in the abdominal area to check for changes that might suggest a tumor can produce abdominal tenderness, which in turn reinforces the belief that there is a tumor. You might also suggest that increasingly seeking reassurance from medical professionals or family is likely to increase anxiety. Conversely, decreasing or stopping activities such as medical reassurance-seeking might result in an initial increase in anxiety, but, over time, the patient is likely to have a decreased focus on health and decreased anxiety.

Helping the primary care provider. Whether you do treat the patient or not, we recommend discussing the following with the patient's PCP. The items are based on a cognitive–behavioral treatment package for hypochondriasis developed by Barsky and Ahern (2004). Although the direct effects of this information alone have not been empirically determined, similar information provided to primary care providers in studies with patients who have somatization disorder produced positive effects (e.g. Smith, Rost, & Kashner, 1995). As such, we believe there is nothing to lose and many benefits to gain.

Helpful management techniques. Shift the focus to ongoing care instead of cure. Manage health anxiety as if it is a chronic disease or illness, minimizing and managing symptoms the best way possible while promoting improved or maintained function in important life domains. Using the following techniques can help to make this shift.

■ Have the patient come in for regular medical visits on a fixed schedule. Doing this separates the patient's symptom status from access to the medical provider. He or she does not have to be symptomatic to have an appointment. Determine an acceptable frequency schedule with the patient and minimize variance in appointments based on symptoms getting better or worse.

■ Because of the nature of anxiety, telling the patient that nothing is wrong with him or her or reassuring him or her is usually not helpful. It is all right to suggest that no progressive or fatal disease is present, but it should also be made clear that a definitive diagnosis or cure may not be possible. The goal is to get the patient to accept that the certainty of being disease-free is impossible and that he or she can shift from looking for this definitive reassurance to managing symptoms and functioning well.

■ If the patient is told a serious disease has been ruled out, explain what might be causing the symptoms. For instance, tell the patient that he or she has a highly sensitive nervous system that leads them to get distressed by symptoms that other patients who have less sensitive systems do not notice. You should also state that the symptoms the patient is experiencing are real and are not imagined or just psychological.

■ Consider that patients with health anxiety benefit from a conservative approach to diagnostic procedures and that excessive testing or intervention can lead the patient to report side effects, new symptoms, and fears. Consider using benign symptom management recommendations and performing a routine physical exam at each appointment as a noninvasive way to assess that symptoms have not changed in any significant manner.

Arrange

We recommend that you and the patient agree to have regularly scheduled appointments. Consider coordinating appointments so the patient sees his or her PCP for a regular physical exam, then sees you directly afterward to continue to target whatever has been agreed on. The number of appointments you have with a patient will likely vary depending on the severity of the health anxiety symptoms. Over time, if symptoms and functioning are improving, it may be helpful to continue to have the patient stick to a fixed interval appointment schedule but increase the amount of time between those appointments. If interventions within primary care have occurred for a period during which you might have expected to see improved functioning and a decrease in symptoms (e.g., three–eight 30-minute consultation appointments; it may take a while for the individual to practice and initiate the multiple skills necessary to decrease symptoms and improve functioning) and little or no change has occurred, a referral to a provider in a specialty mental health clinic who can spend more time with the patient may be warranted.

SUMMARY

Patients with health anxiety have significant distress, suffering, and functional impairment. Preoccupation with having or catching a disease can result in overuse or inappropriate use of the medical system without symptom relief, leaving both PCP and the patient frustrated. Health anxiety symptoms are typically maintained by a combination of thinking errors and avoidance and/or safety behaviors. Cognitive and behavioral interventions are effective, although these treatments have yet to be examined in a primary care setting. Effective behavioral health treatment of patients with health anxiety can be challenging in general and perhaps even more so in the limited time afforded by primary care appointments. At the same time, primary care may be the ideal setting to treat health anxious patients, because they typically have a disease or illness-based view of their problems and may be offended or reluctant to go to a specialty mental health service. Our experience suggests that effective treatment in primary care is likely to include a focus on the patient's symptoms being real, yet benign, with an alternative explanation of what is triggering and/or maintaining symptoms. Explanation of available treatments and patient acceptance for a specific treatment with a focus on functional improvement and symptom management is also important. PCP and behavioral health consultant treatment should be coordinated to include fixed interval appointments focused on symptom management and improvement in functioning as opposed to a "cure" or elimination of symptoms.

References

Abramowitz, J. S., & Braddock, A. E. (2006). Hypochondriasis: Conceptualization, treatment, and relationship to obsessive–compulsive disorder. *Psychiatric Clinics of North America, 29*, 503–519.

Abreu, A. C., & Stuart, S. (2005). Pharmacologic and hormonal treatments for postpartum depression. *Psychiatric Annals, 35*, 569–576.

Agency for Healthcare Research and Quality. (2006). *National healthcare disparities report* (AHRQ Publication No. 07–0012). Rockville, MD: Author.

Ahles, T. A., Wasson, J. H., Seville, J. A., Johnson, D. J., Cole, B. F., Hanscom, B. F., et al. (2006). A controlled trial of methods for managing pain in primary care patients with or without co-occurring psychosocial problems. *Annals of Family Medicine, 4*, 341–350.

Ainsworth, B. E., Haskell, W. L., Leon, A. S., Jacobs, D. R., Jr., Montoye, H. J., Sallis, J. F., et al. (1993). Compendium of physical activities: Classification of energy costs of human physical activities. *Medicine & Science in Sports & Exercise, 25*, 71–80.

Aklin, W. M., & Turner, S. M. (2006). Toward understanding ethnic and cultural factors in the interviewing process. *Psychotherapy: Theory, Research, Practice, Training, 43*, 50–64.

Albert, H. (1999). Psychosomatic group treatment helps women with chronic pelvic pain. *Journal of Psychosomatic Obstetrics and Gynecology, 20*, 216–225.

Alberti, R. E., & Emmons, M. L. (2001). *Your perfect right: Assertiveness and equality in your life and relationships* (8th ed.). Atascadero, CA: Impact Publishers.

Albright, T. L., Parchman, M., Burge, S. K., & the RRNeST Investigators. (2001). Predictors of self-care behavior in adults with type 2 diabetes: An RRNeST study. *Family Medicine, 33*, 354–360.

American Bar Association & American Psychological Association. (2006). *Judicial determination of capacity of older adults in guardianship proceedings.* Retrieved September 1, 2007, from http://www.abanet.org/aging/docs/judges_book_5-24.pdf

American College of Chest Physicians (ACCP)–American Association of Cardiovascular and Pulmonary Rehabilitation (AACVPR) Pulmonary Rehabilitation Guidelines Panel (1997). Pulmonary rehabilitation: Joint AACP/AACVPR evidence-based guidelines. *Chest, 112*, 1363–1396.

American College of Obstetricians and Gynecologist (2004, February 27). *ACOG issues new document on chronic pelvic pain.* Retrieved April 17, 2007, from http://www.acog.org/from_home/publications/press_releases/nr02-27-04-2.cfm

American College of Physicians. (2004). Racial and ethnic disparities in health care: A position paper of the American college of physicians. *Annals of Internal Medicine, 141*, 226–232.

American Diabetes Association. (2007a). Diagnosis and classification of diabetes mellitus. *Diabetes Care, 30*, S42–S47.

American Diabetes Association. (2007b). Nutrition recommendations and interventions for diabetes. *Diabetes Care, 30*, S48–S65.

American Diabetes Association. (2008). Standards of medical care in diabetes—2008. *Diabetes Care, 31*, S12–S54.

American Psychiatric Association. (1994). *Diagnostic and statistical manual of mental disorders* (4th ed.). Washington, DC: Author.

American Psychiatric Association. (2000). *Diagnostic and statistical manual of mental disorders* (4th ed., text rev.). Washington, DC: Author.

American Psychological Association. (2003). *Guidelines for psychological practice with older adults.* Washington, DC: Author.

American Psychological Association. (2006). *Health care of the whole person statement of vision and principles.* Retrieved July 28, 2007, from http://www.apa.org/practice/hcwp_statement.html

American Psychological Association Practice Directorate. (1996). *Models for multidisciplinary arrangements: A state-by-state review of options.* Washington, DC: Author.

Anderson, R. J., Freeland, K. E., Clouse, R. E., & Lustman, P. J. (2001). The prevalence of comorbid depression in adults with diabetes. *Diabetes Care, 24,* 1069–1078.

Anger, J. T., Saigal, C. S., & Litwin, M. S. (2006). The prevalence of urinary incontinence among community dwelling adult women: Results from the National Health and Nutrition Examination Survey. *The Journal of Urology, 175,* 601–604.

Anger, J. T., Saigal, C. S., Stothers, L., Thom, D. H., Rodriguez, L. V., & Litwin, M. S. (2006). The prevalence of urinary incontinence among community dwelling men: Results from the National Health and Nutrition Examination Survey. *The Journal of Urology, 176,* 2103–2108.

Atikeler, M. K., Gecit, I., & Senol, F. A. (2002). Optimum usage of prilocaine–lidocaine cream in early ejaculation. *Andrologia, 34,* 356.

Ayyad, C., & Andersen, T. (2000). Long-term efficacy of dietary treatment of obesity: A systematic review of studies published between 1931 and 1999. *Obesity Reviews, 1,* 113–119.

Baer, J. S., & Lichtenstein, E. (1988). Classification and prediction of smoking relapse episodes: An exploration of individual differences. *Journal of Consulting and Clinical Psychology, 56,* 104–110.

Ball, J., Kearney, B., Wilhelm, K., Dewhurst-Savellis, J., & Barton, B. (2000). Cognitive behaviour therapy and assertion training groups for patients with depression and comorbid personality disorders. *Behavioural and Cognitive Psychotherapy, 28,* 71–85.

Barbach, L. (2000). *For yourself: The fulfillment of female sexuality.* New York: Bantam Doubleday.

Barlow, D. H., Grosset, K. A., Hart, H., & Hart, D. M. (1989). A study of the experience of Glasgow women in the climacteric years. *British Journal of Obstetrics and Gynaecology, 96,* 1192–1197.

Barnes, P. J. (2003). New concepts in chronic obstructive pulmonary disease. *Annual Review of Medicine, 54,* 113–129.

Barsky, A. J., & Ahern, D. K. (2004). Cognitive–behavior therapy of hypochondriasis. *The Journal of the American Medical Association, 291,* 1464–1470.

Barsky, A. J., Ettner, S. L., Horsky, J., & Bates, D. W. (2001). Resource utilization of patients with hypochondriacal health anxiety and somatization. *Medical Care, 39,* 705–715.

Barsky, A. J., Wyshak, G., Klerman, G. L., & Latham, K. S. (1990). The prevalence of hypochondriasis in medical outpatients. *Social Psychiatry and Psychiatric Epidemiology, 25,* 89–94.

Barsky, A. J., Wyshak, G., Latham, K. S., & Klerman, G. L. (1991). Hypochondriacal patients, their physicians, and their medical care. *Journal of General Internal Medicine, 6,* 413–419.

Bartels, S. J., Coakley, E. H., Zubritsky, C., Ware, J., Miles, J. H., & Arean, P. A. (2004). Improving access to geriatric mental health services: A randomized trial comparing treatment engagement with integrated versus enhanced referral are for depression anxiety and at-risk alcohol use. *American Journal of Psychiatry, 161,* 1455–1462.

Bastien, C., Vallieres, A., & Morin, C. M. (2001). Validation of the Insomnia Severity Index as a clinical outcome measure for insomnia research. *Sleep Medicine, 2,* 297–307.

Beardsley, R., Gardocki, G., Larson, D., & Hidalgo, J. (1988). Prescribing of psychotropic medication by primary care physicians and psychiatrists. *Archives of General Psychiatry, 45,* 1117–1119.

Beck, A. T., Guth, D., Steer, R. A., & Ball, R. (1997). Screening for major depression disorders in medical inpatients with the Beck Depression Inventory for Primary Care. *Behaviour Research and Therapy, 35,* 785–791.

Beck, A. T., & Steer, R. A. (1993). *Beck Anxiety Inventory manual.* San Antonio, TX: Psychological Corporation.

Beck, A. T., Steer, R. A., & Brown, G. K. (1996). *Manual for Beck Depression Inventory II (BDI-II).* San Antonio, TX: Psychology Corporation.

Beck, C. T., & Gable, R. K. (2000). Postpartum depression screening scale: Development and psychometric testing. *Nursing Research, 49,* 272–282.

Beck, J. A. (2005). *Cognitive therapy: Basics and beyond.* New York: Guilford Press.

Berkman, L. F., Blumenthal, J., Burg, M., Carney, R. M., Catellier, D., Cowan, M. J., et al. (2003). Effects of treating depression and low perceived social support on clinical events after myocardial infarction: The enhancing recovery in coronary heart disease patients (ENRICHD) randomized trial. *The Journal of the American Medical Association, 289,* 3106–3116.

Betancourt, J. R. (2004). Cultural competence—marginal or mainstream movement? *New England Journal of Medicine, 351,* 953–954.

Betancourt, J. R. (2006). Cultural competency: Providing quality care to diverse populations. *The Consultant Pharmacist, 21,* 988–995.

Betancourt, J. R., Green, A. R., & Carrillo, J. E. (2002, October). *Cultural competence in health care: Emerging frameworks and practical approaches.* New York: The Commonwealth Fund.

Betancourt, J. R., Green, A. R., Carrillo, J. E., & Ananeh-Firempong, O. (2003). Defining cultural competence: A practical framework for addressing racial/ethnic disparities in health and health care. *Public Health Reports, 118,* 293–302.

Beutler, L. E., Harwood, T. M., & Caldwell, R. (2001). Cognitive–behavioral therapy and psychotherapy integration. In K. S. Dobson (Ed.), *Handbook of cognitive behavioral therapies* (2nd ed., pp. 138–170). New York: Guilford Press.

Bisson, J., & Andrew, M. (2005, April 20). Psychological treatment of post-traumatic stress disorder (PTSD). *Cochrane Database of Systematic Reviews, 2,* Article CD003388. Retrieved May 15, 2007, from http://www.cochrane.org/reviews/en/ab003388.html

Blanchard, E. B. (2001). *Irritable bowel syndrome: Psychological assessment and treatment.* Washington, DC: American Psychological Association.

Blanchard, E. B., Jones-Alexander, J., Buckley, T. C., & Forneris, C. A. (1996). Psychometric properties of the PTSD checklist (PCL). *Behaviour Research and Therapy, 34,* 669–673.

Blanchard, E. B., & Scharff, L. (2002). Psychosocial aspects of assessment and treatment of irritable bowel syndrome in adults and recurrent abdominal pain in children. *Journal of Consulting and Clinical Psychology, 70,* 725–738.

Bledsoe, S. E., & Grote, N. K. (2006). Treating depression during pregnancy and postpartum: A preliminary meta-analysis. *Research on Social Work Practice, 16,* 109–120.

Bloom, B., Dey, A. N., & Freeman, G. (2006). Summary health statistics for U.S. children: National health interview survey, 2005. *Vital Health Stat, 10,* 1–84.

Blount, A. (Ed.). (1998). *Integrated primary care.* New York: Norton.

Blount, A. (2003). Integrated primary care: Organizing the evidence. *Families, Systems & Health, 21,* 121–133.

Blount, A., Shoenbaum, M., Kathol, R., Rollman, B. L., Thomas, M., O'Donohue, W., et al. (2007). The economics of behavioral health services in medical settings: A summary of the evidence. *Professional Psychology: Research and Practice, 38,* 290–297.

Blumenthal, J. A., Babyak, M. A., Doraiswamy, M., Watkins, L., Hoffman, B. M., Barbour, K. A., et al. (2007). Exercise and pharmacotherapy in the treatment of major depressive disorder. *Psychosomatic Medicine, 69,* 587–596.

Bobo, W. V., Warner, C. H., & Warner, C. M. (2007). The management of posttraumatic stress disorder (PTSD) in the primary care setting. *Southern Medical Journal, 8,* 797–802.

Bogner, H. R., Morales, K. H., Post, E. P., & Bruce, M. L. (2007). Diabetes, depression, and death: A randomized controlled trial of a depression treatment program for older adults based in primary care (PROSPECT). *Diabetes Care, 30,* 3005–3010.

Bonanno, G. A., Wortman, C. B., Lehman, D. R., Tweed, R. G., Haring, M., Sonnega, J., et al. (2002). Resilience to loss and chronic grief: A prospective study from preloss to 18-months post loss. *Journal of Personality and Social Psychology, 83,* 1150–1164.

Booth, M. L. (2000). Assessment of physical activity: An international perspective. *Research Quarterly for Exercise and Sport, 71,* s114–s120.

Bootzin, R. R., & Epstein, D. R. (2000). Stimulus control. In K. L. Lichstein & C. M. Morin (Eds.), *Treatment of late-life insomnia* (pp. 167–184). Thousand Oaks, CA: Sage Publications.

Borkovec, T. D., Wilkinson, L., Folensbee, R., & Lerman, C. (1983). Stimulus control applications to the treatment of worry. *Behaviour Research and Therapy, 21,* 247–251.

Bower, P., Richards, D., & Lovell, K. (2001). The clinical and cost-effectiveness of self-help treatments for anxiety and depressive disorders in primary care: A systematic review. *British Journal of General Practice, 51,* 838–845.

Boyce, P. M., Talley, N. J., & Balaam, B. (2002). A randomized controlled trial of cognitive behavior therapy, relaxation training, and routine clinical care for the irritable bowel syndrome. *American Journal of Gastroenterology, 98,* 2209–2218.

Boyd, R. C., Le, H. N., & Somberg, R. (2005). Review of screening instruments for postpartum depression. *Archives of Women's Mental Health, 8,* 141–153.

Bradley, R. Greene, J., Russ, E., Dutra, L., & Westen, D. (2005). A multidimensional meta-analysis of psychotherapy for PTSD. *American Journal of Psychiatry, 162,* 214–227.

Brandt, L. J., Bjorkman, D., Fennerty, M. B., Locke, G. R., Olden, K., Peterson, W., et al. (2002). Systematic Review on the management of irritable bowel syndrome in North America. *The American Journal or Gastroenterology, 97,* S7–S26.

Bray, J. H. (1996). Psychologists as primary care practitioners. In R. J. Resnick & R. H. Rozensky (Eds.), *Health psychology through the life span: Practice and research opportunities* (pp. 89–99). Washington, DC: American Psychological Association.

Breastcancer.org. (2006). *All about hot flashes.* Retrieved April 27, 2007, from http://www.breastcancer.org/bey_cope_meno_hotFlash.html

Brewin, C. R., Rose, S., Andrews, B., Green, J., Tata, P., McEvedy, C., et al. (2002). Brief screening instrument for posttraumatic stress disorder. *British Journal of Psychiatry, 181,* 158–162.

Bromberger, J. T., Meyer, P. M., Kravitz, H. M., Sommer, B., Cordal, A., Powell, L., et al. (2001). Psychological distress and natural menopause: A multiethnic community study. *American Journal of Public Health, 91,* 1435–1442.

Brown, R. L., Leonard, T., Saunders, L. A., & Papasouliotis, O. (1998). The prevalence and detection of substance use disorders among inpatients ages 18 to 49: An opportunity for prevention. *Preventive Medicine, 27,* 101–110.

Brown, R. L., & Rounds, L. A. (1995). Conjoint screening questionnaires for alcohol and other drug abuse: Criterion validity in a primary care practice. *Wisconsin Medical Journal, 94,* 135–140.

Brown, T. A., O'Leary, T. A., & Barlow, D. H. (2001). Generalized anxiety disorder. In D. H. Barlow (Ed.), *Clinical handbook of psychological disorders: A step-by-step treatment manual* (pp. 154–208). New York: Guilford Press.

Buist, A. E., Barnett, B. E. W., Milgrom, J., Pope, S., Condon, J. T., Elwood, D. A., et al. (2002). To screen or not to screen-that is the question in perinatal depression. *The Medical Journal of Australia, 177,* S101–S105.

Buist, A., Condon, J., Brooks, J., Speelman, C., Milgrom, J., Hayes, B., et al. (2006). Acceptability of routine screening for perinatal depression. *Journal of Affective Disorders, 93,* 233–237.

Bunker, S. J., Colquhoun, D. M., Esler, M. D., Hickie, I. B., Hunt, D., Jelinek, V. M., et al. (2003). "Stress" and coronary heart disease: Psychosocial risk factors. *Medical Journal of Australia, 178,* 272–276.

Burke, B. L., Arkowitz, H., & Menchola, M. (2003). The efficacy of motivational interviewing: A meta-analysis of controlled clinical trials. *Journal of Consulting and Clinical Psychology, 71,* 843–861.

Burns, R., Nichols, L. O., Martindale-Adams, J., Graney, M. J., & Lummus, A. (2003). Primary care interventions for dementia caregivers: 2-year outcomes from the REACH study. *Gerontologist, 43,* 547–555.

Bush, K., Kivlahan, D. R., McDonell, M. B., Fihn, S. D., & Bradley, K. A. (1998). The AUDIT alcohol consumption questions (AUDIT-C). *Archives of Internal Medicine, 158,* 1789–1795.

Busse, W. W., Kiecolt-Glaser, J. K., Coe, C., Martin, R. J., Weiss, S. T., & Parker, S. R. (1995). NHLBI workshop summary. Stress and asthma. *American Journal of Respiratory and Critical Care Medicine, 151,* 249–252.

Cahill, K., Stead, L. F., & Lancaster, T. (2007, January 24). Nicotine receptor partial agonists for smoking cessation. *Cochrane Database of Systematic Reviews, 1,* Article CD006103. Retrieved September 2, 2007, from http://mrw.interscience.wiley.com/cochrane/clsysrev/articles/CD006103/frame.html

Calfas, K. J., Long, B. J., Sallis, J. F., Wooten, W. J., Pratt, M., & Patrick, K. (1996). A controlled trial of physician counseling to promote the adoption of physical activity. *Preventive Medicine, 25,* 225–233.

Callaghan, G. M., Gregg, J. A., Ortega, E., & Berlin, K. S. (2005). Psychosocial interventions with type 1 and 2 diabetes patients. In W. T. O'Donohue, M. R. Byrd, N. A. Cummings, & D. A. Henderson (Eds.), *Behavioral integrative care: Treatments that work in the primary care setting* (pp. 329–345). New York: Brunner-Routledge.

Camargo, C. A., Jr., Stampfer, M. J., Glynn, R. J., Grodstein, F., Gaziano, J. M., Manson, J. E., et al. (1997). Moderate Alcohol Consumption and Risk for Angina Pectoris or Myocardial Infarction in U.S. Male Physicians. *Annals of Internal Medicine, 126,* 372–375.

Carey, M. P., Wincze, J. P., & Meisler, A. W. (1993). Sexual dysfunction: Male erectile disorder. In D. H. Barlow (Ed.), *Clinical handbook of psychological disorders,* (2nd ed., pp. 442–480). New York: Guilford.

Carr, D. B., Gray, S., Baty, J., & Morris, J. C. (2000). The value of informant versus individual's complaints of memory impairment in early dementia. *Neurology, 55,* 1724–1726.

Carr, R. E. (1998). Panic disorder and asthma: Causes, effects and research implications. *Journal of Psychosomatic Research, 44,* 43–52.

Carrier, S., Brock, G., Kour, N. W., & Lue, T. F. (1993). Pathophysiology of erectile dysfunction. *Urology, 42,* 468–481.

Carrillo, J. E., Green, A. R., & Betancourt, J. R. (1999). Cross-cultural primary care: A patient-based approach. *Annals of Internal Medicine, 130,* 829–834.

Carroll, D., & Seers, K. (1998). Relaxation for the relief of chronic pain: A systematic review. *Journal of Advanced Nursing, 27,* 476–487.

Centers for Disease Control and Prevention. (2000). Cigarette smoking among adults: United States, 1998. *Morbidity and Mortality Weekly Report, 49,* 881–884.

Centers for Disease Control and Prevention. (2001). Physical activity trends—United States 1990–1998, *Morbidity and Mortality Weekly Report, 50,* 166–169.

Centers for Disease Control and Prevention. (2003). Public health and aging: Trends in aging: United States and worldwide. *Morbidity and Mortality Weekly Report, 52,* 101–106.

Centers for Disease Control and Prevention. (2005). *National diabetes fact sheet: General information and national estimates on diabetes in the United States, 2005.* Atlanta, GA: U.S. Department of Health and Human Services, Centers for Disease Control and Prevention.

Centers for Disease Control and Prevention. (2006). Tobacco use among adults: United States, 2005. *Morbidity and Mortality Weekly Report, 55,* 1145–1148.

Centers for Disease Control and Prevention and The Merck Company Foundation. (2007). *The State of Aging and Health in America 2007.* Whitehouse Station, NJ: The Merck Company Foundation.

Chambers, C. V., Markson, L., Diamond, J. J., Lasch, L., & Berger, M. (1999). Health beliefs and compliance with inhaled corticosteroids by asthmatic patients in primary care practices. *Respiratory Medicine, 93,* 88–94.

Chang, J. T., Morton, S. C., Rubenstein, L. Z., Mojica, W. A, Maglione, M., Suttorp, M. J., et al. (2004). Interventions for the prevention of falls in older adults: Systematic review and meta-analysis of randomised clinical trials. *British Medical Journal, 328,* 680–687.

Chang, L., Toner, B. B., Fukudo, S., Guthrie, E., Locke, G. R., Norton, N. J., et al. (2006). Gender, age, society, culture, and the patient's perspective in the functional gastrointestinal disorders. *Gastroenterology, 130,* 1435–1446.

Chaudhuri, R., Livingston, E., McMahon, A. D., Thomson, L., Borland, W., & Thomson, N. C. (2003). Cigarette smoking impairs the therapeutic response to oral corticosteroids in chronic asthma. *American Journal of Respiratory and Critical Care Medicine, 168,* 1308–1311.

Chesson, A. L., Anderson, W. M., Littner, M., Davila, D., Hartse, K., Johnson, S., et al. (1999) Practice parameters for the nonpharmacologic treatment of insomnia. *Sleep, 22,* 1128–1133.

Chobanian, A. V., Bakris, G. L., Black, H. R., Cushman, W. C., Green, I. A., Izzo, J. L., Jr., et al. (2003). Seventh report of the Joint National Committee on Prevention, Detection, Evaluation, and Treatment of High Blood Pressure. *Hypertension, 42,* 1206–1252.

Ciechanowski, P. S., Katon, W. J., Russo, J. E., & Hirsch, I. B. (2003). The relationship of depressive symptoms to symptom reporting, self-care and glucose control in diabetes. *General Hospital Psychiatry, 25,* 246–252.

Clark, R., Tluczek, A., & Wenzel, A. (2003). Psychotherapy for post partum depression: A preliminary report. *American Journal of Orthopsychiatry, 73,* 441–454.

Cole, S. R., Kawachi, I., Liu, S., Gaziano, J. M., Manson, J. E., Buring, J. E., et al. (2001). Time urgency and risk of non-fatal myocardial infarction. *International Journal of Epidemiology, 30,* 363–369.

Comfort, A. (1994). *The new joy of sex.* New York: Crown House Publishing.

Conweil, Y. (2001). Suicide in later life: A review and recommendations for prevention. *Suicide and Life Threatening Behavior, 31*(Suppl.), 32–47.

Cook, J. M., Elhai, J. D., & Areán, P. A. (2005). Psychometric properties of the PTSD checklist with older primary care patients. *Journal of Traumatic Stress, 18,* 371–376.

Cook, N. R., Cutler, J. A., Obarzanek, E., Buring, J. E., Rexrode, K. M., Kumanyika, S. K., et al. (2007). Long term effects of dietary sodium reduction on cardiovascular disease outcomes: Observational follow-up of the trials of hypertension prevention (TOHP). *British Medical Journal, 334,* 885–892.

Coups, E. J., Gaba, A., & Orleans, C. T. (2004). Physician screening for multiple behavioral health risk factors. *American Journal of Preventive Medicine, 27*(Suppl. 1), 34–41.

Cox, J. L., Holden, J. M., & Sagovsky, R. (1987). Detection of postnatal depression: Development of the 10-item Edinburgh postnatal depression scale. *British Journal of Psychiatry, 150,* 782–786.

Coyne, J. C., Schwenk, T. L., & Fechner-Bates, S. (1995). Nondetection of depression by primary care physicians reconsidered. *General Hospital Psychiatry, 16,* 267–276.

Craig, T. K., Boardman, A. P., Mills, K., Daly-Jones, O., & Drake, H. (1993). The south London somatisation study. I: Longitudinal course and the influence of early life experiences. *British Journal of Psychiatry, 163,* 579–588.

Craven, M., & Bland, R. (2006). Better practices in collaborative mental health care: An analysis of the evidence base. *Canadian Journal of Psychiatry, 51*(Suppl 1), 7S–72S.

Crum, R. M., Anthony, J. C., Bassett, S. S., & Folstein, M. F. (1993). Population-based norms for the Mini-Mental State Examination by age and educational level. *The Journal of the American Medical Association, 269,* 2386–2391.

Cuijpers, P., van Straten, A., & Warmerdam, L. (2007). Behavioral activation treatments of depression: A meta-analysis. *Clinical Psychology Review, 27,* 318–326.

Cullen, B., O'Neill, B., Evans, J. J., Coen, R. F., & Lawlor, B. A. (2007). A review of screening tests for cognitive impairment. *Journal of Neurology Neurosurgery and Psychiatry, 78,* 790–799.

Cummings, N. A., Cummings, J. L., & Johnson, J. N. (1997). *Behavioral health in primary care: A guide for clinical integration.* Madison, CT: Psychosocial Press.

Daley, A. J., Macarthur, C., & Winter, H. (2007). The role of exercise in treating postpartum depression: A review of the literature. *Journal of Midwifery & Women's Health, 52,* 56–62.

Dansinger, M. L., Gleason, J. A., Griffith, J. L., Selker, H. P., & Schaefer, E. J. (2005). Comparison of the Atkins, Ornish, Weight Watchers, and Zone Diets for weight loss and heart disease risk reduction: A randomized trial. *The Journal of the American Medical Association, 293*, 43–53.

Dawson, D. A., Grant, B. F., & Li, T. K. (2005). Quantifying the risks associated with exceeding recommended drinking limits. *Alcoholism: Clinical and Experimental Research, 29*, 902–908.

Deacon, B., Lickel, J., & Abramowitz, J. S. (2008). Medical utilization across the anxiety disorders. *Journal of Anxiety Disorders, 22*, 344–350.

Devine, E. C. (1996). Meta-analysis of the effects of psychoeducational care in adults with asthma. *Research in Nursing & Health, 19*, 367–376.

Devine, E. C., & Pearcy, J. (1996). Meta-analysis of the effects of psychoeducational care in adults with chronic obstructive pulmonary disease. *Patient Education and Counseling, 29*, 167–178.

Diabetes Control and Complications Trial Research Group. (1993). The effect of intensive treatment of diabetes on the development and progression of long-term complications in insulin-dependent diabetes mellitus. *New England Journal of Medicine, 329*, 977–986.

Diabetes Prevention Program Research Group. (2002). Reduction in the incidence of type 2 diabetes with lifestyle intervention or metformin. *New England Journal of Medicine, 346*, 393–403.

Di Castelnuovo, A., Rotondo, S., Iacoviello, L., Donati, M. B., & de Gaetano, G. (2002). Meta-analysis of wine and beer consumption in relation to vascular risk. *Circulation, 105*, 2836–2844.

DiLillo, V., Siegfried, N. J., & West, D. S. (2003). Incorporating motivational interviewing into behavioral obesity treatment. *Cognitive and Behavioral Practice, 10*, 120–130.

DiMatteo, R. M., Giordani, P. J., Lepper, H. S., & Croghan, T. W. (2002). Patient adherence and medical treatment outcomes: A meta-analysis. *Medical Care, 40*, 794–811.

Dobmeyer, A. C. (2004). Women's health interventions in primary care OB/GYN. In C. L. Hunter (Chair), *The next big step: Translating specialty behavioral medicine interventions to primary medical settings across the life span*. Seminar conducted at the meeting of the Society of Behavioral Medicine, Baltimore, MD.

Dobson, K. S. (1989). A meta-analysis of efficacy of cognitive therapy for depression. *Journal of Consulting and Clinical Psychology, 57*, 414–419.

Doherty, D. E., Belfer, M. H., Brunton, S. A., Fromer, L., Morris, C. M., & Snader, T. C. (2006). Chronic obstructive pulmonary disease: Consensus recommendations for early diagnosis and treatment. *Journal of Family Practice, 56*(Suppl.), S1–S24.

Donnan, P. T., MacDonald, T. M., & Morris, A. D. (2002). Adherence to prescribed oral hypoglycaemic medication in a population of patients with Type 2 diabetes: A retrospective cohort study. *Diabetic Medicine, 19*, 279–284.

Drossman, D. A. (1994). Struggling with the controlling patient. *American Journal of Gastroenterology, 89*, 1441–1446.

Drossman, D. A., (2006). The functional gastrointestinal disorders and the Rome III process. *Gastroenterology, 130*, 1377–1390.

Drossman, D. A., Li, A., Andruzzi, E., Temple, R. D., Talley, N. J., Thompson, W. G., et al. (1993). U.S. householder survey of functional gastrointestinal disorders: Prevalence, sociodemography, and health impact. *Digest of digestive Science, 38*, 1569–1580.

Drossman, D. A., & Thompson, G. (1992). The irritable bowel syndrome: Review and a graduated multi-component treatment approach. *Annals of Internal Medicine, 116*, 1009–1016.

Dunkel, D., & Glaros, A. G. (1978). Comparison of self-instructional and stimulus control treatments for obesity. *Cognitive Therapy and Research, 2*, 75–78.

Dusseldorp, E., van Elderen, T., Maes, S., Meulman, J., & Kraaij, V. (1999). A meta-analysis of psycho-educational programs for coronary heart disease patients. *Health Psychology, 18*, 506–519.

Eaton, W. W. (2002). Epidemiologic evidence on the comorbidity of depression and diabetes. *Journal of Psychosomatic Research, 53*, 903–906.

Eaton, W. W., Smith, C., Ybarra, M., Muntaner, C., & Tien, A. (2004). Center for Epidemiological Studies Depression Scale: review and revision (CESD and CESD-R). In M. E. Maruish (Ed.), *The use of psychological testing for treatment planning and outcomes assessment: Volume 3 (Instruments for adults)* (pp. 363–377). Mahwah, NJ: Lawrence Erlbaum

Ebrahim, S., Beswick, A., Burke, M., & Davey Smith, G. (2006, October 18). Multiple risk factor interventions for primary prevention of coronary heart disease. *Cochrane Database of Systematic Reviews, 4*, Article CD001561. Retrieved August 5, 2007, from http://mrw.interscience.wiley.com/cochrane/clsysrev/articles/CD001561/frame.html

Eckel, R. H. (2006). Preventive cardiology by lifestyle intervention: Opportunity and/or challenge? Presidential address at the 2005 American Heart Association scientific sessions. *Circulation, 113*, 2657–2661.

Eckel, R. H., & Krauss, R. M. (1998). American Heart Association call to action: Obesity as a major risk factor for coronary heart disease. *Circulation, 97*, 2099–2100.

Edinger, J. D., & Sampson, W. S. (2003). A primary care "friendly" cognitive behavioral insomnia therapy. *Sleep, 26,* 177–182.

Eiser, A. R., & Ellis, G. (2007). Viewpoint: Cultural competence and the African American experience with health care: The case for specific content in cross-cultural education. *Academic Medicine, 82,* 176–183.

Elkin, I., Shea, T., Watkins, J. T., Imber, S. D., Sotsky, S. M., Collins, J. F., et al. (1989). National Institute of Mental Health Treatment of Depression Collaborative Research Program: General effectiveness of treatments. *Archives of General Psychiatry, 46,* 971–982.

Elley, C. R., Kerse, N., Arroll, B., & Robinson, E. (2003). Effectiveness of counselling patients on physical activity in general practice: Cluster randomised controlled trial. *British Medical Journal, 326,* 793–798.

Elmer, P. J., Obarzanek, E., Vollmer, W. M., Simons-Morton, D., Stevens, V. J., Young, D. R., et al. (2006). Effects of comprehensive lifestyle modification on diet, weight, physical fitness, and blood pressure control: 18-month results of a randomized trial. *Annals of Internal Medicine, 144,* 485–495.

Emery, C. F., Schein, R. L., Hauck, E. R., & MacIntyre, N. R. (1998). Psychological and cognitive outcomes of a randomized trial of exercise among patients with chronic obstructive pulmonary disease. *Health Psychology, 17,* 232–240.

Engle, G. L. (1977, April 8). The need for a new medical model: A challenge for biomedicine. *Science, 196,* 129–136.

Engel, J. M., Rapoff, M. A., & Pressman, A. R. (1992). Long-term follow-up of relaxation training for pediatric headache disorders. *Headache, 32,* 152–156.

Evans, J., Heron, J., Francomb, H., Oke, S., & Golding, J. (2001). Cohort study of depressed mood during pregnancy and after childbirth. *British Medical Journal, 323,* 257–260.

Expert Committee on the Diagnosis and Classification of Diabetes Mellitus. (1997). Report of the expert committee on the diagnosis and classification of diabetes mellitus. *Diabetes Care, 20,* 1183–1197.

Faith, M. S., Fontaine, K. R., Cheskin, L. J., & Allison, D. B. (2000). Behavioral approaches to the problems of obesity. *Behavior Modification, 24,* 459–493.

Falicov, C. J. (2001). The cultural meaning of money: The case of Latinos and Anglo Americans. *American Behavioral Scientist, 45,* 313–328.

Fallon, B. A. (2001). Pharmacological strategies for hypochondriasis. In V. Starcevic & D. R. Lipsitt (Eds.), *Hypochondriasis: Modern perspectives on an ancient malady* (pp. 329–351). New York: Oxford University Press.

Fallon, B. A., Schneier, F. R., Marshall, R., Campeas, R., Vermes, D., Goetz, D., et al. (1996). The pharmacotherapy of hypochondriasis. *Psychopharmacology Bulletin, 32,* 607–611.

Farrell, S., Kampert, J. B., Kohl, H. W., Barlow, C. E., Macera, C. A., Paffenbarger, R. S., et al. (1998). Influences of cardiorespiratory fitness levels and other predictors on cardiovascular disease mortality in men. *Medicine and Science in Sports and Exercise, 30,* 899–905.

Fine, L. J., Philogene, G. S., Gramling, R., Coups, E. J., & Sinha, S. (2004). Prevalence of multiple chronic disease risk factors: 2001 National Health Interview Survey. *American Journal of Preventive Medicine, 27*(Suppl. 1), 18–24.

Finger, W. W. (2007). Medications and sexual health. In L. VandeCreek, F. L. Peterson, Jr., & J. W. Bley (Eds.), *Innovations in clinical practice: Focus on sexual health* (pp. 47–61). Sarasota, FL: Professional Resource Press.

Finkelstein, E. A., Ruhm, C. J., & Kosa, K. M. (2005). Economic causes and consequences of obesity. *Annual Review of Public Health, 26,* 239–257.

Fiore, M., Bailey, W., Cohen, S., Dorfman, S., Goldstein, M., Gritz, E., et al. (2000). *Treating tobacco use and dependence. Clinical practice guideline.* Rockville, MD: U.S. Department of Health and Human Services, Public Health Service.

Fiore, M. C., Jaén C. R., Baker, T. B., Bailey, W. C., Benowitz, N. L., Curry, S. J., et al. (2008). *Treating tobacco use and dependence: 2008 Update. Clinical practice guideline.* Rockville, MD: U.S. Department of Health and Human Services, Public Health Service.

Fisher, L., & Glasgow, R. E. (2007). A call for more effectively integrating behavioral and social science principles into comprehensive diabetes care. *Diabetes Care, 30,* 2746–2749.

Fisher, L., Glasgow, R. E., Mullan, J. T., Skaff, M. M., & Polonsky, W. H. (2008). Development of a brief diabetes distress screening instrument. *Annals of Family Medicine, 6,* 246–252.

Fishman, S. M., & Kreis, P. (2002). The opioid contract. *The Clinical Journal of Pain, 18,* S70–S75.

Fleming, M., & Manwell, L. B. (1999). Brief intervention in primary care settings: A primary treatment method for at-risk, problem, and dependent drinkers. *Alcohol Research & Health, 23,* 128–137.

Florence, J. A., & Yeager, B. F. (1999). Treatment of type 2 diabetes mellitus. *American Family Physician, 59,* 2835–2844.

Folstein, M. F., Folstein, S. E., & McHugh, P. R. (1975). Mini-mental state: A practical method for grading the cognitive state of patients for the clinician. *Journal of Psychiatric Research, 12,* 189–198.

Frank, R. G., McDaniel, S. H., Bray, J. H., & Heldring, M. (Eds.). (2003). *Primary care psychology*. Washington, DC: American Psychological Association.

Freedland, K. E., Lustman, P. J., Carney, R. M., & Hong, B. A. (1992). Underdiagnosis of depression in patients with coronary artery disease: The role of nonspecific symptoms. *International Journal of Psychiatry in Medicine, 22,* 221–229.

Freedman, R. R. (2001). Physiology of hot flashes. *American Journal of Human Biology, 13,* 453–464.

Freedman, R. R., & Roehrs, T. A. (2006). Effects of REM sleep and ambient temperature on hot flash-induced sleep disturbance. *Menopause, 13,* 576–583.

Freedman, R. R., & Woodward, S. (1992). Behavioral treatment of menopausal hot flushes: Evaluation by ambulatory monitoring. *American Journal of Obstetrics & Gynecology, 167,* 436–439.

Friday, N. (1998). *Men in love.* New York: Dell.

Friday, N. (1998). *My secret garden: Women's sexual fantasies.* New York: Pocket Books.

Friedman, M., & Rosenman, R. H. (1959). Association of specific overt behavior pattern with blood and cardiovascular findings: Blood cholesterol level, blood clotting time, incidence of arcus, senilis, and clinical coronary artery disease. *The Journal of the American Medical Association, 169,* 1286–1296.

Friedmann, P. D., McCullough, D., Chin, M. H., & Saitz, R. (2000). Screening and intervention for alcohol problems. A national survey of primary care physicians and psychiatrists. *Journal of General Internal Medicine, 15,* 84–91.

Fries, J., Koop, C., & Beadle, C. (1993). Reducing health care costs by reducing the need and demand for medical services. *The New England Journal of Medicine, 329,* 321–325.

Furukawa, T. A., Watanabe, N., & Churchill, R. (2007, January 24). Combined psychotherapy plus antidepressants for panic disorder with or without agoraphobia. *Cochrane Database of Systematic Reviews, 1,* Article CD004364. Retrieved May 15, 2007, from http://mrw.interscience.wiley.com/cochrane/clsysrev/articles/CD004364/frame.html

Gagné M., A. (2005). What is collaborative mental health care? An introduction to the collaborative mental health care framework. *Canadian Collaborative Mental Health Initiative.* Retrieved September 12, 2008 from http://www.ccmhi.ca/en/products/series_of_papers.html

Gallagher-Thompson, D., & Coon, D. W. (2007). Evidence-based psychological treatments for distress in family caregivers of older adults. *Psychology and Aging, 22,* 37–51.

Gallo, J. J., Zubritsky, C., Maxwell, J., Nazar, M., Bogner, H. R., Quijano, L. M., et al. (2004). Primary care clinicians evaluate integrated and referral models of behavioral health care for older adults: Results from a multisite effectiveness trial (PRISM-E). *Annals of Family Medicine, 2,* 305–309.

Galuska, D. A., Will, J. C., Serdula, M. K., & Ford, E. S. (1999). Are health professionals advising obese patients to lose weight? *The Journal of the American Medical Association, 282,* 1576–1578.

Gambescia, N., & Weeks, G. (2006). Treatment of erectile dysfunction. In J. E. Fisher & W. T. O'Donohue (Eds.), *Practitioner's guide to evidence-based psychotherapy* (pp. 284–290). New York: Springer Publishing Company.

Gambescia, N., & Weeks, G. (2007). Sexual dysfunction. In N. Kazantzis & L. L'Abate (Eds.), *Handbook of homework assignments in psychotherapy: Research, practice, and prevention* (pp. 351–368). New York: Springer Publishing Company.

Gannon, L., Hansel, S., & Goodwin, J. (1987). Correlates of menopausal hot flushes. *Journal of Behavioral Medicine, 10,* 277–285.

Ganz, P. A., Greendale, G. A., Petersen, L., Zibecchi, L., Kahn, B., & Belin, T. R. (2000). Managing menopausal symptoms in breast cancer survivors: Results of a randomized controlled trial. *Journal of the National Cancer Institute, 92,* 1054–1064.

Gardner, C. D., Kiazand, A., Alhassan, S., Kim, S., Stafford, R. S., Balise, R. R., et al. (2007). Comparison of the Atkins, Zone, Ornish, and LEARN diets for change in weight and related risk factors among overweight premenopausal women: The A to Z weight loss study: A randomized trial. *The Journal of the American Medical Association, 297,* 969–977.

Gatchel, R. J., & Oordt, M. S. (2003). *Clinical health psychology and primary care: Practical advice and clinical guidance for successful collaboration.* Washington DC: American Psychological Association.

Gatchel, R. J., & Turk, D. C. (1996). *Psychological approaches to pain management: A practitioner's handbook.* New York: Guilford Press.

Gaynes, B. N., Gavin, N., Meltzer-Brody, Lohr, K. N., Swinson, T., Gartlehner, G., et al. (2005). *Perinatal depression: Prevalence, screening accuracy, and screening outcomes* (Evidence report/technology assessment No. 119. AHRQ publication No. 05-E006-2). Rockville, MD: Agency for Health Care Research and Quality.

Germain, A., Moul, D. E., Franzen, P. L., Miewald, J. M., Reynolds, C. F., Monk, T. H., et al. (2006). Effects of a brief behavioral treatment for late-life insomnia: Preliminary findings. *Journal of Clinical Sleep Medicine, 2,* 403–406.

Germaine, L. M., & Freedman, R. R. (1984). Behavioral treatment of menopausal hot flashes: Evaluation by objective methods. *Journal of Consulting and Clinical Psychology, 52,* 1072–1079.

Gilbody, S., Bower, P., Fletcher, J., Richards, D., & Sutton, A. J. (2006). Collaborative care for depression: a cumulative meta-analysis and review of longer-term outcomes. *Archives of Internal Medicine, 166,* 2314–2321.

Gillies, C. L., Abrams, K. R., Lambert, P. C., Cooper, N. J., Sutton, A. J., Hsu, R. T., et al. (2007). Pharmacological and lifestyle interventions to prevent or delay type 2 diabetes in people with impaired glucose tolerance: Systematic review and meta-analysis. *British Medical Journal, 334,* 299–307.

Glasgow, R. E., Fisher, L., Skaff, M., Mullan, J., & Toobert, D. J. (2007). Problem solving and diabetes self-management: Investigation in a large, multiracial sample. *Diabetes Care, 30,* 33–37.

Glasgow, R. E., Funnell, M. M., Bonomi, A. E., Davis, C., Beckham, V., & Wagner, E. H. (2002). Self-management aspects of the improving chronic illness care breakthrough series: Implementation with diabetes and heart failure teams. *Annals of Behavioral Medicine, 24,* pp. 80–87.

Glasgow, R. E., Nelson, C. C., Strycker, L. A., & King, D. K. (2006). Using RE-AIM metrics to evaluate diabetes self-management support interventions. *American Journal of Preventive Medicine, 30,* 67–73.

Glasgow, R. E., & Nutting, P. A. (2004). Diabetes. In L. J. Haas (Ed.), *Handbook of primary care psychology* (pp. 299–311). New York: Oxford University Press.

Glasgow, R. E., & Strycker, L. A. (2000). Preventive care practices for diabetes management in two primary care samples. *American Journal of Preventive Medicine, 19,* 9–14.

Glassman, A. H., O'Connor, C. M., Califf, R. M., Swedberg, K., Schwartz, P., Bigger, J. T., Jr., et al. (2002). Sertraline treatment of major depression in patients with acute MI or unstable angina: Sertraline antidepressant heart attack randomized. *The Journal of the American Medical Association, 288,* 701–709.

Glazer, H. I., & Laine, C. L. (2006). Pelvic floor muscle biofeedback in the treatment of urinary incontinence. *Applied Psychophysiology and Biofeedback, 31,* 187–201.

Global Initiative for Chronic Obstructive Lung Disease (GOLD). (2006). *Executive summary: Global strategy for the diagnosis, management, and prevention of COPD.* Retrieved July 20, 2007, from http://www.goldcopd.org/

Golden, S. H., Lazo, M., Carnethon, M., Bertoni, A. G., Schreiner, P. J., Diez Roux, A. V., et al. (2008). Examining a bidirectional association between depressive symptoms and diabetes. *The Journal of the American Medical Association, 2999,* 2751–2759.

Golden, S. H., Lee, H. B., Schreiner, P. J., Roux, A. D., Fitzpatrick, A. L., Szklo, M., et al. (2007). Depression and type 2 diabetes mellitus: The multiethnic study of atherosclerosis. *Psychosomatic Medicine, 69,* 529–536.

Goldstein, M. G., Whitlock, E. P., & DePue, J. (2004). Multiple behavioral risk factor interventions in primary care: Summary of research evidence. *American Journal of Preventive Medicine, 27*(Suppl. 2), 61–79.

Goodwin, R. D., Kroenke, K., Hoven, C. W., & Spitzer, R. L. (2005). Major depression, physical illness, and suicidal ideation in primary care. *Psychosomatic Medicine, 65,* 501–505.

Goodwin, R. D., Olfson, M., Shea, S., Lantigua, R. A., Carrasquilo, O., Gameroff, M. J., & Weissman, M. M. (2003). Asthma and mental disorders in primary care. *General Hospital Psychiatry, 25,* 479–483.

Gordon, S., & Waldo, M. (1984). The effects of assertiveness training on couples' relationships. *American Journal of Family Therapy, 12,* 73–77.

Gottman, J., & Silver, N. (1999). *The seven principles for making marriage work: A practical guide from the country's foremost relationship expert.* New York: Three Rivers.

Gray, G. V., Brody, D. S., & Johnson, D. (2005). The evolution of behavioral primary care. *Professional Psychology: Research and Practice, 36,* 123–129.

Gregg, J., & Saha, S. (2006). Losing culture on the way to competence: The use and misuse of culture in medical education. *Academic Medicine, 81,* 542–547.

Grigsby, A. B., Anderson, R. J., Freedland, K. E., Clouse, R. E. & Lustman, P. J. (2002). Prevalence of anxiety in adults with diabetes: A systematic review. *Journal of Psychosomatic Research, 53,* 1053–1060.

Gronbaek, M., Becker, U., Johansen, D., Gottschau, A., Schnohr, P., Hein, H. O., et al. (2000). Types of alcohol consumed and mortality from all causes, coronary heart disease, and cancer. *Annals of Internal Medicine, 133,* 411–419.

Guell, R., Resqueti, V., Sangenis, M., Morante, F., Martorell, B., Casan, P., et al. (2006). Impact of pulmonary rehabilitation on psychosocial morbidity in patients with severe COPD. *Chest, 129,* 899–904.

Hajek, P., Stead, L. F., West, R., Jarvis, M., & Lancaster, T. (2005, January 24). Relapse prevention interventions for smoking cessation. *Cochrane Database of Systematic Reviews, 1,* CD003999. Retrieved September 2, 2007, from the Cochrane Library Database at http://mrw.interscience.wiley.com/cochrane/clsysrev/articles/CD003999/frame.html

Hannestad, Y. S., Rortveit, G., Sandvik, H., & Hunaskaar, S. (2000). A community based epidemiological survey of female urinary incontinence: The Norwegian EPICONT study. *Journal of Clinical Epidemiology, 53,* 1150–1157.

Hartmann, U., Schedlowski, M., & Kruger, T. H. (2005). Cognitive and partner-related factors in rapid ejaculation: Differences between dysfunctional and functional men. *World Journal of Urology, 23,* 93–101.

Harvan, J. R., & Cotter, V. T. (2006). An evaluation of dementia screening in the primary care setting. *Journal of the American Academy of Nurse Practitioners, 18,* 351–360.

Haskell, W. L., Lee, I., Pate, R. R., Powell, K. E., Blair, S. N., Franklin, B. A., et al. (2007). Physical activity and public health: Updated recommendation for adults from the American College of Sports Medicine and the American Heart Association. *Medicine & Science in Sports & Exercise, 39,* 1423–1434.

Hatano, Y. (1993). Use of pedometer for promoting daily walking exercise. *Journal of the International Council for Health, Physical Education, Recreation, Sport and Dance, 29,* 4–8.

Havranek, E. P. (2006). Prevalence of depression in chronic heart failure. In E. Molinari, A. Compare, & G. Parati (Eds.), *Clinical psychology and heart disease* (pp. 100–108). Milan: Springer.

Hayes, S. C., & Strosahl, K. D. (Eds.). (2004). *A practical guide to acceptance and commitment therapy.* New York: Springer Publishing Company.

Hayes, S. C., Strosahl, K. D., & Wilson, K. G. (1999). *Acceptance and commitment therapy: An experiential approach to behavior change.* New York: Guildford Press.

Haynes, R. B., Yao, X., Degani, A., Kripalani, S., Garg, A., & McDonald, H. P. (2005, October 19). Interventions for enhancing medication adherence. *Cochrane Database of Systematic Reviews, 4,* Article CD000011. Retrieved August 5, 2007, from http://mrw.interscience.wiley.com/cochrane/clsysrev/articles/CD003999/frame.html

Hays, P. A. (2008). *Addressing cultural complexities in practice* (2nd ed.) Washington, DC: American Psychological Association.

Hay-Smith, E. J. C., & Dumoulin, C. (2006, January 25). Pelvic floor muscle training versus no treatment, or inactive control treatments, for urinary incontinence in women. *Cochrane Database of Systematic Reviews, 1,* Article CD005654. Retrieved August 15, 2007, from http://www.cochrane.org/reviews/en/ab005654.html

Heiman, J. (2000). Orgasmic disorders in women. In S. R. Leiblum & R. C. Rosen (Eds.), *Principles and practice of sex therapy* (3rd ed., pp. 118–153). New York: Guilford.

Heiman, J., & LoPiccolo, J. (1988). *Becoming orgasmic: A sexual and personal growth program for women.* New York: Simon & Schuster.

Hill, N. S. (2006). Pulmonary rehabilitation. *Proceedings of the American Thoracic Society, 3,* 66–74.

Hing, E., Cherry, D. K., & Woodwell, D. A. (2006). *National ambulatory medical care survey: 2004 summary. Advance Data from Vital and Health Statistics, 374,* 1–33.

Hogan, B. E., Linden, W., & Najarian B. (2002). Social support interventions: Do they work? *Clinical Psychology Review, 22,* 381–440.

Holsinger, T., Deveau, J., Boustani, M., & Williams, J. W. (2007). Does this patient have dementia? *The Journal of the American Medical Association, 297,* 2391–2404.

Holzmeister, L. (2006). *The diabetes carbohydrate and fat gram guide* (3rd ed.). Alexandria, VA: American Diabetes Association.

Horowitz, M. J., Wilner, N., & Alvarez, W. (1979). Impact of Event Scale: A measure of subjective stress. *Psychosomatic Medicine, 41,* 209–218.

Hughes, J. R., Stead, L. F., & Lancaster, T. (2007, January 24). Antidepressants for smoking cessation. *Cochrane Database of Systematic Reviews, 1,* Article CD000031. Retrieved September 2, 2007, from http://mrw.interscience.wiley.com/cochrane/clsysrev/articles/CD000031/frame.html

Hultquist, C. N., & Albright, C., & Thompson, D. L. (2005). Comparison of walking recommendations in previously inactive women. *Medical & Science in Sports & Exercise, 37,* 676–683.

Hunot, V., Churchill, R., Teixeira, V., & Silva de Lima, M. (2007, January 24). Psychological therapies for generalised anxiety disorder. *Cochrane Database of Systematic Reviews, 1,* Article CD001848. Retrieved May 15, 2007, from http://www.cochrane.org/reviews/en/ab001848.html

Hunter, M. S., & Liao, K. L. M. (1996). Evaluation of a four-session cognitive–behavioral intervention for menopausal hot flushes. *British Journal of Health Psychology, 1,* 113–125.

Hurlbert, D. F. (1991). The role of assertiveness in female sexuality: A comparative study between sexually assertive and sexually nonassertive women. *Journal of Sex and Marital Therapy, 17,* 183–190.

Iestra, J. A., Kromhout, D., van der Schouw, Y. T., Grobbee, D. E., Boshuizen, H. C., & van Staveren, W. A. (2005). Effect size estimates of lifestyle and dietary changes on all-cause mortality in coronary artery disease patients: A systematic review. *Circulation, 112,* 924–934.

Institute for Healthcare Improvement. (2007). *Patient centered care: General.* Retrieved May 12, 2007, from http://www.ihi.org/IHI/Topics/PatientCenteredCare/PatientCenteredCareGeneral

Institute of Medicine. (2002a). *Report brief. Speaking of health: Assessing health communications strategies for diverse population.* Retrieved May 12, 2007, from http://www.iom.edu/CMS/3775/4471/15432.aspx

Institute of Medicine. (2002b). *Unequal treatment: Confronting racial and ethnic disparities in health care.* Washington, DC: National Academies Press.

Irvin, J. H., Domar, A. D., Clark, C., Zuttermeister, P. C., & Friedman, R. (1996). The effects of relaxation response training on menopausal symptoms. *Journal of Psychosomatic Obstetrics & Gynecology, 17,* 202–207.

Irwin, M. R., Cole, J. C., & Nicassio, P. M. (2006). Comparative meta-analysis of behavioral interventions for insomnia and their efficacy in middle-aged adults and in older adults 55+ years of age. *Health Psychology, 25,* 3–14.

Isaacson, J. H. (2000). Preventing prescription drug abuse. *Cleveland Clinic Journal of Medicine, 67,* 473–475.

Isaacson, J. H., Hopper, J. A., Alford, D. P., & Parran, T. (2005). Prescription drug use and abuse: Risk factors, red flags, and prevention strategies. *Postgraduate Medicine, 118,* 19–26.

Isler, W. C., Hunter, C., Isler, D. E., & Peterson, A. (2003, March). *Minimal contact intervention for insomnia in primary care.* Poster session presented at the annual meeting of the Society of Behavioral Medicine, Salt Lake City, UT.

Jacobson, N. S. (1978). A stimulus control model of change in behavioral couples' therapy: Implications for contingency contracting. *Journal of Marriage and Family Counseling, 4,* 29–34.

Jakicic, J. M., Clark, K., Coleman, E., Donnelly, J. E., Foreyt, J., Melanson, E., et al. (2001). American College of Sports Medicine position stand. Appropriate intervention strategies for weight loss and prevention of weight regain for adults. *Medicine & Science in Sports & Exercise, 33*(12), 2145–2156.

Jamieson, D. J., & Steege, J. F. (1996). The prevalence of dysmenorrheal, dyspareunia, pelvic pain, and irritable bowel syndrome in primary care practices. *Obstetrics and Gynecology, 87,* 55–58.

Januzzi, J. L., Jr., Stern, T. A., Pasternak, R. C., & DeSanctis, R. W. (2000). The influence of anxiety and depression on outcomes of patients with coronary artery disease. *Archives of Internal Medicine, 160,* 1913–1921.

Johns, M. W. (1991). A new method for measuring daytime sleepiness: The Epworth Sleepiness scale. *Sleep, 14,* 540–545.

Johns, M. W. (2000). Sensitivity and specificity of the multiple sleep latency test (MSLT), the maintenance of wakefulness test and the Epworth sleepiness scale: Failure of the MSLT as a goal standard. *Journal of Sleep Research, 9,* 5–11.

Johnson, S. B., & Carlson, D. N. (2004). Medical regimen adherence: Concepts, assessment, and interventions. In T. J. Boll, J. M. Raczynski, & L. C. Leviton (Eds.), *Handbook of clinical health psychology* (pp. 329–354). Washington, DC: American Psychological Association.

Jost, B. C., & Grossberg, G. T. (1996). The evolution of psychiatric symptoms in Alzheimer's disease: A natural history study. *Journal of the American Geriatric Society, 44,* 1078–1081.

Joynt, K. E., & O'Connor, C. M. (2005). Lessons from SADHART, ENRICHD, and other trials. *Psychosomatic Medicine, 67,* S63–S66.

Kahn, E. B., Ramsey, L. T., Brownson, R. C., Heath, G. W., Howze, E. H., Powell, K. E., et al. (2002). The effectiveness of interventions to increase physical activity: A systematic review. *American Journal of Preventive Medicine, 22*(Suppl. 4), 73–107.

Kannel, W. B. (1996). Blood pressure as a cardiovascular risk factor. *The Journal of the American Medical Association, 275,* 1571–1576.

Karlin, B. E., & Fuller, J. D. (2007). Meeting the mental health needs of older adults: Implications for primary care practice. *Geriatrics, 62,* 26–35.

Katon, W. J., Russo, J. E., Von Korff, M., Lin, E. H. B., Ludman, E., & Ciechanowski, P. S. (2008). Long-term effects on medical costs of improving depression outcomes in patients with depression and diabetes. *Diabetes Care, 31,* 1155–1159.

Katz, S., Ford, A. B., Moskowitz, R. W., Jackson, B. A., & Jaffe, M. W. (1963). Studies of illness in the aged. The index of ADL: A standardized measure of biological and psychological function. *The Journal of the American Medical Association, 185,* 914–919.

Keating, G. M., & Siddiqui, M. A. A. (2006). Varenicline: A review of its use as an aid to smoking cessation therapy. *CNS Drugs, 20,* 945–960.

Kelly, M. P., Strassbert, D. S., & Kircher, J. R. (1990). Attitudinal and experiential correlates of anorgasmia. *Archives of Sexual Behavior, 19,* 165–172.

Kennedy, T., Jones, R., Darnley, S., Seed, P., Wessely, S., & Trudie, C. (2005). Cognitive behavior therapy in addition to antispasmodic treatment for irritable bowel syndrome in primary care: Randomized controlled trial. *British Medicine Journal, 331*(435), 1–6.

Kessler, R. C., Chiu, W. T., Demler, O., Merikangas, K. R., & Walters, E. E. (2005). Prevalence, severity, and comorbidity of 12-month DSM-IV disorders in the national comorbidity survey replication. *Archives of General Psychiatry, 62,* 617–627.

Kessler, R. C., Chiu, W. T., Jin, R., Ruscio, A. M., Shear, K., & Walters, E. E. (2006). The epidemiology of panic attacks, panic disorder, and agoraphobia in the national comorbidity survey replication. *Archives of General Psychiatry, 63,* 415–424.

Kessler, R. C., Sonnega, A., Bromet, E., Hughes, M., & Nelson, C. (1995). Posttraumatic stress disorder in the national comorbidity survey. *Archives of General Psychiatry, 52,* 1048–1060.

Kessler, R., & Stafford, D. (2008). Introduction. In R. Keesler & D. Stafford (Eds.), *Collaborative medicine case studies: Evidence in Practice* (pp. 3–8). New York: Springer.

Kilbourne, A. M., Reynolds, C. F., Good, C. B., Sereika, S. M., Justice, A. C., & Fine, M. J. (2005). How does depression influence diabetes medication adherence in older adults. *American Journal of Geriatric Psychiatry, 13,* 202–210.

Kincade, S. (2007). Evaluation and treatment of acute low back pain. *American Family Physician, 75,* 1181–1192.

King, A. C., Haskell, W. L., Young, D. R., Oka, R. K., & Stefanick, M. L. (1995). Long-term effects of varying intensities and formats of physical activity on participation rates, fitness, and lipoproteins in men and women aged 50 to 65 years. *Circulation, 91,* 2596–2604.

Kolb, D. A., & Boyatzis, R. E. (1970). Goal-setting and self-directed behavior change. *Human Relations, 23,* 439–457.

Kop, W. J. (1999). Chronic and acute psychological risk factors for clinical manifestation of coronary artery disease. *Psychosomatic Medicine, 61,* 476–487.

Kop, W. J., & Ader, D. N. (2006). Depression in coronary artery disease: Assessment and treatment. In E. Molinari, A. Compare, & G. Parati (Eds.), *Clinical psychology and heart disease* (pp. 109–119). Milan: Springer.

Kreuter, M. W., Scharff, D. P., Brennan, L. K., & Lukwago, S. N. (1997). Physician recommendations for diet and physical activity: Which patients get advised to change? *Preventive Medicine, 26,* 825–833.

Kroenke, K., & Mangelsdorff, A. D. (1989). Common symptoms in ambulatory care: Incidence, evaluation, therapy, and outcome. *American Journal of Medicine, 86,* 262–266.

Kroenke, K., Spitzer, R. L., & Williams, J. B. (2001). The PHQ-9: Validity of a brief depression severity measure. *Journal of General Internal Medicine, 16,* 606–613.

Kroenke, K., Spitzer, R. L., & Williams, J. B. (2003). The Patient Health Questionnaire-2: Validity of a two-item depression screener. *Medical Care, 41,* 1284–1292.

Kroenke, K., Spitzer, R. L., Williams, J. B. W., Monahan, P. O., & Löwe, B. (2007). Anxiety disorders in primary care: Prevalence, impairment, comorbidity, and detection. *Annals of Internal Medicine, 146,* 317–325.

Kunik, M. E., Braun, U., Stanley, M. A., Wristers, K., Molinary, V., Stoebner, D., et al. (2001). One session cognitive behavioural therapy for elderly patients with chronic obstructive pulmonary disease. *Psychological Medicine, 31,* 717–723.

Labott, S. M. (2004). COPD and other respiratory diseases. In P. M. Camic & S. J. Knight (Eds.), *Clinical handbook of health psychology: A practical guide to effective interventions* (2nd ed., pp. 59–74). Cambridge, MA: Hogrefe & Huber.

Lackner, J. M., Mesmer, C., Morley, S., Dowzer, C., & Hamilton, S. (2004). Psychological treatments for irritable bowel syndrome: A systematic review and meta-analysis. *Journal of Consulting and Clinical Psychology, 72,* 1100–1113.

Lancaster T., & Stead, L. F. (2005, April 20). Individual behavioural counselling for smoking cessation. *Cochrane Database of Systematic Reviews, 2,* Article CD001292. Retrieved September 2, 2007, from http://mrw.interscience.wiley.com/cochrane/clsysrev/articles/CD001292/frame.html

Lang, A. J., Laffaye, C., Satz, L. E., Dresselhaus, T. R., & Stein, M. B. (2003). Sensitivity and specificity of the PTSD checklist in detecting PTSD in female veterans in primary care. *Journal of Traumatic Stress, 16,* 257–264.

Lang, F. R., & Carstensen, L. L. (1994). Close emotional relationships in late life: Further support for proactive aging in the social domain. *Psychology and Aging, 9,* 315–324.

Lange, J. T., Lange, C. L., & Cabaltica, R. B. G. (2000). Primary care treatment of posttraumatic stress disorder. *American Family Physician, 62,* 1035–1040.

Lapierre, S., Dubeú, M., Bouffard, L., & Alain, M. (2007). Addressing suicidal ideations through the realization of meaningful personal goals. *Crisis, 28,* 16–25.

Larkin, K. T. (2005). *Stress and hypertension: Examining the relation between psychological stress and high blood pressure.* New Haven, CT: Yale University Press.

Laumann, E. O., Paik, A., & Rosen, R. C. (1999). Sexual dysfunction in the United States: Prevalence and predictors. *The Journal of the American Medical Association, 281,* 537–544.

Lawton, M. P., & Brody, E. M. (1969). Assessment of older people: Self-maintaining and instrumental activities of daily living. *The Gerontologist, 9,* 179–186.

Leahy, R. L. (2003). *Cognitive therapy techniques: A practitioner's guide.* New York: Guilford Press.

Lee, C. D., Blair, S. N., & Jackson, A. S. (1999). Cardiorespiratory fitness, body composition, and all-cause and cardiovascular disease mortality in men. *American Journal of Clinical Nutrition, 69,* 373–380.

Lesperance, F., & Frasure-Smith, N. (2000). Depression in patients with cardiac disease: A practical review. *Journal of Psychosomatic Research, 48,* 379–391.

Lett, H. S., Blumenthal, J. A., Babyak, M. A., Strauman, T. J., Robins, C., & Sherwood, A. (2005). Social support and coronary heart disease: Epidemiologic evidence and implications for treatment. *Psychosomatic Medicine, 67,* 869–878.

Leverence, R. R., Williams, R. L., Sussman, A., Crabtree, B. F., & RIOS Net Clinicians. (2007). Obesity counseling and guidelines in primary care: A qualitative study. *American Journal of Preventive Medicine, 32,* 334–339.

Levy, R. L., Olden, K. W., Naliboff, B. D., Bradley, L. A., Francisconi, C., Drossman, D. A., et al. (2006). Psychosocial aspects of the functional gastrointestinal disorders. *Gastroenterology, 130,* 1447–1458.

Lewington, S., Clarke, R., Qizilbash, N., Peto, R., & Collins, R. (2002). Age-specific relevance of usual blood pressure to vascular mortality. *The Lancet, 360,* 1903–1913.

Lewis, R. W., Fugl-Meyer, K. S., Bosch, R., Fugl-Meyer, A. R., Laumann, E. O., Lizza, E., et al. (2004). Epidemiology/risk factors of sexual dysfunction. *Journal of Sexual Medicine, 1,* 35–40.

Li, C., Friedman, B., Conwell, Y., & Fiscella, K. (2007). Validity of the Patient Health Questionnaire 2 (PHQ-2) in identifying major depression in older patients. *Journal of the American Geriatric Society, 55,* 596–602.

Lichtenstein, A. H., Appel, L. J., Brands, M., Carnethon, M., Daniels, S., Franch, H. A., et al. (2006). Diet and lifestyle recommendations revision 2006: A scientific statement from the American Heart Association Nutrition Committee. *Circulation, 114*(1), 82–96.

Lin, E. H., Katon, W., Von Korff, M., Bush, T., Lipscomb, P., Russo, J., et al. (1991). Frustrating patients: Physician and patient perspectives among distressed high users of medical services. *Journal of General Internal Medicine, 6,* 241–246.

Lindau, S. T., Schumm, L. P., Laumann, E. O., Levinson, W., O'Muircheartaigh, C. A., & Waite, L. J. (2007). A study of sexuality and health among older adults in the United States. *The New England Journal of Medicine, 357,* 762–774.

Lloyd, C., Smith, J., & Weinger, K. (2005). Stress and diabetes: A review of the links. *Diabetes Spectrum, 18,* 121–127.

Logsdon, M. C., Wisner, K., Billings, D. M., & Shanahan, B. (2006). Raising the awareness of primary care providers about postpartum depression. *Issues in Mental Health Nursing, 27,* 59–73.

Lohr, J. M., Tolin, D. F., & Lilienfeld, S. O. (1998). Efficacy of Eye Movement Desensitization and Reprocessing: Implications for behavior therapy. *Behavior Therapy, 29,* 123–156.

Longo, L. P., Parran, T., Johnson, B., & Kinsey, W. (2000). Addiction: Part II. Identification and management of the drug-seeking patient. *American Family Physician, 61,* 2401–2408.

Longstreth, G. F., Thompson, W. G., Chey, W. D., Houghton, L. A., Mearin, F., & Spiller, R. C. (2006).

Functional bowel disorders. *Gastroenterology, 130,* 1480–1491.

The Look AHEAD Research Group. (2006). The Look AHEAD study: A description of the lifestyle intervention and the evidence supporting it. *Obesity, 14,* 737–752.

LoPiccolo, J., & Stock, W. E. (1986). Treatment of sexual dysfunction. *Journal of Consulting and Clinical Psychology, 54,*158–167.

Lowe, B., Kroenke, K., & Grafe, K. (2005). Detecting and monitoring depression with a two-item questionnaire (PHQ-2). *Journal of Psychosomatic Research, 58,* 163–171.

Lucan, S. C., & Katz, D. L. (2006). Factors associated with smoking cessation counseling at clinical encounters: The Behavioral Risk Factor Surveillance System (BRFSS) 2000. *American Journal of Health Promotion, 21,* 16–23.

Lue, T. F., Giuliano, F., Montorsi, F., Rosen, R. C., Andersson, K., Althof, S., et al. (2004). Summary of the recommendations on sexual dysfunctions in men. *Journal of Sexual Medicine, 1,* 6–24.

Lustman, P. J., Penckofer, S. M., & Clouse, R. E. (2007). Recent advances in understanding depression in adults with diabetes. *Current Diabetes Reports, 7,* 114–122.

MacDonald, R., Fink, H. A., Huckabay, C., Monga, M., & Wilt, T. J. (2007). Pelvic floor muscle training to improve urinary incontinence after radical prostatectomy: A systematic review of effectiveness. *BJU International, 100,* 76–81.

Management of Major Depressive Disorder Working Group. (2000). *VHA/DoD Clinical practice guideline for management of major depressive disorder in adults.* Washington, DC: Department of Veterans Affairs.

Mannino, D., M., Homa, D. M., Akinbami, L. J., Ford, E. S., & Redd, S. C. (2002). Chronic obstructive pulmonary disease surveillance—United States, 1971–2000. *Respiratory Care, 47,* 1184–1199.

Manuck, S. B. (1994). Cardiovascular reactivity in cardiovascular disease: "Once more unto the breach." *International Journal of Behavioral Medicine, 1,* 4–31.

Masters, W. H., & Johnson, V. E. (1970). *Human sexual inadequacy.* Boston: Little, Brown.

Masters, W., Johnson, V., & Kolodny, R. (1995). *Human sexuality.* New York: HarperCollins.

Mathias, S. D., Kuppermann, M., Liberman, R. F., Lipschutz, R. C., & Steege, J. F. (1996). Chronic pelvic pain: Prevalence, health-related quality of life and economic correlates. *Obstetrics & Gynecology, 87,* 321–327.

Mayo Clinic (2005, July 19). *Menopause.* Retrieved April 26, 2007, from http://www.mayoclinic.com/health/menopause/DS00119

McAlpine, D. D., & Wilson, A. R. (2007). Trends in obesity-related counseling in primary care 1995–2004. *Medical Care, 45,* 322–329.

McCaig, L. F., & Nawar, E. W. (2006). National hospital ambulatory medical care survey: 2004 emergency department summary. *Advance Data from Vital and Health Statistics, 372,* 1–29.

McCarthy, B. W. (2001). Relapse prevention strategies and techniques with erectile dysfunction. *Journal of Sex and Marital Therapy, 27,* 1–8.

McCoy, P. M., & Nathan, P. (2007). Effectiveness of cognitive behavior therapy for diagnostically heterogeneous groups: a benchmarking study. *Journal of Consulting and Clinical Psychology, 75,* 344–350.

McDonald, J. S., & Elliott, M. L. (2001). Gynecologic pain syndromes. In J. D. Loeser, S. H. Butler, R. Chapman, & D. C. Turk (Eds.), *Bonica's management of pain* (pp. 1415–1447). Philadelphia, PA: Lippincott Williams & Wilkins.

McIntosh, A., Cohen, A., Turnbull, N., Esmonde, L., Dennis, P., Eatock, J., et al. (2004). *Clinical guidelines and evidence review for panic disorder and generalised anxiety disorder.* Sheffield, England: University of Sheffield/London: National Collaborating Centre for Primary Care.

McKnight, T. L. (2006). *Obesity management in family practice.* New York: Springer Publishing Company.

McMahon, C. G., Abdo, C., Incrocci, L, Perelman, M., Rowland, D., Waldinger, M., et al. (2004). Disorders of orgasm and ejaculation in men. *Journal of Sexual Medicine, 1,* 58–65.

McMahon, C. G., & Touma, K. (1999). Treatment of early ejaculation with paroxetine hydrochloride as needed: 2 single-blind placebo controlled crossover studies. *Journal of Urology, 161,* 1826–1830.

McNally, R. J. (2003). *Remembering trauma.* Cambridge, MA: Harvard University Press.

McQuaid, J. R., Stein, M. B., Laffaye, C., & McCahill, M. E. (1999). Depression in a primary care clinic: The prevalence and impact of an unrecognized disorder. *Journal of Affective Disorders, 55,* 1–10.

Meltzer-Brody, S., Churchill, E., & Davidson, J. R. T. (1999) Derivation of the SPAN, a brief diagnostic screening test for posttraumatic stress disorder. *Psychiatry Research, 88,* 63–70.

Melzack, R., & Wall, P. (1965, November 19). Pain mechanisms: A new theory. *Science, 150,* 971–979.

Merlijn, V. P. B. M., Hunfeld, J. A. M., van der Wouden, J. C., Hazebroek-Kampschreur, A. A. J. M., van Suijlekom-Smit, L. W. A., Koes, B. W., et al. (2005). A cognitive–behavioral program for adolescents with chronic pain: A pilot study. *Patient Education and Counseling, 59,* 126–134.

Meston, C. M., Hull, E., Levin, R. J., & Sipski, M. (2004). Disorders of orgasm in women. *Journal of Sexual Medicine, 1,* 66–68.

Metz, M. E., & McCarthy, B. W. (2003). *Coping with premature ejaculation: Overcome PE, please your partner, and have great sex.* Oakland, CA: New Harbinger.

Metz, M. E., & McCarthy, B. W. (2004). *Coping with erectile dysfunction: How to regain confidence and enjoy great sex.* Oakland, CA: New Harbinger.

Middleton, K. R., & Hing, E. (2006). National hospital ambulatory medical care survey: 2004 outpatient department summary. *Advance Data from Vital and Health Statistics, 373,* 1–27.

Miller, W. R., & Rollnick, S. (2002). *Motivational interviewing* (2nd ed.). New York: Guilford Press.

Miller, W. R., & Wilbourne, P. L. (2002). Mesa grande: A methodological analysis of clinical trials of treatments for alcohol use disorders. *Addiction, 97,* 265–277.

Miller, W. R., Zweben, J., & Johnson, W. R. (2005). Evidence-based treatment: Why, what, where, when and how? *Journal of Substance Abuse Treatment, 29,* 267–276.

Millner, V. S., & Ullery, E. K. (2002). A holistic treatment approach to male erectile disorder. *The Family Journal: Counseling and Therapy for Couples and Families, 10,* 443–447.

Milstein, R., & Slowinski, J. (1999). *The sexual male: Problems and solutions.* New York: Norton.

Mokdad, A. H., Ford, E. S., Bowman, B. A., Dietz, W. H., Vinicor, F., Bales, V. S., et al. (2003). Prevalence of obesity, diabetes, and obesity-related health risk factors, 2001. *The Journal of the American Medical Association, 289,* 76–79.

Mokdad, A. H., Marks, J. S., Stroup, D. F., & Gerberding, J. L. (2004). Actual causes of death in the United States, 2000. *The Journal of the American Medical Association, 291,* 1238–1245.

Morin, C. M., Bootzin, R. R., Buysse, D. J., Edinger, J. D., Espie, C. A., & Lichstein, K. L. (2006). Psychological and behavioral treatment of insomnia: Update of the recent evidence (1998–2004). *Sleep, 29,* 1398–1414.

Morin, C. M., Colecchi, C., Stone, J., Sood, R., & Brink, D. (1999). Behavioral and pharmacological therapies for late-life insomnia: A randomized controlled trial. *The Journal of the American Medical Association, 281,* 991–999.

Morin, C. M., & Espie, C. A. (2003). *Insomnia: A clinical guide to assessment and treatment.* New York: Kluwer Academic/Plenum Publishers.

Morin, C. M., Hauri, P. J., Espie, C. A., Spielman, A. J., Buysse, D. J., & Bootzin, R. R. (1999). Non-pharmacologic treatment of chronic insomnia. *Sleep, 22,* 1134–1156.

Morley, S., Eccleston, C., & Williams, A. (1999). Systematic review and meta-analysis of randomized controlled trials of cognitive behaviour therapy and behaviour therapy for chronic pain in adults, excluding headache. *Pain, 80,* 1–13.

Moye, J., Armesto, J. C., & Karel, M. J. (2005). Evaluating capacity of older adults in rehabilitation settings: Conceptual models and clinical challenges. *Rehabilitation Psychology, 50,* 207–214.

Moye, J., Gurrera, R. J., Karel, M. J., Edelstein, B., & O'Connell, C. (2006). Empirical advances in the assessment of the capacity to consent to medical treatment: Clinical implications and research needs. *Clinical Psychology Review, 26,* 1054–1077.

Murray, C. J. L., & Lopez, A. D. (Eds.). (1996). *The global burden of disease: A comprehensive assessment of mortality and disability for diseases, injuries, and risk factors in 1990 and projected to 2020:* Vol. 1 of Global Burden of Disease and Injury Series. Cambridge, MA: Harvard University Press.

Murray, L., & Carothers, A. D. (1990). The validation of the Edinburgh Postnatal Depression Scale on a community sample. *British Journal of Psychiatry, 157,* 288–290.

Musselman, D. L., Evans D. L., & Nemeroff, C. B. (1998). The relationship of depression to cardiovascular disease. *Archives of General Psychiatry, 55,* 580–592.

National Asthma Education and Prevention Program. (2007). *Expert panel report 3: Guidelines for the diagnosis and management of asthma* (National Institutes of Health Publication No. 07-4051). Retrieved August 8, 2007, from http://www.nhlbi. nih.gov/guidelines/asthma/asthgdln.pdf

National Center for Health Statistics. (2007a). *Incontinence by age, residence, sex, and race/ethnicity: Medicare Beneficiaries, 1992–2003.* Retrieved May 15, 2007, from http://www.cdc.gov/nchs/agingact.htm

National Center for Health Statistics. (2007b). *Visits to office-based physicians: Distribution by physician specialty, age, sex, and race. United States, Selected Years, 1975–2004.* Retrieved May 15, 2007, from http://www.cdc.gov/nchs/agingact.htm

National Cholesterol Education Program. (2002). *Third report on the expert panel on detection, evaluation, and treatment of high blood cholesterol in adults* (NIH Publication No. 02-5215). Retrieved January 6, 2007, from http://www.nhlbi.nih.gov/guidelines/cholesterol/atp3_rpt.htm

National Institute for Clinical Excellence. (2004). *Depression: Management of depression in primary and secondary care* (National Clinical Practice Guideline No. 26). Retrieved September 20, 2008, from http://www.nice.org.uk/nicemedia/pdf/cg23fullguideline.pdf

National Institute for Clinical Excellence. (2005). *Posttraumatic stress disorder: Management of PTSD in adult and children in primary and secondary care* (National Clinical Practice Guideline no 23). Retrieved May 15, 2007, from http://guidance.nice.org.uk/CG26/guidance/pdf/English

National Institute for Health and Clinical Excellence (2006). *Urinary incontinence: The management of urinary incontinence in women* (National Clinical Practice Guideline no. 40). Retrieved June 15, 2007, from http://www.nice.org.uk/nicemedia/pdf/cg40 fullguideline.pdf

National Institute of Diabetes and Digestive and Kidney Diseases. (2005). *National Diabetes Statistics fact sheet: General information and national estimates on diabetes in the United States, 2005.* Bethesda, MD: U.S. Department of Health and Human Services, National Institute of Health.

National Institutes of Health. (1991). Gastrointestinal surgery for severe obesity: Consensus Development Conference Panel. *Annals of Internal Medicine, 115,* 956–961

National Institutes of Health (2000). *The practical guide: Identification, evaluation, and treatment of overweight and obesity in adults* (NIH Publication No. 00-4084). Retrieved January 15, 2007, from http://www.nhlbi.nih.gov/guidelines/obesity/prctgd_c.pdf

National Institutes of Health/National Heart, Lung, and Blood Institute. (1998). *Clinical guidelines on the identification, evaluation, and treatment of overweight and obesity in adults.* Retrieved September 20, 2008, from www. nhlbi.nih.gov/gov/guidelines/obesity/ob_gdlns.pdf

National Institute on Alcohol Abuse and Alcoholism. (2000). *Tenth specialreport to the U.S. congress on alcohol abuse and alcoholism* (NIH publication no. 974017). Rockville, MD: Author.

National Institute on Alcohol Abuse and Alcoholism. (2007a). *Helping patients who drink too much: A clinician's guide* (NIH publication no. 07-3769). Rockville, MD: Author.

National Institute on Alcohol Abuse and Alcoholism. (2007b). *State of the science report on the effects of moderate drinking.* Rockville, MD: Department of Health and Human Services.

National Institute on Drug Abuse. (2005). *Research report series: Prescription drugs abuse and addiction* (NIH publication no. 05-4881). Rockville, MD: Author.

National Institute on Drug Abuse. (2006). *NIDA info facts: Prescription pain and other medications.* Retrieved March 24, 2007, from http://www.nida.nih.gov/PDF/Infofacts/PainMed06.pdf

National Kidney and Urologic Diseases Information Clearinghouse. (2005). *Erectile dysfunction.*

(National Institutes of Health Publication No. 06-3923). Bethesda, MD: Author.

Nelson, H. D., Haney, E., Humphrey, L., Miller, J., Nedrow, A., Nicolaidis, C., et al. (2005). Management of menopause-related symptoms. *Agency for Healthcare Research and Quality: Evidence Report/Technology Assessment, 120,* 1–6.

Nelson, M. E., Rejeski, W. J., Blair, S. N., Duncan, P. W., Judge, J. O., King, A. C., et al. (2007). Physical activity and public health in older adults: Updated recommendation from the American College of Sports Medicine and the American Heart Association. *Medicine & Science in Sports & Exercise, 39,* 1435–1445.

Newman, S., Steed, L., & Mulligan, K. (2004). Self-management interventions for chronic illness. *The Lancet, 364,* 1523–1537.

Nichols, G. A., & Brown, J. B. (2003). Unadjusted and adjusted prevalence of diagnosed depression in type 2 diabetes. *Diabetes Care, 26,* 744–749.

Nici, L., Donner, C., Wouters, E., Zuwallack, R., Ambrosino, N., Bourbeau, J., et al. (2006). American Thoracic Society/European Respiratory Society Statement on Pulmonary Rehabilitation. *American Journal of Respiratory Critical Care Medicine, 173,* 1390–1413.

Nield, L., Moore, H. J., Hooper, L., Cruickshank, J. K., Vyas, A., Whittaker, V., et al. (2007). Dietary advice for treatment of type 2 diabetes mellitus in adults. *Cochrane Database of Systematic Reviews, 3,* Article CD004097. Retrieved March 5, 2008, from http://mrw.interscience.wiley.com/cochrane/clsysrev/articles/CD004097/frame.html

Nisenson, L. G., Pepper, C. M., Schwenk, T. L., & Coyne, J. C. (1998). The nature and prevalence of anxiety disorders in primary care. *General Hospital Psychiatry, 20,* 21–28.

Norman, S. A., Lumley, M. A., Dooley, J. A., & Diamond, M. P. (2004). For whom does it work? Moderators of the effects of written emotional disclosure in a randomized trial among women with chronic pelvic pain. *Psychosomatic Medicine, 66,* 174–183.

Norris, S. L., Engelgau, M. M., & Narayan, K. M. V. (2001). Effectiveness of self-management training in type 2 diabetes: A systematic review of randomized controlled trials. *Diabetes Care, 24,* 561–587.

Norris, S. L., Grothaus, L. C., Buchner, D. M., & Pratt, M. (2000). Effectiveness of physician-based assessment and counseling for exercise in a staff model HMO. *Preventive Medicine, 30,* 513–523.

Norris, S. L., Zhang, X., Avenell, A., Gregg, E., Schmid, C. H., & Lau, J. (2005). Long-term non-pharmacological weight loss interventions for adults with prediabetes. *Cochrane Database of Systematic Reviews, 2,* Article CD005270. Retrieved March 5, 2008, from http://mrw.interscience.wiley.com/cochrane/clsysrev/articles/CD005270/frame.html

Nowell, P. D., Mazumdar, S., Buysse, D. J., Dew, M. A., Reynolds, C. F., & Kupfer, D. J. (1997). Benzodiazepines and zolpidem for chronic insomnia. *The Journal of the American Medical Association, 278,* 2170–2177.

Noyes, R. (2001). Hypochondriasis: Boundaries and comorbidities. In G. J. G. Asmundson, S. Taylor, & B. J. Cox (Eds.), *Health anxiety: Clinical and research perspectives on hypochondriasis and related conditions* (pp. 132–160). New York: John Wiley & Sons.

Núñez, A. E. (2000). Transforming cultural competence into cross-cultural efficacy in women's health education. *Academic Medicine, 75,* 1071–1080.

Nusbaum, M. R. H., & Hamilton, C. D. (2002). The proactive sexual health history. *American Family Physician, 66,* 1705–1712.

O'Donohue, W. T., Byrd, M. R., Cummings, N. A., & Henderson, D. A. (Eds.). (2005). *Behavioral integrative care: Treatments that work in the primary care setting.* New York: Brunner-Routledge.

Ogden, C. L., Carroll, M. D., Curtin, L. R., McDowell, M. A., Tabak, C. J., & Flegal, K. M. (2006). Prevalence of overweight and obesity in the United States, 1999–2004. *The Journal of the American Medical Association, 295,* 1549–1555.

O'Hara, M. W., & Swain, A. M. (1996). Rates and risk of postpartum depression: A meta-analysis. *International Review of Psychiatry, 8,* 37–54.

Okazaki, S., & Tanaka-Matsumi, J. (2006). Cultural consideration in cognitive–behavioral assessment. In H. A. Hays & G. Y. Iwamasa (Eds.), *Culturally responsive cognitive–behavioral therapy: Assessment, practice, and supervision* (pp. 247–266). Washington, DC: American Psychological Association.

Osterberg, L., & Blaschke, T. (2005). Adherence to medication. *New England Journal of Medicine, 353,* 487–497.

Ott, C. H., Lueger, R. J., Kelber, S. T., & Prigerson, H. G. (2007). Spousal bereavement in older adults: Common, resilient, and chronic grief with defining characteristics. *The Journal of Nervous and Mental Disease, 195,* 332–341.

Paasche-Orlow, M. (2004). The ethics of cultural competence. *Academic Medicine, 79,* 347–350.

Padwal, R., Li, S. K., & Lau, D. C. W. (2003, October 20). Long-term pharmacotherapy for obesity and overweight. *Cochrane Database of Systematic Reviews, 4,* Article CD004094. Retrieved September 2, 2007, from http://mrw.interscience.wiley.com/cochrane/clsysrev/articles/CD004094/frame.html

Paffenbarger, R. S., Hyde, R. T., Wing, A. L., & Hsieh, C. C. (1986). Physical activity, all-cause mortality, and longevity of college alumni. *New England Journal of Medicine, 314,* 605–613.

Palmer, C. (2005). Exercise as a treatment for depression in elders. *Journal of the American Academy of Nurse Practitioners, 17,* 60–66.

Parchman, M. L., Romero, R. L., & Pugh, J. A. (2006). Encounters by patients with type 2 diabetes— complex and demanding: An observational study. *Annals of Family Medicine, 4,* 40–45.

Parks, S. M., & Novielli, K. D. (2000). A practical guide to caring for caregivers. *American Family Physician, 62,* 2613–2622.

Pate, R. R., Pratt, M., Blair, S. N., Haskell, W. L., Macera, C. A., Bouchard, C., et al. (1995). Physical activity and public health: A recommendation from the Centers for Disease Control and Prevention and the American College of Sports Medicine. *The Journal of the American Medical Association, 273,* 402–407.

Pauwels, R. A., & Rabe, K. F. (2004). Burden and clinical features of chronic obstructive pulmonary disease (COPD). *The Lancet, 364,* 613–620.

Peak, C. J. (2008). Planning care in the clinical, operational and financial worlds. In R. Keesler & D. Stafford (Eds.), *Collaborative medicine case studies: Evidence in practice* (pp. 25–38). New York: Springer.

Perelman, M. A. (2006). A new combination treatment for premature ejaculation: A sex therapist's perspective. *Journal of Sexual Medicine, 3,* 1004–1012.

Perri, M. G., Martin, A. D., Leermakers, E. A., Sears, S. F., & Notelovitz, M. (1997). Effects of group- versus home-based exercise training in healthy older men and women. *Journal of Consulting and Clinical Psychology, 65,* 278–285.

Peterson, F. L., & Fuerst, D. E. (2007). Assessment and treatment of erection dysfunction. In L. VandeCreek, F. L. Peterson, Jr., & J. W. Bley (Eds.), *Innovations in clinical practice: Focus on sexual health* (pp. 119–134). Sarasota, FL: Professional Resource Press.

Peyrot, M., & Rubin, R. R. (2007). Behavioral and psychosocial interventions in diabetes: A conceptual review. *Diabetes Care, 30,* 2433–2440.

Piasecki, T. M. (2006). Relapse to smoking. *Clinical Psychology Review, 26,* 196–215.

Pincus, H. A., Tanielian, T. L., Marcus, S. C., Olfson, M., Zarin, D. A., Thompson, J., et al. (1998). Prescribing trends in psychotropic medications: Primary care, psychiatry, and other medical specialties. *The Journal of the American Medical Association, 279,* 526–531.

Pleis, J. R., & Lethbridge-Cejku, M. (2006). Summary health statistics for U.S. adults: National Health Interview Survey, 2005. *Vital Health Stat, 10,* 1–153.

Polonsky, D. C. (2000). Premature ejaculation. In S. R. Leiblum & R. C. Rosen (Eds.), *Principles and practice of sex therapy* (3rd ed., pp. 305–332). New York: Guilford Press.

Polonsky, W. H., Fisher, L., Earles, J., Dudl, R. J., Lees, J., Mullan, J., et al. (2005). Assessing psychosocial stress in diabetes. *Diabetes Care, 28,* 626–631.

Poston, W. S. C., Haddock, C. K., Pinkston, M. M., Pace, P., Reeves, R. S., Karakoc, N., et al. (2006). Evaluation of a primary care-oriented brief counseling intervention for obesity with and without orlistat. *Journal of Internal Medicine, 260,* 388–398.

Potter, M. B., Vu, J. D., & Croughan-Minihane, M. (2001). Weight management: What patients want from their primary care physicians. *Journal of Family Practice, 50,* 513–518.

Prigerson, H. G., Frank, E., Kasl, S. V., Reynolds, C. F., III, Anderson, B., Zubenko, G. S., et al. (1995). Complicated grief and bereavement-related depression as distinct disorders: Preliminary empirical validation in elderly bereaved spouses. *American Journal of Psychiatry, 152,* 22–30.

Prins, A., Ouimette, P., Kimerling, R., Cameron, R. P., Hugelshofer, D. S., Shaw-Hegwer, J., et al. (2003). The primary care PTSD screen (PC-PTSD): Development and operating characteristics. *Primary Care Psychiatry, 9,* 9–14.

Prochaska, J. O., & DiClemente, C. C. (1983). Stages of processes of self-change of smoking: Toward an integrative model of change. *Journal of Consulting and Clinical Psychology, 51,* 390–395.

Prochaska, J. O., & Velicer, W. F. (1997). The transtheoretical model of health behavior change. *American Journal of Health Promotion, 12,* 38–48.

Pronk, N. P., & Wing, R. R. (1994). Physical activity and long-term maintenance of weight loss. *Obesity Research, 2,* 587–599.

Qaseem, A., Vijan, S., Snow, V., Cross, J. T., Weiss, K. B., & Owens, D. K. (2007). Glycemic control and type 2 diabetes mellitus: The optimal hemoglobin A1c targets. A guidance statement from the American College of Physicians. *Annals of Internal Medicine, 147,* 417–422.

Qualls, S. H., Segal, D., Norman, S., Niederehe, G., & Gallagher-Thompson, D. (2002). Psychologists in practice with older adults: Current patterns, sources of training, and need for continuing education. *Professional Psychology: Research and Practice, 33,* 435–442.

Ranney, L., Melvin, C., Lux, L., McClain, E., & Lohr, K. N. (2006). Systematic review: Smoking cessation intervention strategies for adults and adults in special populations. *Annals of Internal Medicine, 145,* 845–856.

Rapkin, A. J. (1990). Neuroanatomy, neurophysiology, and neuropharmacology of pelvic pain. *Clinical Obstetrics and Gynecology, 33,* 119–129.

Regev, L. G., Zeiss, A., & Zeiss, R. (2006). Orgasmic disorders. In J. E. Fisher & W. T. O'Donohue (Eds.), *Practitioner's guide to evidence-based psychotherapy* (pp. 469–477). New York: Springer Publishing Company.

Rehm, J., Room, R., Graham, K., Monteiro, M., Gmel, G., & Sempos, C. T. (2003). The relationship of average volume of alcohol consumption and patterns of drinking to burden of disease: An overview. *Addiction, 98,* 1209–1228.

Reid, M. C., Fiellin, D. A., & O'Connor, P. G. (1999). Hazardous and harmful alcohol consumption in primary care. *Archives of Internal Medicine, 159,* 1681–1689.

Richard, D. C. S., & Lauterbach, D. (2007). *Handbook of exposure therapies.* Burlington, MA: Academic Press.

Ridgeway, N. A., Harvill, D. R., Harvill, L. M., Falin, T. M., Forester, G. M., & Gose, O. D. (1999). Improved Control of Type 2 Diabetes Mellitus: A Practical Education/Behavior Modification Program in a Primary Care Clinic. *Southern Medical Journal, 92,* 667–672.

Riecher-Rössler, A., & Hofecker Fallapour, M. (2003). Postpartum depression: Do we still need this diagnostic term? *Acta Psychiatrica Scandinavica, 108*(Suppl. 418), 51–56.

Ries, A. L. (2005). Pulmonary rehabilitation and COPD. *Seminars in Respiratory and Critical Care Medicine, 26,* 133–141.

Ries, A. L., Bauldoff, G. S., Carlin, B. W., Casaburi, R., Emery, C. F., Mahler, D. A., et al. (2007). Pulmonary rehabilitation: Joint ACCP/AACVPR evidence-based clinical practice guidelines. *Chest, 131,* 4S–42S.

Riley, A., & Riley, E. (1999). Relevant issues in diagnosis and management of psychosexual disorders. *Primary Care Psychiatry, 5,* 161–165.

Robinson, P. J., & Reiter, J. T. (2007). *Behavioral consultation and primary care: A guide to integrating services.* New York: Springer Publishing Company.

Robinson, P., Wischman, C., & Vento, A. D. (1996). *Treating depression in primary care: a manual for primary care and mental health providers.* Reno, NV: Context Press.

Rollnick, S., Mason, P., & Butler, C. (1999). *Health behavior change: A guide for practitioners.* London: Churchill Livingstone.

Rosal, M. C., Ockene, J. K., Luckmann, R., Zapka, J., Goins, K. V., Saperia, G., et al. (2004). Coronary heart disease multiple risk factor reduction: Providers perspectives. *American Journal of Preventive Medicine, 27,* 54–60.

Rosamond, W., Flegal, K., Friday, G., Furie, K., Go, A., Greenlund, K., et al. (2007). Heart disease and stroke statistics—2007 update: A report from the American Heart Association statistics committee and stroke statistics committee. *Circulation, 115,* e69–e171.

Rosen, R. C., & Leiblum, S. R. (1995). Treatment of sexual disorders in the 1990s: An integrated approach. *Journal of Consulting and Clinical Psychology, 63,* 877–890.

Rosen, R. C., Leiblum, S. R., & Spector, I. P. (1994). Psychologically based treatment for male erectile disorder: A cognitive–interpersonal model. *Journal of Sex and Marital Therapy, 20,* 67–85.

Rosqvist, J. (2005). *Exposure treatments for anxiety disorders: A practioner's guide to concepts, methods, and evidence-based practice.* New York: Routledge.

Roy-Byrne, P. P., Craske, M. G., Stein, M. B., Sullivan, G., Bystritsky, A., Katon, W., et al. (2005). A randomized effectiveness trial of cognitive–behavioral therapy and medication for primary care panic disorder. *Archives of General Psychiatry, 62,* 290–298.

Roy-Byrne, P. P., Davidson, K. W., Kessler, R. C., Asmundson, G. J. G., Goodwin, R. D., Kubzansky, L., et al. (2008). Anxiety disorders and comorbid medical illness. *General Hospital Psychiatry, 30,* 208–225.

Rozanski, A., Blumenthal, J. A., & Kaplan, J. (1999). Impact of psychological factors on the pathogenesis of cardiovascular disease and implications for therapy. *Circulation, 99,* 2192–2217.

Rudd, M. D., Joiner, T., & Rajab, M. H. (2001). *Treating suicidal behavior: An effective, time-limited approach.* New York: Guilford Press.

Ruff, G. A., & St. Lawrence, J. S. (1985). Premature ejaculation: Past research progress, future directions. *Clinical Psychology Review, 5,* 627–639.

Sabatino, C. P., & Basinger, S. L. (2000). Competency: Reforming our legal fictions. *Journal of Mental Health and Aging, 6,* 119–143.

Sacks, F. M., Svetkey, L. P., Vollmer, W. M., Appel, L. J., Bray, G. A., Harsha, D., et al. (2001). Effects on blood pressure of reduced dietary sodium and the dietary approaches to stop hypertension (DASH) diet. *New England Journal of Medicine, 344,* 3–10.

Salkovskis, P. M., Rimes, K. A., Warwick, H. M. C., & Clark, D. M. (2002). The health anxiety inventory: Development and validation of scales for the measurement of health anxiety and hypochondriasis. *Psychological Medicine, 32,* 843–853.

Salkovskis, P. M., & Warwick, H. M. C. (2001). Making sense of hypochondriasis: A cognitive model of health anxiety. In G. J. G. Asmundson, S. Taylor, & B. J. Cox (Eds.), *Health anxiety: Clinical and research perspectives on hypochondriasis and related conditions* (pp. 46–64). New York: John Wiley & Sons.

Salkovskis, P. M., Warwick, H. M. C., & Deale, A. C. (2003). Cognitive–behavioral treatment for severe and persistent health anxiety (hypochondriasis). *Brief Treatment and Crisis Intervention, 3,* 353–367.

Salthouse, T. A. (2004). What and when of cognitive aging. *Current Directions in Psychological Science, 13,* 140–144.

Salthouse, T. A. (2006). Mental exercise and mental aging: Evaluating the validity of the "use it or lose it" hypothesis. *Perspectives on Psychological Science, 1,* 68–87.

Saltzman, E., Anderson, W., Apovian, C. M., Boulton, H., Chamberlain, A., Cullum-Dugan, D., et al. (2005). Criteria for patient selection and multidisciplinary evaluation and treatment of the weight loss surgery patient. *Obesity Research, 13,* 234–243.

Sanford, S. D., Lichstein, K. L., Durrence, H. H., Riedel, G. W., Taylor, D. J., & Bush, A. J. (2006). The influence of age, gender, ethnicity, and insomnia on Epworth sleepiness scores: A normative US population. *Sleep Medicine, 7,* 319–326.

Scheidt, S. (1996). A whirlwind tour of cardiology for the mental health professional. In R. Allan & S. Scheidt (Eds.), *Heart and mind: The practice of cardiac psychology* (pp. 15–62). Washington, DC: American Psychological Association.

Schneider, P. L., Crouter, S. E., & Bassett, D. R. (2004). Pedometer measures of free-living physical activity: Comparison of 13 models. *Medicine & Science in Sports & Exercise, 36,* 331–335.

Schochat, T., Umphress, J., Israel, A., & Ancoli-Israel, S. (1999). Insomnia in primary care patients. *Sleep, 22,* S359–S365.

Schols, A. M., Slangen, J., Volovics, L., & Wouters, E. F. (1998). Weight loss is a reversible factor in the prognosis of chronic obstructive pulmonary disease. *American Journal of Respiratory and Critical Care Medicine, 157,* 1791–1797.

Schulberg, H. C., Katon, W., Simon, G. E., & Rush, A. J. (1998). Treating major depression in primary care practice: An update of the agency for health care policy and research practice guidelines. *Archives of General Psychiatry, 55,* 1121–1127.

Schulberg, H. C., Raue, P. J., & Rollman, B. L. (2002). The effectiveness of psychotherapy in treating depressive disorders in primary care practice: Clinical and cost perspectives. *General Hospital Psychiatry, 24,* 203–212.

Schwartz, S. M., Trask, P. C., & Ketterer, M. W. (1999). Understanding chest pain: What every psychologist should know. *Journal of Clinical Psychology in Medical Settings, 6,* 333–351.

Sears, S. F., Todaro, J. F., Lewis, T. S., Sotile, W., & Conti, J. B. (1999). Examining the psychosocial impact of implantable cardioverter defibrillators: A literature review. *Clinical Cardiology, 22,* 481–489.

Segraves, R. T. (2003). Pharmacological management of sexual dysfunction: Benefits and limitations. *CNS Spectrums, 8,* 225–229.

Seitz, D. P. (2005). Screening mnemonic for generalized anxiety disorder. *Canadian Family Physician, 51,* 1340–1342.

Semans, J. H. (1956). Premature ejaculation: New approach. *Southern Medical Journal, 49,* 353–358.

Shadel, W. G., & Niaura, R. (2003). Brief behavioral treatment. In D. B. Abrams, R. Niaura, R. A. Brown, K. M. Emmons, M. G. Goldstein, & P. M. Monti (Eds.), *The tobacco dependence treatment handbook* (pp. 101–117). New York: Guilford Press.

Shapiro, F. (1989) Eye movement desensitization: A new treatment for posttraumatic stress disorder. *Journal of Behavior Therapy and Experimental Psychiatry, 20,* 211–217.

Sharp, L. K., & Lipsky, M. S. (2002). Screening for depression across the lifespan: A review of measures for use in primary care settings. *American Family Physician, 66,* 1001–1008.

Shaw, E., Levitt, C., Wong, S., & Kaczorowski, J. (2006). Systematic review of the literature on postpartum care: Effectiveness of postpartum support to improve maternal patenting, mental health, quality of life, and physical health. *BIRTH, 33,* 210–220.

Sherbourne, C. D., Hays, R. D., Ordway, L., DiMatteo, M. R., & Kravitz, R. L. (1992). Antecedents of adherence to medical recommendations: Results from the medical outcomes study. *Journal of Behavioral Medicine, 15,* 447–469.

Shiina, A., Nakazato, M., Mitsumori, M., Koizumi, H., Shimizu, E., Fujisaki, M., et al. (2005). An open trial of outpatient group therapy for bulimic disorders: Combination program of cognitive behavioral therapy with assertive training and self-esteem enhancement. *Psychiatry and Clinical Neurosciences, 59,* 690–696.

Shoup, R., Dalsky, G., Warner, S., Davies, M., Connors, M., Khan, M., et al. (1997). Body composition and health-related quality of life in patients with obstructive airway disease. *European Respiratory Journal, 10,* 1576–1580.

Shulman, K. I. (2000). Clock drawing: Is it the ideal screening test? *International Journal of Geriatric Psychiatry, 15,* 548–561.

Silagy, C., Lancaster, T., Stead, L., Mant, D., & Fowler, G. (2004, July 19). Nicotine replacement therapy for smoking cessation. *Cochrane Database of Systematic Reviews, 3,* Article CD000146. Retrieved September 2, 2007, from http://mrw.interscience.wiley.com/cochrane/clsysrev/articles/CD000146/frame.html

Simon, G. E., Katon, W. J., Lin, E. H., Rutter, C., Manning, W. G., Von Korff, M., et al. (2007). Cost-effectiveness of systematic depression treatment among people with diabetes mellitus. *Archives of General Psychiatry, 64,* 65–72.

Simons, J. S., & Carey, M. P. (2001). Prevalence of sexual dysfunctions: Results from a decade of research. *Archives of Sexual Behavior, 30,* 177–219.

Sivertsen, B., Omvik, S., Pallesen, S., Bjorvatn, B., Havik, O. E., Kvale, G., et al. (2006). Cognitive behavioral therapy vs zopiclone for treatment of chronic primary insomnia in older adults: A randomized controlled trial. *The Journal of the American Medical Association, 295,* 2851–2858.

Skultety, K. M., & Zeiss, A. (2006). The treatment of depression in older adults in the primary care setting: An evidence-based review. *Health Psychology, 6,* 665–674.

Smith, D. (2002, January). Psychologists now eligible for reimbursement under six new health and behavior codes. *Monitor on Psychology, 33,* 19.

Smith, D. E., Heckemeyer, C. M., Kratt, P. P., & Mason, D. A. (1997). Motivational interviewing to improve adherence to a behavioral weight-control program for older obese women with NIDDM: A pilot study. *Diabetes Care, 20,* 53–54.

Smith, G. R., Rost, K., & Kashner, T. M. (1995). A trial of the effect of a standardized psychiatric consultation on health outcomes and costs in somatizing patients. *Archives of General Psychiatry, 52,* 238–243.

Smith, M. T., & Wegener, S. T. (2003). Measures of sleep: The Insomnia Severity Index, Medical Outcomes Study (MOS) Sleep Scale, Pittsburgh Sleep Diary (PSD), and Pittsburgh Sleep Quality Index (PSQI). *Arthritis and Rheumatism, 49,* S184–S196.

Smith S., & Trinder, J. (2001). Detecting insomnia: Comparison of four self-report measures of sleep in a young adult population. *Journal of Sleep Research, 10,* 229–235.

Smitherman, T. A., Kendzor, D. E., Grothe, K. B., & Dubbert, P. M. (2007). Promoting physical activity changes in primary care settings: A review of cognitive and behavioral strategies. *American Journal of Lifestyle Medicine, 1,* 397–409.

Spanier, J. A., Howden, C., W., & Jones, M. P. (2003). A systematic review of alternative therapies in the irritable bowel syndrome. *Archives of Internal Medicine, 163,* 265–274.

Spann, S. J., Nutting, P. A., Galliher, J. M., Peterson, K. A., Pavlik, V. N., Dickinson, L. M., et al. (2006). Management of type 2 diabetes in the primary care setting: A practice-based research network study. *Annals of Family Medicine, 4,* 23–31.

Spitzer, R. L., Kroenke, K., Linzer, M., Hahn, S. R., Williams, J. B., deGruy, F. V., III, et al. (1995). Health-related quality of life in primary care patients with mental disorders. Results from the PRIME-MD 1000 study. *The Journal of the American Medical Association, 274,* 1511–1517.

Spitzer, R. L., Kroenke, K., Williams, J. B. W., & Löwe, B. (2006). A brief measure for assessing generalized anxiety disorder: The GAD-7. *Archives of Internal Medicine, 166,* 1092–1097.

Spitzer, R. L., Yanovski, S. Z., Wadden, T. A., Marcus, M. D., Stunkard, A. J., Devlin, M., et al. (1993). Binge eating disorder: Its further validation in a multisite study. *International Journal of Eating Disorders, 13,* 137–153.

Stanley, M. A., Hopko, D. R., Diefenbach, G. J., Bourland, S. L., Rodriguez, H., & Wagener, P. (2003). Cognitive behavior therapy for late-life generalized anxiety disorder in primary care: Preliminary findings. *American Journal of Geriatric Psychiatry, 11,* 92–96.

Stanley, M. A., Roberts, R. E., Bourland, S. L., & Novy, D. M. (2001). Anxiety disorders among older primary care patients. *Journal of Clinical Geropsychology, 7,* 105–116.

Stanton, A. L. (1987). Determinants of adherence to medical regimens by hypertensive patients. *Journal of Behavioral Medicine, 10,* 377–394.

Stathopoulou, G., Powers, M. B., Berry, A. C., Smits, J. A. J., & Otto, M. W. (2006). Exercise interventions for mental health: A quantitative and qualitative review. *Clinical Psychology: Science and Practice, 13,* 179–193.

Stead, L. F., & Lancaster, T. (2005, April 20). Group behaviour therapy programmes for smoking cessation. *Cochrane Database of Systematic Reviews, 2,* Article CD001007. Retrieved September 2, 2007, from http://mrw.interscience.wiley.com/cochrane/clsysrev/articles/CD001007/frame.html

Stein, D. J., Ipser, J. C., & Seedat, S. (2006, January 25). Pharmacotherapy for post traumatic stress disorder (PTSD). *Cochrane Database of Systematic Reviews, 1,* Article CD002795. Retrieved May 15, 2007, from http://mrw.interscience.wiley.com/cochrane/clsysrev/articles/CD006239/frame.html

Stein, M. B., Kirk, P., Prabhu, V., Grott, M., & Terepa, M. (1995). Mixed anxiety-depression in a primary care clinic. *Journal of Affective Disorders, 34,* 79–84.

Stein, M. B., Roy-Byrne, P. P., McQuaid, J. R., Laffaye, C., Russo, J., McCahill, M., et al. (1999). Development of a brief diagnostic screen for panic disorder in primary care. *Psychosomatic Medicine, 61,* 359–364.

Steinman, L. E., Frederick, J. T., Prohaska, T., Satariano, W. A., Dornberg-Lee, S., Fisher, R., et al. (2007). Recommendations for treating depression in community-based older adults. *American Journal of Preventive Medicine, 33,* 175–181.

Stevenson, D. W., & Delprato, D. J. (1983). Multiple component self-control program for menopausal hot flashes. *Journal of Behavior Therapy & Experimental Psychiatry, 14,* 137–140.

Stewart, M., Brown, J. B., Boon, H., Galajda, J., Meredith, L., & Sangster, M. (1999). Evidence on patient–doctor communication. *Cancer Prevention and Control, 3*, 25–30.

Stewart, S. H., & Watt, M. C. (2001). Assessment of health anxiety. In G. J. G. Asmundson, S. Taylor, & B. J. Cox (Eds.) *Health anxiety: Clinical and research perspectives on hypochondriasis and related conditions* (pp. 95–131). New York: John Wiley & Sons.

Strosahl, K., & Robinson, P. (2008). The primary care behavioral health model: Applications to prevention, acute care and chronic condition management. In R. Keesler & D. Stafford (Eds.), *Collaborative medicine case studies: Evidence in practice* (pp. 85–95). New York: Springer.

Substance Abuse and Mental Health Services Administration. (2006). *Results from the 2005 National Survey on Drug Use and Health: National findings* (Office of Applied Studies, NSDUH Series H-30, DHHS Publication No. SMA 06-4194). Rockville, MD: Author.

Surwit, R. S., & Schneider, M. S. (1993). Role of stress in the etiology and treatment of diabetes mellitus. *Psychosomatic Medicine, 55*, 380–393.

Surwit, R. S., van Tilburg, M. A. L., Zucker, N., McCaskill, C. C., Parekh, P., Feinglos, M. N., et al. (2002). Stress management improves long-term glycemic control in type 2 diabetes. *Diabetes Care, 25*, 30–34.

Swartzman, L. C., Edelberg, R., & Kemmann, E. (1990). Impact of stress on objectively recorded menopausal hot flushes and on flush report bias. *Health Psychology, 9*, 529–545.

Symonds, T., Roblin, D., Hart, K., & Althof, S. (2003). How does premature ejaculation impact a man's life? *Journal of Sex and Marital Therapy, 29*, 361–370.

Takigawa, N., Tada, A., Soda, R., Takahashi, S., Kawata, N., Shibayama, T., et al. (2007). Comprehensive pulmonary rehabilitation according to severity of COPD. *Respiratory Medicine, 101*, 326–332.

Talcott, G. W., Russ, C. R., & Dobmeyer, A. (2001, October). *Integrating behavioral health providers into primary care in the USAF: The behavioral health optimization project.* Paper presented at the Behavioral Healthcare Tomorrow Conference, Washington, DC.

Talley, N. J., Zinsmeister, A. R., Van Dyke, C., & Melton, L. J. (1991). Epidemiology of colonic symptoms and the irritable bowel syndrome. *Gastroenterology, 101*, 927–934.

Tanaka-Matsumi, J., Seiden, D. Y., & Lam, K. N. (1996). The culturally informed functional assessment (CIFA) interview: A strategy for cross-cultural behavioral practice. *Cognitive and Behavioral Practice, 3*, 215–233.

Tangalos, E. G., Smith, G. E., Ivnik, R. J., Petersen, R. C., Kokmen, E., Kurland, L. T., et al. (1996). The Mini-Mental State Examination in general medical practice: Clinical utility and acceptance. *Mayo Clinic Proceedings, 71*, 829–837.

Taylor, S., & Asmundson, G. J. G. (2004). *Treating health anxiety: A cognitive–behavioral approach.* New York: Guilford Press.

Taylor, S., & Asmundson, G. J. G., & Coons, M. (2005). Current directions in the treatment of hypochondriasis. *Journal of Cognitive Psychotherapy, 19*, 285–304.

The Look AHEAD Research Group. (2006). The Look AHEAD study: A description of the lifestyle intervention and the evidence supporting it. *Obesity, 14*, 737–752.

Thomson, N. C., Chaudhuri, R., & Livingston, E. (2004). Asthma and cigarette smoking. *European Respiratory Journal, 24*, 822–833.

Thornton, M., & Travis, S. S. (2003). Analysis of the reliability of the Modified Caregiver Strain Index. *Journal of Gerontology Series B: Psychological Sciences Social Sciences, 58*, S127–132.

Tombaugh, T. N., & McIntyre, N. J. (1992). The Mini-Mental State Examination: A comprehensive review. *Journal of the American Geriatrics Society, 40*, 922–935.

Toner, B. B., Segal, Z. V., Emmott, S. D., & Myran, D. (2000). *Cognitive–behavioral treatment of irritable bowel syndrome: The brain–gut connection.* New York: Guilford Press.

Toobert, D. J., Hampson, S. E., & Glasgow, R. E. (2000). The summary of diabetes self-care activities measure. *Diabetes Care, 23*, 943–950.

Toomey, T. C., Hernandez, J. T., Gittelman, D. F., & Hulka, J. F. (1994). Relationship of sexual and physical abuse to pain and psychological assessment variables in chronic pelvic pain patients. *Pain, 53*, 105–109.

Topolski, T. D., LoGerfo, J., Patrick, D. L., Williams, B. Walwick, J., & Patrick, M. B. (2006). The rapid assessment of physical activity (RAPA) among older adults. *Preventing Chronic Disease, 3.* Retrieved September 3, 2007, from http://www.pubmedcentral.nih.gov/articlerender.fcgi?artid=1779282

Trumper, A., & Appleby, L. (2001). Psychiatric morbidity in patients undergoing heart, heart and lung, or lung transplantation. *Journal Psychosomatic Research, 50*, 103–105.

Tully, M. A., Cupples, M. E., & Young, I. S. (2004). Promoting physical activity in primary care: How to get over the hurdles? *The Ulster Medical Journal, 73*, 1–3.

Turk, D. C., & Monarch, E. S. (2002). Biopsychosocial perspective on chronic pain. In D. C. Turk & R. J. Gatchel (Eds.), *Psychological approaches to pain management: A practitioner's handbook* (2nd ed., pp. 3–29). New York: Guilford Press.

Tyrer, P., Seivewright, H., & Behr, G. (1999). A specific treatment for hypochondriasis? *The Lancet, 353,* 672–673.

University of Washington Health Promotion Research Center. (n.d.) *Rapid Assessment Physical Activity Scale (RAPA).* Retrieved September 2, 2007 from http://depts.washington.edu/hprc/docs/rapa_03_06.pdf

U.S. Department of Health and Human Services. (1996). *Physical activity and health: A report of the Surgeon General.* Atlanta, GA: U.S. Department of Health and Human Services, Centers for Disease Control and Prevention, National Center for Chronic Disease Prevention and Health Promotion.

U.S. Department of Health and Human Services. (1999). *Mental health: A report of the Surgeon General.* Rockville, MD: National Institutes of Health, National Institute of Mental Health.

U.S. Department of Health and Human Services. (2000, November). *Healthy people 2010: Understanding and improving health and objectives for improving health* (2nd ed.). Washington, DC: Government Printing Office.

U.S. Department of Health and Human Services. (2004a). *The seventh report of the Joint National Committee on Prevention, Detection, Evaluation, and Treatment of High Blood Pressure* (NIH Publication No. 04–5230). Retrieved January 6, 2007, from http://www.nhlbi.nih.gov/guidelines/hypertension/jnc7full.pdf

U.S. Department of Health and Human Services. (2004b). *The Health Consequences of Smoking: A Report of the Surgeon General.* Atlanta, GA: U.S. Department of Health and Human Services, Centers for Disease Control and Prevention, National Center for Chronic Disease Prevention and Health Promotion, Office on Smoking and Health.

U.S. Department of Health and Human Services. (2005). *Your guide to lowering your cholesterol with TLC* (NIH Publication No. 06-5235). Retrieved January 6, 2007, from http://www.nhlbi.nih.gov/health/public/heart/chol/chol_tlc.pdf

U.S. Department of Health and Human Services. (2006). *Your Guide to Lowering Your Blood Pressure with DASH* (NIH Publication No. 06-4082). Retrieved January 6, 2007, from http://www.nhlbi.nih.gov/health/public/heart/hbp/dash/new_dash.pdf

U.S. Department of Health and Human Services & U.S. Department of Agriculture. (2005). *Dietary Guidelines for Americans, 2005* (6th ed.). Washington, DC: U.S. Government Printing Office.

U.S. Food and Drug Administration. (n.d.). *Alternatives to High-Sodium Foods.* Retrieved January 15, 2007, from http://www.fda.gov/fdac/foodlabel/sodtabl.html

U.S. Preventive Services Task Force. (2002a). Behavioral counseling in primary care to promote physical activity: Recommendation and rationale. *Annals of Internal Medicine, 137,* 205–207.

U.S. Preventive Services Task Force. (2002b). Screening for depression: Recommendations and rationale. *Annals of Internal Medicine, 136,* 760–764.

U.S. Preventive Services Task Force. (2004). Screening and behavioral counseling interventions in primary care to reduce alcohol misuse. *Annals of Internal Medicine, 140,* 554–556.

van Boeijen, C. A, van Oppen, P. van Balkom, A. J. L. M., Visser, S., Kempe, P. T., Blankenstein, N., et al. (2005). Treatment of anxiety disorders in primary care: A randomized controlled trial. *British Journal of General Practice, 55,* 763–769.

van Lankveld, J. (1998). Bibliotherapy in the treatment of sexual dysfunctions: A meta-analysis. *Journal of Consulting and Clinical Psychology, 66,* 702–708.

van Schaik, D. J. F., Klijn, A. F., van Hout, H. P. J., van Marwijk, H. W. J., Beekman, A. T. F., de Haan, M., et al. (2004). Patients' preferences in the treatment of depressive disorder in primary care. *General Hospital Psychiatry, 26,* 184–189.

Vasan, R. S., Beiser, A., Seshadri, S., Larson, M. G., Kannel, W. B., D'Agostino, R. B., et al. (2002). Residual lifetime risk for developing hypertension in middle-aged women and men: The Framingham Heart Study. *The Journal of the American Medical Association, 287,* 1003–1010.

Vermeire, E., Wens, J., Van Royen, P., Biot, Y., Hearnshaw, H., & Lindenmeyer, A. (2005, February 23). Interventions for improving adherence to treatment recommendations in people with type 2 diabetes mellitus. *Cochrane Database of Systematic Reviews,2,* Article CD003638. Retrieved March 5, 2008, from http://mrw.interscience.wiley.com/cochrane/clsysrev/articles/CD003638/frame.html

Vitaliano, P. P., Zhang, J., & Scanlan, J. M. (2003). Is caregiving hazardous to one's physical health? A meta-analysis. *Psychological Bulletin, 129,* 946–972.

Vogt, F., Hall, S., & Marteau, T. M. (2005). General practitioners' and family physicians' negative beliefs and attitudes towards discussing smoking cessation with patients: A systematic review. *Addiction, 100,* 1423–1431.

Von Korff, M. (1999). Pain management in primary care: An individualized stepped-care approach. *Psychological Factors in Pain, 22,* 360–373.

Von Korff, M., Balderson, B. H., Saunders K., Miglioretti, D. L., Lin, E. H., Berry, S., et al. (2005). A trial of an activating intervention for chronic back pain in primary care and physical therapy settings. *Pain, 13,* 323–330.

Wadden, T. A., Brownell, K. D., & Foster, G. D. (2002). Obesity: Responding to the Global Epidemic. *Journal of Consulting and Clinical Psychology, 70,* 510–525.

Wakefield, J. C. (1987). Sex bias in the diagnosis of primary orgasmic dysfunction. *American Psychologist, 42,* 464–471.

Waldinger, M. D., Zwinderman, A. H., & Olivier, B. (2001). Antidepressants and ejaculation: A double-blind, randomized, placebo-controlled, fixed-dose study with paroxetine, sertraline, and nefazodone. *Journal of Clinical Psychopharmacology, 21,* 293–297.

Walling, M. K., O'Hara, M. W., Reiter, R. C., Milburn, A. K., et al. (1994). Abuse history and chronic pain in woman: II a multivariate analysis of abuse and psychological morbidity. *Obstetrics & Gynecology, 84,* 200–206.

Walters, J. T. R., Bisson, J. I., & Shepherd, J. P. (2007). Predicting posttraumatic stress disorder: Validation of the Trauma Screening Questionnaire in victims of assault. *Psychological Medicine, 37,* 143–150.

Warshaw, H. S., & Kulkarni, K. (2004). *Complete guide to carb counting* (2nd ed.). Alexandria, VA: American Diabetes Association.

Warwick, H. M., Clark, D. M., Cobb, A. M., & Salkovskis, P. M. (1996). A controlled trial of cognitive–behavioral treatment of hypochondriasis. *British Journal of Psychiatry, 169,* 189–195.

Weeks, S. K., McGann, P. E., Michaels, T. K., & Penninx, B. W. (2003). Comparing Various Short-Form Geriatric Depression Scales Leads to the GDS-5/15, *Journal of Nursing Scholarship, 35,* 133.

Wehr, S. H., & Kaufman, M. E. (1987). The effects of assertive training on performance in highly anxious adolescents. *Adolescence, 22,* 195–205.

Weiss, B. D. (1998). Diagnostic evaluation of urinary incontinence in geriatric patients. *American Family Physician, 57,* 2675–2684.

Weiss, D., & Marmar, C. (1997). The Impact of Event Scale-Revised. In J. Wilson & T. Keane (Eds.), *Assessing psychological trauma and PTSD* (pp. 168–190). New York: Guildford Press.

Weissman, A. M., Levy, B. T., Hartz, A. J., Bentler, S., Donohue, M., Ellingrod, V. L., et al. (2005). Pooled analysis of antidepressant levels in lactating mothers, breast milk, and nursing infants. *American Journal of Psychiatry, 161,* 1066–1078.

Wesner, R. B., & Noyes, R. (1991). Imipramine: An effective treatment for illness phobia. *Journal of Affective Disorders, 22,* 43–48.

Wesselmann, U. (2001). Chronic pelvic pain. In D. C. Turk & R. Melzack (Eds.). *Handbook of Pain Assessment* (2nd ed., pp. 567–578). New York: Guilford Press.

Westman, E. C., Behm, F. M., Simel, D. L., & Rose, J. E. (1997). Smoking behavior on the first day of a quit attempt predicts long-term abstinence. *Archives of Internal Medicine, 157,* 335–340.

Wetherell, J. L., Sorrell, J. T., Thorp, S. R., & Patterson, T. L. (2005). Psychological interventions for late-life anxiety: A review and early lessons from the CALM study *Journal of Geriatric Psychiatry and Neurology, 18,* 72–82.

Whelton, P. K., He, J., Appel, L. J., Cutler, J. A., Havas, S., Kotchen, T. A., et al. (2002). Primary prevention of hypertension: Clinical and public health advisory from the National High Blood Pressure Education Program. *The Journal of the American Medical Association, 288,* 1882–1888.

White, A. R., Rampes, H., & Campbell, J. L. (2006, January 25). Acupuncture and related interventions for smoking cessation. *Cochrane Database of Systematic Reviews, 1,* Article CD000009. Retrieved September 2, 2007, from http://mrw.interscience. wiley.com/cochrane/clsysrev/articles/CD000009/ frame.html

Whitlock, E. P., Orleans, C. T., Pender, N., & Allan, J. (2002). Evaluating primary care behavioral counseling interventions: An evidence-based approach. *American Journal of Preventive Medicine, 22,* 267–284.

Whitlock, E. P., Polen, M. R., Green, C. A., Orleans, C. T., & Klein, J. (2004). Behavioral counseling interventions in primary care to reduce risky/ harmful alcohol use by adults: A summary of the evidence for the U.S. preventive services task force. *Annals of Internal Medicine, 140,* 558–569.

Wijma, K., Melin, A., Nedstrand, E., & Hammar, M. (1997). Treatment of menopausal symptoms with applied relaxation: A pilot study. *Journal of Behavior Therapy & Experimental Psychiatry, 28,* 251–261.

Wilde, B. E., Sidman, C. L., & Corbin, C. B. (2001). A 10,000-step count as a physical activity target for sedentary women. *Research Quarterly for Exercise and Sport, 72,* 411–414.

Williams, M., Budavari, A., Olden, K. W., & Jones, M. P. (2005). Psychosocial assessment of functional gastro-intestinal disorders in clinical practice. *Journal of Clinical Gastroenterology, 39,* 847–857.

Williams, P. M., Goodie, J. L., & Motisinger, C. D. (2008). Treating eating disorders in primary care. *American Family Physician, 77,* 187–195.

Willis, S. L., Tennstedt, S. L., Marsiske, M., Ball, K., Elias, J., & Koepke, K. M. (2006). Long-term effects of cognitive training on everyday functional outcomes in older adults. *The Journal of the American Medical Association, 296,* 2805–2814.

Wilson, J. F. (2007). Posttraumatic stress disorder needs to be recognized in primary care. *Annals of Internal Medicine, 146,* 617–620.

Wing, R. R. (1997). Behavioral approaches to the treatment of obesity. In G. Bray, C. Bouchard, & P. T. James (Eds.), *Handbook of obesity* (pp. 855–873). New York: Marcel Dekker.

Wing, R. R., & Polley, B. A. (2001). Obesity. In A. Baum, T. A. Revenson, & J. E. Singer (Eds.), *Handbook of health psychology* (263–279). Mahwah, NJ: Erlbaum.

Wolf, N. J., & Hopko, D. R. (2008). Psychosocial and pharmacological interventions for depressed adults in primary care: A critical review. *Clinical Psychology Review, 28,* 131–161.

Yamamoto, S., Mogi, N., Umegaki, H., Suzuki, Y., Ando, F., Shimakata, H., et al. (2004). The clock drawing test as a valid screening method for mild cognitive impairment. *Dementia and Geriatric Cognitive Disorders, 18,* 172–179.

Yeager, D. E., Magruder, K. M., Knapp, R. G., Nicholas, J. S., & Frueh, B. C. (2007). Performance characteristics of the posttraumatic stress disorder checklist and SPAN in veterans' affairs primary care settings. *General Hospital Psychiatry, 29,* 294–301.

Yesavage, J. A., Brink, T. L., Rose, T. L., Lum, O., Huang, V., Adey, M. B., et al. (1983). Development and validation of a geriatric depression screening scale: A preliminary report. *Journal of Psychiatric Research, 17,* 37–49.

Yohannes, A. M., Baldwin, R. C., & Connolly, M. J. (2000). Mood disorders in elderly patients with chronic obstructive pulmonary disease. *Reviews in Clinical Gerontology, 10,* 193–202.

Zettle, R. D. (2004). ACT with affective disorders. In S. C. Hayes & K. D. Strosahl (Eds.), *A practical guide to acceptance and commitment therapy* (pp. 77–102). New York: Springer Publishing Company.

Ziegelmann, J. P., Luszczynska, A., Lippke, S., & Schwarzer, R. (2007). Are goal intentions or implementations better predictors of health behavior? A longitudinal study in orthopedic rehabilitation. *Rehabilitation Psychology, 52,* 97–102.

Zijlstra, G. A. R., van Haastregt, J. C. M., van Rossum, E., van Eijk, J. T. M., Yardley, L., & Kempen, G. I. J. M. (2007). Interventions to reduce fear of falling in community-living older people: A systematic review. *Journal of the American Geriatrics Society, 55,* 603–615.

Zilbergeld, B. (1992). *The new male sexuality.* New York: Bantam Books.

Index

A1c. *See* Glycated hemoglobin

AACVPR. *See* American Association of Cardiovascular and Pulmonary Rehabilitation

AAFP. *See* American Academy of Family Physicians

ABC model, 48

Acceptance and commitment therapy (ACT), 72

Accommodation, 15, 223

ACCP (American College of Chest Physicians), 139

Acculturation level, 59

ACE-R (Addenbrooke's Cognitive Examination-Revised), 215

Acetaminophen, 190

ACOG (American College of Obstetricians and Gynecologists), 229

ACT (acceptance and commitment therapy), 72

Activities of Daily Living (ADLs), 215

Activity, pacing of, 176–178. *See also* Physical activity

Acute pain, 172

ADA. *See* American Diabetes Association

Addenbrooke's Cognitive Examination-Revised (ACE-R), 215

Addictive medications, 192

Adherence to treatment regimens, 43–49
    and asthma, 147–151
    and CVD, 157, 158, 165, 167
    social/environmental factors affecting, 58

ADLs (Activities of Daily Living), 215

Advise phase, 6

African Americans
    diabetes among, 113
    mistrust of, 57

Agency for Health Care Policy and Research Guidelines, 66

Agency for Healthcare Research and Quality, 19

Agree phase, 6

AIM (American in Motion) program, 108

Airflow, 144

Alaska Natives, diabetes among, 113

Alcohol abuse, 186, 190

Alcohol consumption
    and CVD, 156, 157, 167
    and diabetes, 115
    and erectile dysfunction, 196, 201
    and menopause, 233, 236
    mistakes/assumptions about, 187
    reducing, 188, 189
    sexual problems caused by, 202
    and sleep problems, 89
    stopping, 188, 189

Alcohol dependence, 183, 186, 190

Alcohol misuse, 183–190
    5A's model of treating, 183–190
    advising about, 186–187
    assessment of, 184–186
    defined, 183
    and dependence, 190
    interventions for, 188–189
    and specialized mental healthcare, 183

Alcohol screening, 184–186

Alcohol Use Disorders Identification Test (AUDIT), 184–186

Alcohol Use Disorders Identification Test-Consumption (AUDIT-C), 184, 186

Allergies, 152

Allergy medication, 202

Alli, 102

All-or-nothing thinking, 41

Alpha-glucosidase inhibitors, 114

Alprazolam, 190

Alprostadil, 196

Alzheimer's Association, 216

American Academy of Family Physicians (AAFP), 19, 56, 108

American Association of Cardiovascular and Pulmonary Rehabilitation (AACVPR), 139–140

American Bar Association, 216

American College of Chest Physicians (ACCP), 139

American College of Obstetricians and Gynecologists (ACOG), 229

American College of Physicians, 19, 56

American College of Sports Medicine, 107

American Diabetes Association (ADA), 113, 114, 122, 123

American Heart Association, 107, 156, 159

American Indians, diabetes among, 113

American in Motion (AIM) program, 108

American Psychological Association (APA), 31, 216

American Thoracic Society (ATS), 143

Anafranil, 240

AND I C REST screen, 73

Anesthetics, 204

Anger, CVD and, 158, 168

ANS (Autonomous Nervous System Questionnaire), 78

Antepartum depression, 225–229

Anticholinergics, 138

Anticonvulsant medication, 202

Antidepressants
    for depression, 68, 71
    for premature ejaculation, 204
    sexual problems caused by, 202, 208

Antihistamines, 74

Anxiety
    and asthma, 146
    and COPD, 138, 142
    and CVD, 158, 168

About the Authors

Christopher L. Hunter, Ph.D., ABPP, works out of the Office of Health Affairs/TRICARE Management Activity as the Department of Defense program manager for behavioral health in primary care. He is board certified in clinical health psychology and has launched several behavioral health consultation services in family and internal medicine clinics in major medical centers. He also has extensive experience training psychology interns, social workers, and licensed psychologists to start and work in integrated behavioral health consultation services. He has conducted numerous national presentations and workshops on integrated care, is a graduate of the University of Memphis, and resides in Arlington, Virginia.

Jeffrey L. Goodie, Ph.D., ABPP, is an assistant professor in the Department of Family Medicine at the Uniformed Services University of the Health Sciences in Bethesda, Maryland. He is board certified in clinical health psychology and has served as a behavioral health consultant in family and internal medicine, and obstetrics clinics, as well as trained, supervised, and provided consultation for other behavioral health providers working in primary care. He has published research, conducted workshops, and presented at national and international conferences about integrated primary care. He earned his doctoral degree from West Virginia University.

Mark S. Oordt, Ph.D., ABPP, is a licensed clinical psychologist living in San Antonio, Texas. He is board certified in clinical health psychology and is the author (with Robert J. Gatchel) of *Clinical Health Psychology and Primary Care: Practical Advice and Clinical Guidance for Successful Collaboration* (American Psychological Association, 2003). He has provided consultation and training to numerous medical facilities on the integration of behavioral health services into primary care clinics, and he has served on the training faculties of psychology internship and postdoctoral fellowship training programs. Dr. Oordt has authored articles and chapters in the areas of suicide risk management, disease management, and military psychology.

Anne C. Dobmeyer, PhD., ABPP, is director of the clinical health psychology service at Wright-Patterson Medical Center, Wright-Patterson Air Force Base, Ohio, and is board certified in clinical health psychology. She has established fully integrated primary care services in family and internal medicine, and women's health clinics in three major medical centers. Additionally, she has trained and supervised psychology interns, social workers, and psychologists in providing integrated primary care services. Her integrated primary care publications and presentations have focused on training models and outcome evaluation for integrated services. Dr. Dobmeyer is a graduate of Utah State University and resides with her family in Dayton, Ohio.